NUTRITION AND THE BRAIN

Volume 7

Nutrition and the Brain Series

Series Editors: Richard J. Wurtman
Judith J. Wurtman

Nutrition and the Brain

Volume 7

Food Constituents Affecting Normal and Abnormal Behaviors

Editors

Richard J. Wurtman, M.D.
Professor of Neuroendocrine Regulation
Department of Applied
Biological Sciences
Massachusetts Institute of Technology
Cambridge, Massachusetts

Judith J. Wurtman, Ph.D.
Research Associate
Department of Applied
Biological Sciences
Massachusetts Institute of Technology
Cambridge, Massachusetts

Raven Press ■ New York

Raven Press, 1140 Avenue of the Americas, New York, New York 10036

Made in the United States of America

Library of Congress Cataloging-in-Publication Data
Main entry under title:

Food constituents affecting normal and abnormal
  behaviors.

  (Nutrition and the brain ; v. 7)
  Includes bibliographies and index.
  1. Brain—Diseases—Nutritional aspects.   2. Mental
illness—Nutritional aspects.   3. Food—Composition.
4. Human behavior—Nutritional aspects.   5. Brain
chemistry.   I. Wurtman, Richard J., 1936–
II. Wurtman, Judith J.   III. Series.   [DNLM:
1. Appetite Disorders—chemically induced.   2. Behavior
—drug effects.   3. Brain—metabolism.   4. Dietary
Carbohydrates.   5. Dietary Proteins.   W1 NU8632 v. 7 /
WL 300 F686]
QP376.N86   vol. 7   599'.0188 s   85-25608
[RC386.2]   [616.89'1]
ISBN 0-88167-142-8

Preface

The general theme of this volume is the effects of particular food constituents on behavior. Those constituents discussed are, for the most part, compounds—like carbohydrates and proteins—whose consumption causes known neurochemical changes which are compatible with their behavioral actions.

For more than three decades it has been a canon of brain science that a drug that alters the levels or actions of a particular brain neurotransmitter can thereby modify any type of behavior that is mediated by neurons releasing that transmitter. Only a short extension of this doctrine is required in order to predict that a food constituent which mimics the drug's neurochemical effect will also produce similar behavioral changes. The behaviors now recognized as capable of being influenced by food constituents include some things people do normally (like feel sleepy or hungry, or express vigilance, or choose among foods) and some that are pathologic (like the affective manifestations of clinical depression or the carbohydrate-craving sometimes associated with obesity or bulimia). Indeed, the fact that food constituents can modify such behaviors has spawned interest in using these compounds as though they were drugs, by administering them in pure form and large doses, alone or along with drugs whose actions they might potentiate, or side-effects ameliorate. A "desirable" behavioral change might be to increase the likelihood that a normal phenomenon will occur (for example, sleepiness at night, or alertness during the day), or to decrease the intensity of an abnormal feeling or action (like sadness in depression, or involuntary movements in tardive dyskinesia). The requirement that a food constituent's putative behavioral effect be associated with a demonstrated neurochemical action, in animals, before being taken seriously provides investigators with an objective criterion for evaluating anecdotes purporting to illustrate such behavioral effects: If animals receiving the food constituent fail to demonstrate any detectable change in brain composition, then one might appropriately be skeptical about its propensity to affect the behavior of humans.

In keeping with traditions established in prior volumes of this series, all authors who have contributed chapters to this volume are themselves active investigators in the fields that they describe. Dr.. Spring has pioneered developing sensitive and specific tests for demonstrating behavioral responses of normal people to actual foods; Dr. Young has explored the fate and biochemical effects of tryptophan *in vivo*, and related these findings to tryptophan's efficacy in depression; Dr. van Praag and his associates have tested possible precursor-based therapies for depression directed towards both serotonin- and catecholamine-releasing neurons; Dr. Rosenthal and his NIMH colleagues have provided the initial clinical descriptions of a variant of depression, the "seasonal affective disorder syndrome," which is associated with both affective and appetitive pathologies; Drs. Pirke and Ploog have characterized metabolic abnormalities that are often associated with—and may be etiologically related to—anorexia nervosa; and Dr. Pardridge—who also contributed chapters to volumes I and V of this series—has identified the particular blood-brain barrier transport systems that allow dietary aspartame to increase brain phenylalanine levels.

The sequence of chapters in this volume starts with the description of the behavioral effects of neurochemically active foods and nutrients in normal people. The next two chapters describe attempts to use tryptophan—an amino acid whose effect on the brain is similar to that of dietary carbohydrate—to treat depression when given alone, along with tyrosine, or in the form of 5-hydroxytryptophan. (The extensive discussion of the tryptophan-depression relationship in this volume reflects both the preponderance of publications on this subject in the literature dealing with the use of nutrients to treat behavioral diseases, and its absence from earlier volumes.) The volume then focuses on the inappropriate uses of foods—presumably for their neurochemical effects—by patients whose psychopathologies are affective (seasonal depression) or primarily appetitive (bulimia; anorexia nervosa; types of obesity). The last chapter discusses a newly-marketed but widely-used food additive, aspartame; consumption of large doses of this sweetener changes the chemical composition of the brain (elevating brain phenylalanine in humans, tyrosine in rats) and may also modify certain behaviors in susceptible populations: Inclusion of this topic reflects both its applicability as a paradigm for studying how food constituents can affect neurotransmitters and behavior, and its great current interest. (Additional information about the safety evaluation of aspartame's effects that preceded its introduction into the food supply was provided in a chapter in Volume VI of this series.)

In one way or another, all of the chapters in this volume touch on the brain neurons that make serotonin from tryptophan, and on the property of these neurons to make more of their neurotransmitter after consumption of carbohydrate-rich meals. This property still seems paradoxical: Why should a meal that contains no tryptophan—that is, one rich in carbohydrate but lacking protein—elevate brain tryptophan and serotonin levels, while a meal which includes tryptophan [within protein] has no effect (or even the opposite effect)?

The answer relates to two special properties of trytophan—its plasma levels are not substantially reduced by insulin, and it tends to be the scarcest amino acid in most dietary proteins—plus the fact that circulating tryptophan must compete with other "large neutral amino acids" for transport into the brain. (Plasma levels of these competitors *are* lowered by insulin, and these amino acids *are* abundant in dietary proteins.) The fact that a carbohydrate-rich meal thus raises the "plasma tryptophan ratio" (to other large neutral amino acids) while a high-protein meal has the opposite effect allows serotonergic neurons to "sense" food-induced changes in plasma composition, and to inform the rest of the brain about the composition of the foods currently being digested and absorbed (that is, their carbohydrate-to-protein ratio). One use to which the brain puts this information is the maintenance of nutritional balance, decreasing the likelihood, for example, that a carbohydrate-rich, protein-poor breakfast will be followed by a lunch of similar composition.

One disadvantage of this coupling of serotonin release to plasma composition is that numerous other functions of serotoninergic neurons thereby become hostage to food intake: Perhaps eating the "wrong" food increases the likelihood of an undesirable behavior (like sleepiness after a carbohydrate-rich lunch, as described by Spring); perhaps the depressed patient chooses to overeat carbohydrate-rich snacks and becomes obese (as discussed by Rosenthal and Heffernan) precisely because these foods amplify serotonergic neurotransmission, just like most anti-depressant drugs; perhaps overconsumption of aspartame—which, as discussed by Pardridge, tastes like sugar but has opposite effects on brain serotonin synthesis—can increase the dieter's cravings for carbohydrates. Serotonergic neurons may turn out to be unique among neurons in their capacity to respond to real foods. Only future research will tell.

This volume will be of interest to investigators working in nutrition, metabolism, psychology, neuroscience, pharmacology, and toxicology, as well as to psychiatrists, internists, neurologists, and to people who counsel patients with obesity and eating disorders.

Provincetown, Massachusetts　　　　　　　　　　　　　　Richard J. Wurtman
August 1985　　　　　　　　　　　　　　　　　　　　　Judith J. Wurtman

Contents

Contributors

Margaret M. Heffernan   *Clinical Psychobiology Branch, National Institutes of Mental Health, 9000 Rockville Pike, Bethesda, Maryland 20205*

C. Lemus   *Department of Psychiatry, Albert Einstein College of Medicine, Montefiore Medical Center, New York, New York 10467*

William M. Pardridge   *Department of Medicine, UCLA School of Medicine, Los Angeles, California 90024*

Karl M. Pirke   *Max-Planck-Institut für Psychiatrie, Kraepelin Strasse 10, 8000 München 40, Federal Republic of Germany*

Detlev Ploog   *Max-Planck-Institut für Psychiatrie, Kraepelin Strasse 10, 8000 München 40, Federal Republic of Germany*

Norman E. Rosenthal   *Unit of Outpatient Services, Clinical Psychobiology Branch, National Institutes of Mental Health, 9000 Rockville Pike, Bethesda, Maryland 20205*

Bonnie Spring   *Department of Psychology, Texas Tech University, Lubbock, Texas 79409*

H. M. van Praag   *Department of Psychiatry, Albert Einstein College of Medicine, Montefiore Medical Center, New York, New York 10467*

S. N. Young   *Department of Psychiatry, McGill University, 1033 Pine Avenue West, Montreal, Quebec, Canada H3A 1A1*

NUTRITION AND THE BRAIN

Volume 7

Nutrition and the Brain, Vol. 7, edited by
R. J. Wurtman and J. J. Wurtman. Raven Press,
New York © 1986.

Effects of Foods and Nutrients on the Behavior of Normal Individuals

Bonnie Spring

Department of Psychology, Texas Tech University, Lubbock, Texas 79409

I. INTRODUCTION

Although much is known about the long-term behavioral consequences of malnutrition, the acute effects of food consumption in adequately nourished individuals have only recently begun to be studied. This chapter reviews current findings concerning the effects of foods and food constituents on the behavior of normal children and adults. Consistencies and contradictions in the research literature are noted and discussed, and important future directions are suggested.

Research on diet–behavior relationships has been prompted by several factors. One impetus stems from popular beliefs about the effects of certain food constituents (e.g., sugar) on activity levels and mood. Controlled investigations in the laboratory have been undertaken to test the validity of anecdotal observations. A second impetus derives from the work of applied psychologists seeking to determine the timing and composition of meals that can optimize performance in the workplace or the classroom.

A third important influence stems from the demonstration that certain food constituents that are neurotransmitter precursors can alter the synthesis and release of brain neurotransmitters (172,173). These findings raised the possibility that foods might produce changes in behavior by altering the levels of brain neurotransmitters that are associated with various psychological functions.

Not all neurotransmitters are influenced by the availability of their precursors in the diet. The work of Wurtman and his collaborators at the Massachusetts Institute of Technology indicates that several conditions must be in effect for precursor control of neurotransmitter synthesis to occur. First, plasma levels of the neurotransmitter precursor must covary with the intake of foods. There cannot be a feedback mechanism that maintains plasma levels of the precursor within a constant, narrow range. Second, the precursor must be able to cross the blood-brain barrier. Third, the transport mechanism that carries nutrients from the blood to the brain must not be completely saturated, so that it can become more saturated when plasma levels of the precursor rise. Fourth, the enzyme that catalyzes the conversion of precursor to neurotransmitter must be of low affinity. At ordinary nutrient concentrations, the enzyme must bind the nutrient relatively poorly and function inefficiently at changing its chemical structure. Under such conditions, the amount of precursor available is the rate-limiting factor in neurotransmitter synthesis. If precursor concentrations increase, the activity of the enzyme increases, and more neurotransmitter can be synthesized. Finally, there cannot be feedback inhibition of the catalytic enzyme when the level of neurotransmitter rises.

All five conditions are met for the amino acid tryptophan, from which the brain synthesizes the monoamine neurotransmitter serotonin. Much of this chapter concerns behavioral consequences of interventions that influence brain serotonin. Precursor control has also been demonstrated, under certain conditions, for the catecholamine neurotransmitters norepinephrine (NE) and dopamine (DA) and for acetylcholine, histamine, and glycine.

The essential amino acid tryptophan cannot be synthesized by humans or other mammals. Since the body's nutritional supply of tryptophan is obtained from dietary protein, it might seem that a protein meal would elevate brain tryptophan or serotonin. However, the opposite occurs. Brain tryptophan and serotonin decline after a protein-rich meal. This paradox occurs because protein contains very little tryptophan (1–1.6%) in comparison with the other large neutral amino acids: leucine, isoleucine, valine, tyrosine, and phenylalanine (25%). Since all the large neutral amino acids compete for access to the same carrier molecules for transport across the blood-brain barrier, the brain influx of tryptophan declines relative to its competitors after a high-protein meal.

As one effect of a protein-containing meal is to lower brain tryptophan and serotonin, another can be to elevate brain tyrosine (63). Since tyrosine is the precursor to the catecholamine neurotransmitters, brain catecholamine synthesis might be expected to increase following a protein-rich meal. Indeed, increases in brain tyrosine can enhance catecholamine synthesis (62), especially under certain conditions, such as when organisms are stressed (12).

Paradoxically, a meal lacking protein but rich in carbohydrates increases brain tryptophan and serotonin synthesis, even though such a meal contains no tryptophan. In organisms that have been fasting, a carbohydrate-rich, protein-poor meal brings about a rise in the ratio of plasma tryptophan to the other large neutral amino acids. In humans who have fasted since breakfast and eaten a carbohydrate test meal for lunch, the rise in the plasma tryptophan ratio is evident regardless of whether the test meal has consisted primarily of sucrose or starch (103). The change in the plasma tryptophan ratio comes about because the carbohydrate meal triggers insulin secretion. Insulin causes most of the amino acids other than tryptophan to leave the bloodstream and be taken up into muscle. In animals that have fasted overnight, the insulin secretion triggered by a carbohydrate causes a 40 to 60% fall in plasma leucine, isoleucine, and valine and a 15 to 30% fall in plasma tyrosine. Plasma tryptophan levels do not fall, because tryptophan binds to albumin molecules as insulin strips away the free fatty acids, which are usually albumin bound. Consequently, brain influx of tryptophan is increased, and synthesis and release of brain serotonin are also accelerated, insofar as the latter are assessed by cerebrospinal fluid (CSF) 5-hydroxyindoleacetic acid (5-HIAA) (51,52).

For a test meal to reliably elevate brain serotonin, it must be not only carbohydrate rich, but also protein poor. A meal need only contain some protein in order to impede the brain influx of tryptophan. As compared to a single meal without any protein, a test meal with 18% protein significantly decreases brain tryptophan and significantly increases brain valine, leucine, and tyrosine in rats (63). Consequently, a meal containing only 18% protein is sufficient to reverse the carbohydrate-induced rise in brain tryptophan in rats (63). The minimum proportion of protein needed to offset the effects of carbohydrate on brain tryptophan in humans remains to be established.

In addition to the catecholamines, it is also possible to increase the synthesis and release of brain acetylcholine by administering a precursor, choline (26,87). A similar result can be achieved by administering lecithin (phosphatidylcholine), a phospholipid that is the major dietary source of choline and that can be broken down into choline (90). Just as a meal rich in lecithin elevates blood choline and neuronal acetylcholine, deprivation of dietary choline brings about a fall in plasma choline (9). However, the extent to which brain neurons actually increase their release of acetylcholine when more precursor is made available depends on the firing frequency of the target neurons. Choline acetyltransferase (CAT), the enzyme that catalyzes the synthesis of acetylcholine from its precursors choline and acetyl coenzyme A, is more sensitive to additional precursor in neurons that are firing rapidly. In addition, among patients with Alzheimer's disease, for whom the possibility of treatment with acetylcholine precursors has been of considerable interest, an added complication is that CAT can be reduced in the hippocampus and cerebral cortex by as much as 90% (11,42).

II. METHODOLOGIC ISSUES

A. Research Design

Three primary research designs have been used in diet–behavior research: cross-sectional methods, repeated measures or within-subjects designs, and correlational studies. Each is best suited to particular questions and exigencies, and each has associated strengths and limitations. One issue that crosscuts all the designs is the need to estimate in advance of the experiment the approximate magnitude of the diet–behavior relationship. This can be done by employing preliminary analyses of effect size and statistical power (28) so that final sample sizes are sufficient to provide a valid test of research hypotheses. When the experiment is completed, it is also useful to define the characteristics of population subgroups who prove to be more than normally sensitive to nutrients so that these individuals can be studied further.

1. Cross-Sectional Designs

Cross-sectional or between-group comparison designs are occasionally the only ethically defensible method for human research. An example is the natural experiment involving exposure to hazardous substances that can occur in foods (47a,167). In one study that was both retrospective and cross-sectional, Valcuikas et al. (159) studied Michigan farmers exposed to high levels of polybrominated biphenyl (PBB) through its inadvertent introduction into the food chain several years earlier. When the Michigan subjects were compared to a comparable population in Wisconsin, the target population showed an increased incidence of symptoms suggestive of neurological disturbance. In addition, memory was impaired on laboratory procedures (15). Since it would not have been justifiable to expose healthy people to PBB and to test memory before and after exposure, the research might have stopped here. In doing so, it would have been inferred that the experimental and control groups were comparable in all major respects, and that the between-group differences were attributable to PBB exposure.

Brown et al. (16), however, undertook a study of chemical plant workers with much greater exposure and higher body concentrations of PBB. The chemical workers, despite their higher PBB concentrations, exceeded the Michigan farmers on memory performance, even though the two groups were matched on educational and occupational parameters. The disconfirming evidence suggests that the memory disturbance observed in the Michigan farmers is associated with a third confounding variable rather than with exposure to PBB. One plausible factor is psychological distress (anxiety and depression), which was correlated more highly with memory impairment in the Michigan sample than were measures of PBB concentrations.

The PBB example illustrates the major problem associated with cross-sectional designs. The experimental and control groups may differ in performance on the dependent measure because they also differ in some important respect other than exposure to the target substance. In other words, the experimental and control groups may differ not only on the independent variable (group membership) and the dependent variable (target behavior), but also on a third extraneous variable, such as depression.

The problem of third variables that are confounded with group membership is exacerbated in the use of intact groups that were assigned to conditions by nature rather than by the experimenter. The same difficulty plagues correlational studies of diet–behavior associations. Might certain personality or psychological characteristics be associated with the decision to work in or live near a chemical plant, to consume a certain diet, or to file a major lawsuit for health damages? How might these factors affect the performances under investigation? Such difficulties are lessened when subjects are randomly assigned to be exposed to different nutrients, as is done in most experimental studies of diet–behavior relationships. Even so, the problem of inadvertent systematic bias remains, and randomly assigned groups must also be tested for signs of nonequivalence that could potentially explain the results.

The PBB example also illustrates several possible solutions to the problem of third variables. One is to match groups on suspected confounding variables, such as age, education, socioeconomic status, and gender. A second is to test for within-group correlation of behavioral variables with biological variables that presumably account for the results (e.g., plasma concentrations of amino acids, glucose, insulin, or alternative explanatory variables, e.g., corticosteroids). The third and most important strategy is to replicate or seek disconfirming evidence from independently derived samples.

Cross-sectional designs also present advantages in cases other than experiments of nature. One is the instance in which a researcher seeks to identify population subgroups who may prove especially sensitive to nutrient effects. This strategy is especially appropriate in the early stages of research on a nutrient when there is a need to assess the sensitivity of various demographic groups. For example, in an initial study of the behavioral effects of carbohydrates, Spring et al. (151) compared males to females and younger to older individuals. Results suggested that females and older individuals might prove more sensitive than their male and younger counterparts. An important component of any experimental approach, but especially of cross-sectional studies, is the examination of extreme outliers or of population subgroups who depart from the group mean. These individuals score in a direction that indicates unusual over- or underresponsiveness to nutrients. It can be important to replicate the findings for outliers to see if their deviance persists. If so, the characteristics of these subgroups may provide a basis for generating useful hypotheses about unusual food sensitivities (168a).

Cross-sectional designs may also be favored over repeated measurements protocols when the novelty of a procedure is inherently important. For example, Grunberg (76) tested whether cigarette smoking differentially affects consumption of foods varying in taste and caloric content. He presented subjects with a selection of foods differing in taste, calories, and nutrient composition. The subjects' assigned task was to rate the foods on various dimensions of taste. Although the experiment appeared to be concerned with taste perception, the actual dependent variable was the amount consumed from each specific food. Grunberg et al. (77) found that cigarette smoking preferentially affects the consumption of sweet-tasting, high-calorie foods. Had the exact procedure been repeated with smokers smoking and not smoking, extraneous factors, such as familiarity or boredom, might have influenced food selection and limited the generalizability of results. In real life, the individual who craves a sweet, high-calorie food but who has on the previous evening consumed a large quantity of chocolate candy, now has the option of switching to cake. This option is not available in a repeated measurements protocol involving restricted food choices.

2. Repeated Measurements Design

The inherent variability among individuals reduces the statistical power of cross-sectional designs and necessitates large sample sizes so that extraneous variability will average out as "noise." Variability among individuals is reduced when subjects serve as their own controls and are tested under several experimental conditions.

The elimination diet is one repeated measures design that was used in evaluating the Feingold (49) hypothesis. After baseline testing, the putative offending agents are removed from the child's diet to see whether improvement results. These substances are then reinstated to see whether problem behaviors return. Assessments are usually conducted in naturalistic settings with ratings made by parents and teachers. The major advantage of the elimination approach is that it assesses nutrient effects on actual behavior problems that prove most troublesome to the child and to those in the surrounding environment. A major disadvantage is that it is difficult to conduct elimination studies in a double-blind fashion. The enthusiasm of family members about the new diet may generate expectancy effects and self-fulfilling prophecies (134). A second disadvantage is that it may prove difficult to assess the effects of eliminating single food constituents. For example, a diet that eliminates food additives will also exclude 86% of products high in sucrose and 45% of products low in sucrose (126).

The second major within-subjects approach is the double-blind, placebo-controlled trial, sometimes called the challenge approach. Challenge studies provide the most compelling evidence about diet–behavior relationships. Target substances and control substances that are inert or that exert distinctly different effects are presented in counterbalanced order, followed by tests of their acute behavioral effects. Challenge studies permit evaluation of order effects and the time course of short-term behavioral changes. Assessments are often made in a laboratory and are more intrusive than naturalistic observations, so that generalizability outside the laboratory may be an issue.

Order and sequence effects can be troublesome in repeated measurements designs. For example, in a study of activity levels, Behar et al. (7) found that children were significantly quieter on the third day of testing than on the first and grew quieter over the course of each test session. Covariance analyses can often be used to equalize the pre-drug levels of performance on different test days. However, complexities of interpretation can arise if groups initially differing in baseline scores come to score identically under the common influence of the laboratory procedures (150).

Order effects can wreak particular havoc with tests of information processing. Since performance is more variable and more influenced by subject characteristics on the initial days of testing, it is wise to administer practice sessions until a stable level of performance has been attained. However, it may be that the early stages of learning are of particular interest. In this case, it will be necessary to administer parallel test forms across test sessions, although these can be a challenge to construct. For example, in studies of memory, it is possible to assemble word lists that are matched on word frequency, imagery, and associative strength and yet still to have lists that vary in difficulty. The dual solutions to this problem are pilot testing and counterbalancing of test forms. An added consideration is that the memory of items from previous lists can intrude and interfere with responses to subsequent lists when the interval between lists is too short. One further issue related to order effects is the fact that tests may be performed differently early and later in the course of practice. Processing operations may require considerable cognitive effort and may be performed sequentially early in testing. Later on, processing may become automatic, allowing leftover cognitive resources to perform several operations simultaneously (86,144). Practice testing can minimize but may not thoroughly eliminate the effect of such changes.

3. Correlational Designs

Correlational designs are useful primarily for generating hypotheses about diet–behavior relationships. Such hypotheses can be tested subsequently in experimental designs. In the correlational approach, behavioral characteristics of individual subjects are examined in relation to their eating habits. Prinz and co-workers (125,126) have effectively used the correlational approach to demonstrate an association between habitual consumption of high-calorie carbohydrates and restless or aggressive behavior in children. The correlational approach requires a large number of subjects, and its chief weakness is its inability to disentangle cause from effect. Correlational findings can also be misleading when they are interpreted to imply cause–effect relationships. For example, it cannot be inferred that carbohydrates cause hyperactive behavior. Alternatively, a tendency toward hyperactivity may cause children to consume many carbohydrates, perhaps even because of their calming effect. Still another possibility is that both the hyperactivity and the heightened carbohydrate intake result from a third variable, such as heightened metabolic rate.

Prinz and Riddle (125) make the point that correlational designs can begin to generate hypotheses about cumulative or chronic effects of diet that are neglected by acute challenge studies. This point is well taken. Habitual food preferences are currently being assessed as an individual difference variable in some research

(1,38). However, one limitation is that food intake records possess substantial limitations as measures of dietary intake (3).

B. Foods Versus Nutrients

1. Studies of Single Nutrients

Studies of single amino acids, such as tryptophan, tyrosine, and choline or lecithin, are analogous to psychopharmacological studies of pure substances. Such protocols are usually both elegant and powerful. For example, Lieberman et al. (102) found a 40% reduction in subjective vigor 2 hr after tryptophan administration. The target amino acid and placebo can usually be packaged in identical-appearing capsules, so that double-blind procedures can be easily maintained. It is worthwhile to perform a midway chemical analysis of the substances, however, since pharmaceutical errors can potentially create chaos for data interpretation (7). One added complexity is the difficulty of establishing with certainty that placebo substances lack behavioral effects (132). For example, valine or leucine placebos can block brain uptake of both tryptophan and tyrosine. Moreover, aspartame, a commonly used placebo in studies on the behavioral effects of sugar, can elevate brain tyrosine (179). Hence it remains possible that some "placebos" can also produce acute behavioral change.

The major limitation of studies of single nutrients is that they are not representative of how people eat. Even denizens of the health food store usually consume amino acid pills along with foods.

2. Studies of Foods

Studies of foods bear a high face validity to the central question in this field: How do ordinary meals affect behavior? For the findings of diet–behavior research to have meaning beyond basic science considerations, this is the question that must ultimately be addressed.

While targeted toward the heart of the problem, studies of foods represent a complex undertaking. First, effects on behavior are usually smaller than those in studies of single nutrients (103,151), so that sizable samples and tight methodologic control may be needed to detect them. Second, dose-response parameters are largely unknown, making it difficult to determine portion sizes for experimental studies. For example, body weight differences between females and males render a standard size test meal a proportionally higher dosage of nutrients for females.

The problem of suitable control conditions for food studies is also a thorny one. A protein food has frequently been used as the control for a carbohydrate meal. Protein lowers the tryptophan ratio, whereas carbohydrate elevates it (103). In addition to lowering brain tryptophan, however, protein can also elevate brain tyrosine under certain conditions. Results thus may reflect an averaging of both effects. Moreover, it appears that a midday meal of any type can produce performance impairments (38). Consequently, important questions for studies of single nutrients are whether they impair performance to a greater extent than a balanced lunch or no lunch.

As in the case of single-nutrient studies, questions arise about the representativeness of test meals comprised of single foods. Findings may not be generally applicable to the behavior of people who eat only three balanced meals per day. However, results may be generalizable to the sizable group of consumers who practice restriced diets or who consume snack foods. The incidence of dietary intake habits largely restricted to single nutrients is not negligible. For example, the Scottish psychiatrist Ian Menzies (110) described a subgroup of children who subsisted on diets comprised almost entirely of fruit drinks, potato chips, cookies, and tea. Many elderly individuals, because of restricted incomes and appetites, also selectively favor carbohydrates and may, for example, practice the "toast for lunch" syndrome (145). Dieters frequently implement the opposite form of restriction, selectively consuming protein and eliminating carbohydrates as a means toward weight loss. Snackers who favor candy bars consume the equivalent of a pure carbohydrate meal, since the amount of protein contained in most sugary snacks is insufficient to block the influx of tryptophan into the brain. Conversely, snackers who prefer cheese consume protein in the absence of carbohydrate.

It is usually not possible to preserve double-blind test conditions in studies of foods. Consequently, psychological factors may dovetail with biological ones in influencing subjects' responses to foods. For example, even when carbohydrate and protein meals have been equated for calories, the dieter may be perturbed about eating a sugary test meal, since such foods are usually off limits to calorie restrictors. A related question concerns how to match test meals in order to make them as equivalent as possible on key psychological parameters. Should matching be based on calories, on volume, or on taste? Efforts to match foods on one set of parameters may cause them to be unmatched on another. For example, in one study that matched protein and carbohydrate meals on calories, the protein meal left subjects feeling more highly satiated (151). In the same study, a preliminary attempt was made to devise milk shakes equated for both volume and calories. This effort was ultimately abandoned because it led to the creation of a highly unpalatable protein concoction.

3. Combination Approach

An interesting new approach combines key aspects of the single-nutrient and the food study paradigms. Young (180) presented subjects with amino acid mixtures that were tryptophan free, balanced, or tryptophan supplemented. All the mixtures were 100 g and contained 15 amino acids in approximately the same proportion found in milk. In addition, the balanced mix contained 2.3 g L-tryptophan, and the tryptophan-supplemented mix included 10.3 g L-tryptophan. Amino acids were served in water, flavored with chocolate syrup and saccharin. This approach permits precise study of known combinations of nutrients in a double-blind fashion. However, palatability remains problematic.

C. Time Parameters

1. Acute Versus Chronic Effects

Questions about time parameters enter into diet–behavior studies in several ways. The first is the nature of the effects that are studied. Research on neurotransmitter precursors has usually focused on acute rather than chronic effects. The exception has been those studies that deplete brain neurotransmitter levels by chronically feeding a nutrient-deficient diet (e.g., ref. 106). Acute effects are of greatest interest because amino acids are rapidly metabolized regardless of whether they are taken in as pure substances or as components of protein. Tissue concentrations do not continue to rise with repeated administration, as they do with lipid-soluble substances. However, some evidence suggests that the chronic effects of administering amino acids might be of interest to study. For example, in normal subjects, Yuwiler et al. (181) found a cumulative increase in early morning plasma serotonin after 8 consecutive days of tryptophan loading (50 mg/kg). After many days of administration, the sleepiness following an acute tryptophan load was also intensified and prolonged. In a possibly related finding, Hartmann et al. (83) found that sleep latencies continued to shorten after cessation of a 7-day period of tryptophan loading. The Hartmann et al. (83) finding of a possible "continuing effect" of tryptophan, like the finding by Yuwiler et al. (181) of intensification of effects later in dosing, suggests that possible chronic effects of amino acid administration may warrant further consideration.

2. Time Course of Acute Behavioral Changes

The time course of acute biochemical changes that are thought to underlly psychological changes is a critical consideration in determining when to administer behavioral tests. The designs of several studies comparing the behavioral effects of carbohydrate and protein meals are based on the hypothesis that behavioral change will parallel fluctuations in the tryptophan ratio. Dependent variables in these studies are administered with a lag of at least 1 hr following a test meal. Differences in the plasma tryptophan ratio following the two kinds of meals served as lunch are significant by this interval and remain so until at least 5 hr later (103). The Lieberman et al. (103) findings also suggested that behavioral differences associated with the two types of lunch are at a maximum 1 to 3 hr after eating and largely gone 4 to 5 hr after the meals. However, in a recent study comparing amino acid mixtures that were balanced, tryptophan-deficient, or tryptophan-rich, Young (180) found some behavioral effects 5 hr after intake.

Young's (180) finding of nutrient-related mood differences 5 hr after test meals is at variance with the failure of Lieberman et al. (103) to find them after this interval. The discrepancies may be related to differences in the nutrients administered, to the fact that subjects in the Lieberman et al. (103) protocol were tested continuously during the 5-hr period following the meals, or to the fact that Young (180) served the food constituents for breakfast rather than lunch. Nonetheless if behavioral differences do arise from brain events paralleling the plasma tryptophan ratio, they should persist for at least 5 hr.

When studies simultaneously assess behavioral and biological parameters, it is conceivable that the stress induced by blood drawing can affect both types of measures. It is preferable methodologically to insert an indwelling catheter some time before the first blood sample is drawn and the first behavioral test administered. The initial discomfort to the subject and the risk of bruising are somewhat increased with a catheter; but the catheter minimizes the discomfort and anxiety that are associated with multiple repeated blood samplings and may reduce the impact of stress on behavioral and biological measures.

3. Breakfast, Lunch, Dinner, or Snacks

It cannot be assumed that foods have identical effects when served at different times of day. In considering the reasons for time-of-day differences in nutrient effects, there are two major categories of explanation. One concerns the association between the duration of fasting and the magnitude of insulin response. For example, a meal served for breakfast after an overnight fast can be expected to produce a greater insulin response than will the same meal served for lunch after a standard breakfast. The reason is that the overnight-fasted subject who is given the test meal for breakfast will have been fasting for at least 12 hr and will have low resting levels of insulin. In contrast, the subject fasting only since breakfast and given a test meal for lunch will have observed a fast only for approximately 5 hr, may still be digesting breakfast, and may already have somewhat elevated levels of insulin. The insulin response to a new meal may be blunted under these conditions.

Extremely long durations of fasting may alter the usual findings for particular meals. For example, Craig (38) has pointed out that the usual post-lunch dip in performance may not be found if the meal reverses a prolonged period of food deprivation. Clearly, there is a need to disentangle the effects of duration of fasting from those due to the timing of meals.

Circadian rhythms afford the second explanation for time-of-day differences in nutrient effects. Many biological and behavioral characteristics display diurnal variation. These include feelings of alertness or drowsiness, body temperature, perceptual search performance, short-term memory efficiency, and secretion of cortisol or potassium. Some of these indicators fluctuate in parallel, and others vary independently. The time course for the various functions and possible underlying mechanisms are still being investigated (53,54). Endogenous diurnal variations in mood and performance constitute the backdrop against which meals will exert their effects. At this point, one can only speculate about whether a performance that is rapidly improving or at its peak diurnal efficiency may be more immune to nutrient-related changes than is a performance on the downswing. These are important questions in need of additional research.

Three other comments are in order about the timing of meals. One is the need to standardize the time taken to consume test foods, for example, by allowing subjects a 30-min interval to finish the meal. Greater variability in the duration of intake may work to obscure the time course of behavioral changes.

A second point concerns a topic that has with few exceptions (33) been largely neglected in research. This is the effect of single-nutrient foods that follow a meal containing mixed nutrients. Examples include sweet-tasting carbohydrates (e.g., candy) or protein-rich foods (e.g., cheese) that may be eaten as desserts or as snacks. In what quantities and at what interval may single-nutrient foods augment or offset the effects of prior meals? Are the behavioral effects of a carbohydrate-rich food different when they follow a protein-rich versus a carbohydrate-rich meal? Do the aftereffects of a sugary dessert differ from those of the same food eaten as an after-dinner snack? These questions warrant additional investigation.

The final issue is related to the phenomenon of snacking. Clinical observations suggest that a subset of patients with eating disorders or depression show cravings for sweet-tasting, carbohydrate-rich foods (41,92,93,133), although formal nutrient analyses remain to be performed. Often patients' cravings occur characteristically at a specific time of day. An unknown but important question is whether foods will produce distinctive effects during time periods when they are craved.

D. Individual Differences

Individuals may differ in their sensitivities to particular nutrients. Some evidence of individual differences does exist in the literature, although findings are in need of replication. For example, it has been suggested that females may be more sensitive than males to nutrient effects (151,176), and that older individuals may be more sensitive than younger ones (151). Another finding has been that adults who score high on extroversion and low on neuroticism on the Eysenck Personality Inventory (48) show the greatest decrements in performance efficiency after lunch (25,39).

Another potentially influential individual difference variable is usual eating habits. Craig (38) found that the post-lunch dip in performance efficiency was exacerbated when subjects ate what was for them an unusually heavy lunch. In another similar demonstration, Adam (1) found that sleep was disrupted when subjects departed from their usual bedtime eating habits. Electrophysiological recordings of sleep detected increased broken sleep when usual bedtime snackers went without an evening snack, as well as when usual noneaters had a nutritional drink prior to bedtime. Caffeine is another food constituent that exerts different effects as a function of habitual patterns of intake (130).

Few data are available on other sources of individual variation that could moderate the response to nutrients, although other factors that warrant investigation include stress, anxiety or depression, obesity or eating disorders, and cigarette smoking.

E. Target Behaviors

The selection of target behaviors for research on nutrient effects has proceeded according to both theoretical and practical considerations. The literature on the behavioral consequences of altering serotoninergic neurotransmission is particularly extensive. Findings reviewed in the next section suggest a role for central nervous system (CNS) serotonin in modulating locomotor activity, aggression, sleep, sensory responses, mood, and performance. An important question in research on tyrosine has concerned its efficacy as a possible treatment for depression. Similarly, choline and lecithin have been examined for their potential to alleviate memory disturbances. Research on the effects of eating or skipping meals has focused more generally on consequences for performance, especially on tests of learning and attention.

There has also been at least one important gap in the literature. Short-term memory has been largely neglected as a dependent measure except in studies of acetylcholine agonists and antagonists.

Another unanswered and intriguing question concerns the relationship between the changes detected by various test indicators. A topic of particular interest concerns the correlation between self-reported mental state and laboratory measures of performance. Under certain conditions, the two are highly intercorrelated. For example, deterioration in mood and cognitive test performance were so highly intercorrelated ($r \geqslant 0.85$) in a study of ranger trainees undergoing 100 hr of sleep deprivation, caloric restriction, and strenuous exercise that Bugge et al. (18) considered mood measures to represent an accurate appraisal of mental efficiency. In a different study, Glenville and Broughton (65) compared self-ratings of sleepiness with performance after eight male subjects underwent a night of sleep deprivation. The authors found correlations ranging from 0.50 to 0.69 between sleepiness on the one hand and vigilance performance and reaction time on the other. Interestingly, measures of short-term memory and handwriting were uncorrelated with drowsiness.

Under some circumstances, subjective and objective indicators may show less parallelism. Rapoport (129) has reviewed evidence suggesting that, for children, subjective reports of mood change may be less sensitive to the effects of dietary substances than they are for adults. She notes that it is unclear whether children actually experience fewer subjective effects or whether they are simply poorer reporters. In contrast, behavioral measures of speech rate, attention span, reaction time, and motor activity often prove quite sensitive to food substances in pediatric populations.

Sleep is an example that may produce variable agreement between subjective and objective measures. In psychiatric populations, correlations between patients' and nurses' estimates of time spent sleeping or waking have been found to range from approximately 0.70 (79) to 0.17 (36). Part of the discrepancy may occur because observers rate sleep primarily on the basis of physical movements, which may be an imperfect indicator of time spent in bed but awake. However, patients with insomnia may also grossly underestimate the amount of sleep they obtain (40). Despite their imperfect correlations, subjective ratings, observer ratings, and electroencephalogram (EEG) measures may each provide important information about nutrient effects on the phenomenology of sleep.

III. GENERAL EFFECTS OF MEALS

Studies on the effects of eating or skipping meals derive from applied considerations about how to optimize performance in the workplace or enhance children's learning.

A. Lunch

Elegant reviews describing circadian rhythms in performance (31) and the effects of lunch (25,38,39) have appeared in the literature from England. At 2:00 in the afternoon, a reduction in work efficiency can be demonstrated under controlled laboratory conditions (10). The 2:00 p.m. dip is also evident in naturalistic contexts in such outcomes as errors made by shift workers, falling asleep at the wheel of an automobile, or compulsive brakings by locomotive drivers (see review by Craig, ref. 38). It seemed possible that the 2:00 p.m. decline in efficiency might represent a post-lunch dip reflecting the behavioral consequences of eating lunch.

Christie and McBrearty (25) undertook three studies of the post-lunch dip. The first traced the changes in pulse rate, oral temperature, and deep body temperature after 20 subjects ate lunch; it also detected increases in pulse rate 1 hr after the meal. The second study, also of 20 individuals, noted increases in capillary blood glucose 1 hr after eating and found no change in deep body temperature. This study also found that self-reported mood activation scores were decreased and deactivation scores increased when sampled 1½ hr after eating. The third study sampled 10 males and 10 females on 2 days 1 week apart. On one day, lunch and coffee were eaten at 1:00 p.m.; on the other day, only coffee was consumed at this time. Conditions were counterbalanced. Self-reported mood deactivation increased significantly 1½ hr after lunch but declined significantly when no lunch was eaten. Performance on a letter cancellation task declined from 1 to 3 hr after lunch and improved during this time without lunch, although differences were significant only for male subjects. Christie and McBrearty (25) also found evidence of an individual difference, such that persons characterized as stable extroverts on the basis of the Eysenck Personality Inventory (48) showed a greater post-lunch dip than neurotic introverts.

Craig et al. (39) conducted a study to evaluate whether post-lunch performance decrements reflected an actual decline in sensory–perceptual sensitivity or a change in motivational, nonsensory decision criteria (71). Forty subjects were randomly assigned to lunch and no-lunch conditions. Subjects assigned to lunch ate a three-course meal free of charge between noon and 1:00 p.m. Coffee and tea were available after the meal but had to be purchased at personal expense. Subjects not given lunch were instead offered a free cup of tea or coffee. Performance was tested 1 hr before and 1 hr after lunch. Subjects viewed the two letters A or B presented for 0.82 sec on 480 trials. They judged which stimulus had been seen and rated their confidence in each judgment. Signal detection analyses indicated that perceptual discrimination efficiency was diminished after subjects ate lunch but was unaffected when they had no lunch. Decision criteria for rating stimuli were unaffected. As in the Christie and McBrearty study (25), stable extroverts showed the greatest dip in perceptual efficiency. It will be important for future studies to more carefully control caffeine consumption, since higher caffeine intake in the no-lunch group could provide an alternative explanation of the results.

Craig (38) also reports a recent unpublished study using a letter cancellation task. Subjects worked for 30 min to put a slash through every E in a passage of prose read before and after lunch. A heavy three-course lunch of approximately 1,000 calories increased errors of omission, whereas a light sandwich lunch of less than 300 calories tended to reduce errors. Effects were minimized when subjects ate their usual size lunch and were maximized when the lunch was unusually large or small.

Craig (38) reviews studies that failed to find a post-lunch dip, especially when the meal ended a very long fast. He also reviews evidence suggesting that the dip may be greatest when the lunch contains a high proportion of carbohydrates.

B. Breakfast

Until recently, the effects found for eating breakfast had been more beneficial than those found for eating lunch, even though the benefits were slight. Except for an enhancement of taste sensitivity (176) and increased memory for distractors (123), both of which were found late in the morning, no advantages of skipping breakfast had been empirically demonstrated. In two crossover studies, Pollitt et al. (122,123) compared the late morning performance of 9- to 11-year-old well-nourished children when they ate or did not eat breakfast following an evening fast. There were 32 children in the first study and 39 in the second. On the breakfast day, a high-carbohydrate breakfast (65–75 g) that also included some protein (12–15 g) and fat (16–20 g) was served between 8:00 and 8:30 a.m. Children engaged in quiet activities from 8:30 to 11:15, when behavioral testing began. In both studies, skipping breakfast increased the number of errors that children made on the Matching Familiar Figures Test (96), which requires children to identify a correct pattern from multiple displayed alternatives. The lower the blood levels of insulin and glucose, the more errors the children made. Performance on the Continuous Performance Test (CPT), a measure of vigilance, was unaffected in the one study in which this was examined. Missing breakfast increased recall of incidental but not central information on the Hagen Central Incidental Test (78). Pollitt et al. (123) attributed the increased recall of incidental information after skipping breakfast to attentiveness to task-irrelevant stimuli due to heightened anxiety. However, another interpretation might be that hunger increases distractibility.

Conners and Blouin (32) conducted a similar study of 10 children tested on two occasions when they ate a mixed-nutrient breakfast at an unspecified time and on two occasions when they skipped breakfast after an overnight fast. On each test day, children were assessed at 9:50 a.m., 11:00 a.m., and 12:10 p.m. Although accuracy of performance on the CPT did not reveal significant effects of skipping breakfast, performance was significantly more variable without breakfast at all three test times. In addition, a trend was observed for arithmetic performance to improve by 11:00 a.m. when children ate breakfast. This practice or familiarization effect was absent when children skipped breakfast.

Although both the studies by Pollitt et al. (122,123) and Conners and Blouin (32) demonstrated somewhat greater advantages of eating rather than skipping breakfast, it is important to note that in both cases, testing commenced at least 2 hr after meals. (This must be surmised for the Conners and Blouin study since breakfast time was unspecified.) Study designs had not been parallel to those demonstrating the post-lunch dip in performance. Hence it remained possible that researchers had failed to administer their measures when a true post-breakfast performance dip was present. The performance dip following lunch is present between 1 and 2 hr after a meal. A post-breakfast dip in performance might also have been observed if testing occurred 1 to 2 hr after the morning meal rather than later. Conversely, it is possible that adverse effects of skipping lunch would be found if testing began 3 hr after mealtime. By this interval, the effects of maintaining a fast may become evident. Stated differently, the adverse effects of skipping breakfast that had been demonstrated may simply have represented the negative consequences of prolonged fasting. Study designs had used too long a meal–test interval to adequately test for post-breakfast decrements. A similar comment was made by Craig (38). Another suggestion offered by Spring et al. (150) was that, since the circadian rhythm for some performance functions begins to take a downswing in the early afternoon (53), performance after lunch might be more vulnerable to disruption by nutrient effects. Craig (38) pointed out that the converse holds true in the morning, when many rhythms are on the upswing and may be relatively immune to disturbance by foods.

Results of the most recent study by Conners et al. (33) suggest that breakfast may also produce a post-meal dip in performance. The Conners et al. (33) study has been the first to compare breakfasts comprised of different nutrients and to examine performance in the 2 hr following meals.

Conners et al. (33) randomly assigned a mixed group of 50 normal and hyperactive children to receive a high-carbohydrate breakfast, a high-protein breakfast, or no breakfast at 8:15 a.m. Children who ate the carbohydrate breakfast performed worse on a test of vigilance than those who fasted. Impairments were significant from 30 min to 4 hr after the meal. Children who ate the carbohydrate breakfast also performed significantly worse than those who ate protein. Although subjects who ate protein displayed somewhat poorer vigilance than those who fasted, it is unclear whether these differences were significant. It is noteworthy that the Conners group also found evidence of a post-breakfast dip as late as 4 hr after eating. The discrepancy from previous results may be due to the fact that their high-carbohydrate breakfast lacked sufficient protein to block the brain uptake of tryptophan.

IV. BEHAVIORAL EFFECTS OF TRYPTOPHAN, CARBOHYDRATES, AND OTHER SEROTONINERGIC INTERVENTIONS

Behavioral research on the effects of carbohydrates is still in its infancy. At this preliminary stage of investigation, it is important to examine which behavioral parameters are most likely to be sensitive to variations in dietary carbohydrates.

To the extent that unbalanced carbohydrate meals exert their effects by enhancing serotonin synthesis, the animal and human literatures on behavioral consequences of manipulating serotonergic neurotransmission are relevant.

A. Activity and Aggression

1. Animal Studies of Motor Activity

The serotonin precursors tryptophan and 5-hydroxytryptophan (5-HTP) usually decrease locomotor activity in rats (111,112,153,166). On the other hand, some researchers have claimed that serotonin precursors can enhance behavioral activation. In rats, serotonin precursors, especially when given with agents that increase CNS serotonin availability [e.g., monoamine oxidase inhibitors (MAOIs), reuptake blockers] can cause signs of activation (69,146). Warbritton et al. (166) have argued convincingly that increased locomotor activity is not among the indices of activation that are triggered by tryptophan. Instead, signs of activation involve autonomic arousal and skeletal muscle hyperactivity (e.g., myoclonus). In humans, by contrast, serotonin precursors can ameliorate posthypoxic intention myoclonus, although they can also exacerbate other types of myoclonus (75,163).

The remaining inconsistent findings concern evidence that a greater dietary intake of carbohydrate relative to protein is associated with increased motor activity in rats. When Chiel and Wurtman (24) fed rats a diet involving increasing ratios of carbohydrate relative to protein, animals showed increased nocturnal activity. Findings were independent of fat content, caloric intake, and weight gain. Similarly, Buckalew and Hickey (17) fed rats solutions containing from 0 to 20% sucrose. Measurements with an activity platform and impulse counter indicated that the rats that consumed more sucrose were significantly more active than those not fed sucrose. The findings by Chiel and Wurtman (24) and Buckalew and Hickey (17) concerning activity level and carbohydrate intake in rats are at variance with data from most experimental studies of human subjects.

2. Animal Studies of Aggression

Findings have consistently demonstrated that muricide (mouse-killing) can be induced in rats by manipulations that reduce serotonergic function. Such manipulations include lesions of the raphe nuclei (70), inhibition of serotonin synthesis by parachlorophenylalanine (PCPA) (139), and maintaining animals on a tryptophan-free diet for 4 to 6 days (60). Moreover, muricide can be reduced by treating rats with L-tryptophan or lithium, which, among other actions, increases serotonin release (156). Serotonin agonists are effective treatments regardless of whether muricide was induced by isolation, thiamine deficiency, or a tryptophan-free diet.

3. Human Studies: Correlational

Prinz et al. (126) studied 28 hyperactive children and 26 nonhyperactive controls aged 4 to 7 years. Mothers kept 7-day food intake records for the children during the week prior to laboratory testing. At the end of the week, children were videotaped in a playroom. Raters blind to the children's diagnostic and dietary characteristics scored the tapes for destructive–aggressive behavior, restlessness, and quadrant changes. Hyperactive children failed to differ from controls in patterns of food intake. For hyperactive children, however, sugar consumption during the prior week was positively correlated 0.45 with rated destruction–aggression, 0.33 with rated restlessness, and was not significantly correlated with quadrant changes. In comparison, for the control children, sugar consumption was positively correlated 0.59 with quadrant changes and was not significantly correlated with either behavior rating.

M. Wolraich, P. J. Stumbo, R. Milich, C. Chenard, and F. Schultz at the University of Iowa (*unpublished manuscript*, 1984) attempted to replicate the Prinz et al. (126) findings. Mothers of 32 hyperactive boys and 26 controls, aged 7 to 12 years, completed 3-day diet records and food frequency interviews. The hyperactive group were of lower socioeconomic status than the controls, and a significantly greater proportion of hyperactive children were on sugar-restricted diets. Sugar-restricted children did not differ from nonrestricted children in dietary content, however, with the result that there were no significant dietary differences between hyperactive children and controls. Partial correlations (controlling for age) between total sugar intake and 37 behavioral and cognitive variables failed to detect any significant correlations within the hyperactive group (the only group for whom behavioral data were available). The higher the ratio of sugar to total calories consumed, however, the higher were free play activity levels (measured by grid crossings and ankle actometer), off task behaviors, and attention shifts (both rated by observers). These correlations ranged from 0.39 to 0.55. Results can be considered to represent only a weak replication of Prinz et al. (126) because of the lack of significant correlations between total sugar intake and behavior. Moreover, as the authors point out, because of the large number of correlations computed, the few significant findings could have emerged by chance alone.

In another recent correlational study, Prinz and Riddle (125) identified 91 healthy caucasian boys aged 4½ to 5½ years. Based on mothers' 7-day food intake records for their children, extreme groups were selected with the 23 highest and 23 lowest sucrose consumers, based on mean daily sucrose intake in grams divided by body weight in kilograms. At the end of the week of food intake recording, a version of the CPT of vigilance was administered. Children were asked to press a lever in response to a slide showing a duck for 500 msec and to refrain from responding to slides showing other animals. The children who were in the habit of eating large quantities of sucrose (averaging 6.65 g/kg) showed significantly lowered sensitivity on the vigilance test. Although these children responded to significantly fewer ducks than the children who usually ate lesser amounts of sugar, they did not overrespond to a related nontarget stimulus (an eagle). Consequently, differences reflect lowered sensitivity to targets rather than impulsive responding to nontargets among children who usually eat much sugar.

Prinz and Riddle (125) compared the two groups of children on other factors in order to evaluate third variables that could explain their correlational findings. Both groups were comparable with respect to family income, family size, child IQ, occupational status, number of children in the family, mother's knowledge of behavioral principles, and child's body weight. Not surprisingly, the children who usually ate much sucrose habitually consumed 30% more carbohydrate than controls but did not differ in protein or fat intake. The absence of a difference in weight is striking, especially in the presence of a highly significant ($p = 0.001$) excess of calories consumed by the high-sucrose children.

Although Prinz et al. (126) hypothesize that sucrose might provoke agitated or aggressive behavior in hyperactive children with attention deficits, they acknowledge that this conclusion cannot validly be drawn from correlational data. Since no information is available about what children ate shortly before testing, it is unclear what foods were influencing their activity levels and vigilance test performance. If food intake was limited in the hours before testing, it is even possible that the children who usually eat much sucrose were in a state of caloric deprivation when they were tested, with this factor explaining their restlessness and poor performance.

Although correlational data cannot delineate the effects of sugar on behavior, they can help to describe the characteristics of individuals who prefer to eat large amounts of sugar. Findings suggest that restless, aggressive children who have difficulties sustaining vigilant attention are prone to eat large quantities of sugar.

The most parsimonious explanation for the correlational findings is that highly active or aggressive children consume excess carbohydrates and calories because of a metabolic need for energy. The absence of a weight difference between high- and low-sucrose-consuming children is consistent with the hypothesis of an increased metabolic rate in hyperactive children.

Alternatively, dietary preference for sugar may be an adaptive means of elevating brain tryptophan in order to help modulate high levels of activity or aggressive behavior. Just as adults learn that drinking caffeine-containing beverages can enhance their level of alertness, highly active or aggressive children may have learned that sugar produces a calming effect on behavior. It is possible that such children eat sugar in order to control and lower their behavioral activation and aggressiveness. The evidence connecting serotonergic hypofunction and aggression in humans is not definitive but is suggestive. First, psychiatric patients with a history of violent behavior show reduced levels of the serotonin metabolite 5-HIAA (14). Second, preliminary reports suggest that tryptophan (116) and lithium (140) may be of some value in treating aggressive behavior. Additional conflicting evidence is reviewed below.

Prinz and Riddle (125) propose that another characteristic of the highly active children who eat large quantities of sugar is that their mothers enforce significantly fewer limits concerning their children's access to the refrigerator or food cabinets. However, there are also conflicting data. For example, Wolraich et al. (*unpublished manuscript*, 1984) found that 60% of mothers of hyperactive children claimed to restrict their children's sugar intake, compared to only 12% of controls. The more fundamental question concerns the problem of whether self-reported parental attitudes reflect parental behavior, and whether either bears a relationship to what children actually eat. Parents who allege to practice sugar restriction appear to have difficulty implementing this policy, since Wolraich et al. found that only 47% are able to restrict their children's sugar intake to below 50 g/day. Moreover, children may thwart their parents' dietary regimens. Wolraich et al. found that hyperactive children reported that they ate more sugar then their parents knew about (126 versus 94 mg).

Again, the picture that emerges from these correlational data is that highly active children with vigilance deficits habitually consume large amounts of sugar. They may do so over their parents' objections or with their consent, but they seem to do so nonetheless. Correlational findings cannot address the question of how sugar affects children's behavior; only experimental designs can answer this question. However, the correlational findings do raise the interesting question of why restless, aggressive children with vigilance deficits apparently find it reinforcing to eat large amounts of sugar.

As already suggested, sugar consumption may meet a metabolic need for calories or engender a desirable, calming effect by enhancing the brain uptake of tryptophan. The need to increase the brain influx of tryptophan might be particularly great among a subgroup of hyperactive children who display alterations of tryptophan metabolism, such that less plasma tryptophan is available for brain uptake (94). However, the existence and nature of alterations in tryptophan metabolism among hyperactive children remain controversial (30,131,170).

4. Experimental Studies of Children

Although correlational research has generated interesting ideas about the relationship between sugar and children's behavior, findings can be misleading if interpreted as more than tentative hypotheses. Indeed, in this case, hypotheses based on correlational data are at variance with results from most experimental research. Experimental designs that can validly assess the effects of sugar on behavior are those in which sugar and a control substance are administered and their behavioral consequences compared at 15, 30, 45, 60, 120, and 180 min after ingestion.

Behar et al. (7) identified 21 boys whose parents responded to a newspaper advertisement seeking children with adverse behavioral reactions to sugar. Nine of the children met criteria for attention deficit disorder with hyperactivity. Eight did not qualify for a psychiatric diagnosis. The remainder presented ambiguous clinical pictures or past episodes of disturbance that had currently resolved. The boys, aged 6½ to 14 years, were medication free for 1 week before the study and were maintained on a high-carbohydrate diet for 3 days prior to testing.

On three different days, a minimum of 48 hr apart, children were fasted overnight. At 8:00 a.m. the following morning, in double-blind fashion, children received drinks containing saccharin placebo or 1.75 g/kg sucrose or glucose. Motor activity was measured cumulatively with an actometer, an acceleration-sensitive device worn on the child's belt that measured movement in counts per hour from 1 to 5 hr after ingestion. An observer also rated impulsive, restless, and inattentive behavior using a 10-item scale at 30 and 60 min and then at hourly intervals thereafter. Actometer counts of movement failed to detect significant changes in activity after either of the sugars as compared to placebo. When the data from both sugars were combined, however, at 3 hr after ingestion, sugar produced a slightly but significantly greater decrease in activity than did placebo, according to actometer counts. The observer rating scale failed to detect this phenomenon, nor did the CPT or a memory test detect other behavioral differences attributable to the test substances.

Ferguson (50) performed two sugar challenge studies. In the first, 12 children, aged 7 to 14 years, were challenged three times with sucrose (at 0.5, 1.0, and 1.5 g/kg) and three times with aspartame. Even though these children were selected because their parents believed they showed adverse responses to sugar, no significant differences were found between the effects of the two challenges on activity levels, observer ratings, or cognitive measures. A second study of 17 preschoolers, aged 3 to 4 years, challenged the children with aspartame or 30 g sucrose. Again, no differences were found on actometer measures, behavioral observations, or cognitive tests, although three boys performed nonsignificantly worse on drawings after the sugar challenge.

Wolraich et al. (171) conducted two studies of hyperactive boys who were admitted to a clinical research center and maintained on a sucrose-free diet for 3 days of testing. Both studies included 16 boys, aged 7 to 12 years in the first study and 8 to 12 years in the second. After a first day of baseline testing, children were challenged in double-blind fashion on the second and third days with a beverage containing either aspartame or 1.75 g/kg sucrose. In the first study, challenges were given 1 hr after lunch. In the second, drinks were given in the morning after an overnight fast. From 30 min after challenge until 3 hr afterward, children were assessed with actometer and observer ratings of playroom activity, with learning, vigilance, and memory tasks and measures of impulsivity. No significant differences between sucrose and aspartame were found on any measure in either study.

Results of these three challenge studies have been impressively consistent in demonstrating either no effect or a slight reduction of activity in comparison with placebo when children consume sugar. A series of studies of psychiatric inpatients performed recently by Conners and his associates (32,33) has detected more variable effects of sugar on behavior.

In a first pilot study, Conners and Blouin (32) studied 13 children hospitalized for severe behavior disorders, anxiety, and attention deficits. After a high-protein breakfast, children were challenged with 50 g sucrose, fructose, or orange juice on alternative days in counterbalanced order. The interval between breakfast and challenge was unspecified. Observers and staff but not children were blind to treatment condition. When compared to juice, both sugars increased observer ratings of total movement and decreased ratings of appropriate behaviors based on 15-sec samplings of behavior in a classroom. Teachers were unable to detect these changes, nor did nurses detect differences when using a ward rating scale. The elapsed time between challenge and behavior ratings was unstated. In commenting on the study, Conners notes that it does not permit conclusions about diet–behavior relationships because dietary control was not maintained and because subjects were not blind to experimental conditions.

In a second study, 37 children who were psychiatric inpatients received 1.25 g/ kg sucrose or fructose or the taste equivalent of aspartame. All subjects received all three treatments after breakfast in counterbalanced order for 1 week for periods ranging from 1 to 21 weeks. Double-blind conditions were maintained, and daily food intake was assessed although not controlled. The intervals between breakfast and challenge, or between challenge and testing, were unspecified, and subjects apparently could eat other snacks during this time. In this study, observer ratings of movement in the classroom indicated that sucrose lowered minor motor activity (restlessness rated while the child sits in a chair) but had no effect on gross motor activity (activity when the child is not seated). In contrast, fructose lowered gross motor activity without affecting minor motor activity. A hierarchical regression analysis was performed to control for the effects of age, baseline behavior rates, and nutrients eaten for breakfast. Results indicated that protein and carbohydrate intake at breakfast explained a greater proportion of the variance in behavior than did the challenge substances (33). When age, baseline behaviors, and breakfast foods (apparently not including snacks) were held constant statistically, the sugar challenge appeared to increase deviant behavior. However, this statistical effect was blocked by a breakfast meal of mixed nutrients including protein.

The Conners et al. (33) findings suggest the need to consider the effects of prior food intake when examining the behavioral consequences of carbohydrate snacks. It is difficult to evaluate the specific findings about carbohydrate effects on behavior because of three sources of variability: the amount of food eaten by the children for breakfast and snacks, its nutrient composition, and the interval between eating and behavioral assessment. Since allowing subjects to choose their own meals and snacks introduces a correlational element into an experimental protocol, the conservative approach is to regard the results as hypothesis generating. Conners et al. (33) introduced the useful technique of hierarchical multiple regression to statistically estimate the impact of both manipulated and nonmanipulated variables. An important next step will be to follow up with experimental manipulations of breakfast constituents and subsequent snacks to see whether the same effects emerge. The design of such a study would optimally involve standard high-protein and high-carbohydrate breakfasts, matched on fat content and eaten after an overnight fast. Food intake would be controlled, challenges given at a fixed interval after breakfast, and behavior measured from 15 min to 3 hr after challenges. Conners et al. (33) have completed such a study of performance effects, but activity was not a dependent variable.

The majority of experimental studies of the effects of sugar on children's behavior have suggested no change or a decrease in activity after sugar consumption. Conners et al. (33) have found both decreases and increases in activity after carbohydrate consumption, with differences possibly explained by what else the child has eaten. The Conners et al. protocol differed from the others in allowing subjects to choose what they ate for breakfast and snacks prior to challenge. Another difference is the fact that the Conners et al. sample were presumably severely disturbed, since they were psychiatric inpatients. In addition, 43% of the sample met criteria for pica (ingesting various kinds of nonfood substances). If an experimental design can replicate the correlational finding suggesting an increase in activity when a sugar challenge follows a high-carbohydrate meal, results will be at variance with other human findings but consistent with rat study findings by Chiel and Wurtman (24) and Buckalew and Hickey (17). A replication study might also examine the intervals between meal and challenge, and between challenge and behavior, since differences from other studies might help explain discrepant results.

5. Experimental Research on Adult Aggression

In a recent study, Young (180) and his colleagues examined the effects of tryptophan depletion on aggression in normal adults. Young administered the tryptophan-free, tryptophan-balanced, and tryptophan-supplemented amino acid mixtures described earlier in this chapter to 36 normal males aged 18 to 30 years. At 8:00 a.m., after an overnight fast, subjects received one of the three mixtures in a cross-sectional design. Five hours later, mood was assessed with a self-report scale. Subjective hostility did not differ among the three groups. Young (180) also used a laboratory test of aggression first introduced by Buss (19). Subjects were encouraged, incorrectly, to believe that they had a partner in the study. They were told that the partner was to be tested for pain sensitivity by rating electric shocks, whereas the subject was to be tested for auditory perception and reaction time. The subject heard tones supposedly selected by the partner. Some of the tones that the partner apparently chose to inflict on the subject were uncomfortably loud. In response to each tone, the subject was to rapidly choose from buttons that allegedly delivered the partner different intensities of shock. Hence the subject had an opportunity to retaliate for the unnecessarily loud noise. The dependent variables were the duration and intensity of shocks intended for the partner. Like the subjective estimate of hostility, the Buss aggression paradigm failed to detect changes in aggression following the amino acid mixtures. However, the study represents a good example of an effort to adapt a procedure from experimental social psychology to the study of diet–behavior relationships.

B. Sensory Responses

1. Animal Studies

Three aspects of sensory responsivity appear to be modulated by serotonin in animals: acoustic startle reflex, temperature regulation, and pain sensitivity. In rats, the acoustic startle reflex is increased by depletion of brain serotonin and decreased by serotonin agonists. Lesions of the raphe nuclei (44) or a tryptophan-free diet (165) heighten startle. Walters et al. (165) found that a 64% depletion of whole-brain serotonin was required to significantly elevate startle amplitudes; a 28% decrease was not sufficient. Dietary L-tryptophan restored startle responses to control levels. Consistent with other findings, serotonin infused into the forebrain via the lateral ventricle depressed startle (43).

Serotonin agonists and antagonists affect body temperature and temperature preferences in immature and grown rats. One possible explanation may be that serotoninergic neurons in the hypothalamus are involved in modulating a thermoregulatory set point. Acute treatment with serotonin precursors lowers body temperature in rats and is associated with preference for higher temperatures. Conversely, depletion of brain serotonin via PCPA elevates body temperature and results in preference for lower temperatures (67,68).

Animal data also suggest serotoninergic involvement in responsivity to pain. Lytle et al. (106) found that a tryptophan-poor corn diet reduced brain serotonin and increased responsiveness to electric shock in rats. Both effects were reversed by an injection of tryptophan.

2. Human Studies

Whereas animal studies suggest that serotonin agonists depress the startle response, lower body temperature, and raise temperature preferences, comparable human data are lacking. Data are available, however, that suggest that tryptophan reduces pain discriminability and enhances pain tolerance in human subjects.

In normal human subjects, Seltzer et al. (138) reduced pain sensitivity by feeding subjects 3 g tryptophan combined with a high-carbohydrate, low-protein, low-fat diet. Lieberman et al. (102) studied the acute effects of tryptophan on thermal and pain perception in normal adults using signal detection methodology. At 7:15 a.m., after an overnight fast, eight male subjects received tryptophan (50 mg/kg) or placebo in a double-blind crossover design. At 9:00 a.m., subjects were tested for their abilities to discriminate among different intensities of thermal stimuli delivered via a Hardy–Wolff–Goodell dolorimeter. Separate assessments were made of P(A), the subjects' sensitivity in discriminating each stimulus intensity, and of B, the subjects' response bias toward describing stimuli as more or less intense. Of five paired stimulus comparisons, tryptophan reduced discriminability for stimuli at 320 versus 270 mcal when compared to placebo. These intensities were rated painful or very painful. Tryptophan did not alter discriminability between the most painful stimuli or among less painful thermal stimuli. Tryptophan did not affect response bias for any stimulus comparison. In discussing these findings, Lieberman et al. (102) point out that morphine and diazepam also fail to reduce discriminability among intensely painful stimuli. Moreover, unlike tryptophan, these drugs affect the attitudinal or response bias aspect of pain perception.

In patients with chronic pain, Sternbach et al. (152) found that tryptophan increased pain tolerance and reduced depression. In five patients with deafferentation pain following rhizotomy and cordotomy, tryptophan alleviated recurrent pain (98). Recently, Seltzer et al. (137) studied 30 patients with chronic maxillo-facial pain who were assigned on a double-blind basis to receive either cellulose placebo or 3 g tryptophan daily combined with a high-carbohydrate, low-protein, low-fat diet. At baseline, week 1, and week 4 of treatment, subjects rated their average pain on a 100-point scale and completed the Magill Pain Inventory (which assesses pain right now), the Beck and Zung Depression Scales, and the Spielberger State-Trait Anxiety Scale. By the end of the treatment month, average pain had decreased to a significantly greater extent with tryptophan (32-point decrease) than with placebo (11-point decrease). However, pain right now, as measured by the Magill Scale, was not differentially affected. Although anxiety and depression also decreased significantly over the 1-month period, tryptophan and placebo did not differ in their effect on mood.

Results suggest that tryptophan, particularly in combination with a carbohydrate-rich, protein-poor meal, could prove advantageous in the treatment of chronic pain. The avenue by which benefits come about, particularly the interplay with psychological distress, remains to be clearly unraveled.

C. Sleep

Several comprehensive reviews have described more than 43 investigations of the effects of tryptophan on sleep (29,81,82). A majority of studies indicate that tryptophan reduces the latency to fall asleep. Sleep onset can be facilitated in daytime as well as evening hours (148). Moreover, an infant formula containing tryptophan reduces sleep latencies in newborns in comparison with a feeding of valine and low carbohydrate (177,178).

There have also been some failures to find sleep-enhancing effects (e.g., refs. 2 and 117). In part, the inconsistent results may reflect differences in dosage. Soporific effects appear to be unreliable with 1 g tryptophan or less. Hartmann (81) originally found a sleepiness-inducing effect of 1 g tryptophan. In a double-blind crossover study of sleep latencies for seven women and five men, however, Adam and Oswald (2) failed to find differences between placebo and 1 g tryptophan, coupled with high- or low-carbohydrate meals.

More recently, Hartmann et al. (83) failed to find evidence that tryptophan surpassed placebo in decreasing subjectively reported sleep latencies. Separate groups of insomniac subjects received either 1 g tryptophan ($n = 29$), 100 mg secobarbital ($n = 22$), 30 mg flurazepam ($n = 22$), or placebo ($n = 22$) 30 min before bedtime for 7 nights. For the 7-day treatment period and a 6-day withdrawal period, subjects estimated time to fall asleep initially and after nighttime awakenings. Neither tryptophan nor secobarbital lessened subjectively reported insomnia in comparison with placebo, a surprising result since secobarbital is generally an effective hypnotic. An unexpected finding was that sleep latencies continued to shorten during the withdrawal period for subjects who had received tryptophan and for no other group. Consequently, by the end of the withdrawal phase, sleep latencies were significantly shorter than pretreatment latencies for subjects in the tryptophan group. In discussing the possible "continuing effect" of tryptophan, Hartmann et al. (83) point to similar trends in several other studies. They raise the possibility that alterations in serotonin receptors or other receptors might occur with long-term administration of tryptophan.

In trying to reconcile discrepant findings concerning tryptophan and sleep, Hartmann and Greenwald (82) suggest several generalizations. First, dosage is an important variable. Effects on sleep latency are unclear or nonexistent with less than 1 g tryptophan. Second, results are mixed with entirely normal subjects. The time to sleep onset is so brief in healthy adults that study designs need to allow ample duration to observe a tryptophan effect. For example, Nicholson and Stone (117) administered tryptophan 20 min before bedtime, and their subjects required only 10 to 12 min on placebo to fall asleep. Thus, to be detected, an effect of tryptophan would have to occur within 30 min. Since tryptophan is not as rapidly absorbed as standard hypnotic drugs, it should be taken approximately 1 hr before bedtime in order for the effects to be detectable. Finally, severely and chronically insomniac patients may prove refractory to the sleep-inducing effects of tryptophan. One suggestion is that such patients may become responsive only after repeated administrations of tryptophan (136a).

A majority of studies have found no dramatic effects of tryptophan in dosages up to 5 g on EEG measures of sleep stages (13,148). Unlike most hypnotics, tryptophan does not reduce rapid eye movement (REM) time or shorten stages 3 and 4 sleep; in fact, it slightly increases the duration of stage 4 sleep. At dosages exceeding 5 g, tryptophan can reduce REM sleep, and findings concerning REM latency are contradictory (82).

D. Mood

1. Depression and Euphoria

Serotonergic deficiencies may play a role in the etiology of some primary affective disorders. The serotonin metabolite 5-HIAA is abnormally low in the lumbar CSF of some depressed patients (4). Moreover, there appears to be a subgroup of affective disorder patients in whom plasma free tryptophan is decreased in relation to competing neutral amino acids (35,114). Based on a review of these data, Van Praag (160) suggests that approximately 40% of depressed patients may have a deficit in central serotonin metabolism.

The efficacy of tryptophan for the treatment of depression is controversial. Both positive and negative results have been reported (34). More promising evidence suggests that L-tryptophan can enhance the antidepressant efficacy of MAOIs (164). Studies of the other serotonin precursor, 5-HTP, have indicated somewhat greater antidepressant efficacy than for L-tryptophan (160).

For both tryptophan and 5-HTP, antidepressant efficacy may be greatest for patients who show biochemical evidence of serotonergic hypofunction. Unfortunately, there are no clear clinical signs that differentiate these patients from non-responsive individuals.

Taken together, the findings suggest that affective disorders are biologically heterogeneous, and that it is probably an oversimplification to regard any treatment as acting on a single neurotransmitter. Nonetheless, some depressions may be associated with evidence of central serotonergic hypofunction and may respond to serotonin precursors. It is also important to note that anxiety and agitation in depressed patients have not been found to be responsive to L-tryptophan (88,104).

Early studies reported that L-tryptophan induced euphoria in normal individuals (119,147), but these findings have not been replicated recently (72,102). On the other hand, recent reports suggest that 5-HTP can have a significant euphoriant effect in normal individuals (127,157).

In an elegant study of 36 normal males, Young and co-workers (cited in ref. 180) administered balanced, tryptophan-supplemented, or tryptophan-depleted amino acid mixtures at 8:00 a.m. after an overnight fast. The investigators tested the prediction that the tryptophan-depleted mixture would induce depression. When tested 5 hr later, subjects who were fed the tryptophan-depleted mixture showed a significant increase in self-reported depression compared to baseline scores. More-over, post-test depression scores for this group were significantly greater than those of the two groups fed the other test mixtures.

The Young group (180) provided converging evidence of depression by means of an interesting procedure. Subjects were asked to proofread and detect errors in typed passages containing mistakes in punctuation and spelling. They did so while hearing different types of distraction played over headphones. The low (easily ignored) distractor involved passages from a statistics text book. A high (hard to ignore) distractor presented eyewitness accounts of the bombing of Hiroshima. A dysphoric distractor presented themes of hopelessness and helplessness. This content should match the mental set held by a depressed person and should be difficult for such an individual to ignore. Subjects showed no differences in proofreading skill when tested at baseline. After the amino acids, the balanced group scored similarly with all three distractors, and the tryptophan-supplemented group actually per-formed best with the dysphoric distractor. The finding of greatest importance was that the tryptophan-depleted subjects were the only group to show significantly impaired performance with the dysphoric as compared to the low distractor. Thus findings from both the self-report mood scales and the proofreading task were consistent with the hypothesis that tryptophan depletion can produce a rapid low-ering of mood in normal male subjects.

Young et al. (180) also presented data demonstrating that the tryptophan-free mixture produced a marked depletion of plasma tryptophan by 5 hr. Given how rapidly the plasma and behavioral changes occurred, results raise an important but highly speculative question. Can human subjects consume foods that deplete plasma tryptophan to this degree, for example, by favoring carbohydrate snacks that are low in protein? Would such diets induce depression in susceptible individuals? Can dietary habits exacerbate the negative mood of the subgroup of depressed individuals who crave carbohydrates (41,92,93,133), or will even the most carbohydrate-rich diet usually provide enough protein to prevent depletion of plasma tryptophan?

2. *Drowsiness and Calmness*

Although much interest has focused on the effects of tryptophan on depression, the most consistent effect of L-tryptophan when administered to normal subjects is to induce drowsiness and to reduce subjective alertness. Greenwood et al. (72) gave normal adult volunteers 5 g L-tryptophan or placebo. When compared to placebo, tryptophan significantly increased self-reported drowsiness, clumsiness, muzziness, and mental slowing assessed by Visual Analogue Mood Scales (VAMS) (55). Effects were maximal 1 hr after ingestion and returned to baseline by 3 hr. In a crossover design, Hartmann et al. (85) gave 4 g L-tryptophan, leucine, or placebo to 12 normal adults, aged 18 to 30 years, at 10:00 p.m. Sleepiness ratings on a 7-point scale taken at 15-min intervals demonstrated that by 60 to 90 min after ingestion, tryptophan induced significantly greater drowsiness than either placebo or leucine. Yuwiler et al. (181) gave subjects L-tryptophan once at 50 mg/kg, once at 100 mg/kg, and for 14 days at 50 mg/kg. At both acute doses, subjects reported increased drowsiness that began approximately 30 min after ingestion and lasted for several hours. More pronounced drowsiness was reported at the higher dose. Lethargy was greater and more enduring with chronic administration, sometimes lasting into the evening.

In a recent study, Lieberman and co-workers (102) compared tryptophan (50 mg/kg) and placebo given in counterbalanced order, double-blind, to 20 healthy men. Substances were given at 6:15 or 7:15 a.m. after an overnight fast. Mood tests were administered 2 hr later. Compared to placebo, tryptophan significantly decreased the alertness factor of the VAMS (151). Tryptophan also increased fatigue and decreased subjective vigor, as measured by the Profile of Mood States (POMS) (108). The reduction in subjective vigor after tryptophan intake was quite large in magnitude: a decrease of 40% compared to placebo. Findings indicate that the ability of tryptophan to induce drowsiness is not confined to the evening hours. A substantial increase in fatigue also follows morning administration.

Clearly, tryptophan induces drowsiness and lowers subjective alertness. Can a carbohydrate-rich, protein-poor meal induce the same effect? The answer seems to be affirmative, although the effect is smaller in magnitude and less reliable. Hartmann et al. (84) recorded self-rated sleepiness at 15-min intervals among 12 normal males and females, aged 20 to 35 years. Subjects consumed six different liquid test meals in counterbalanced order at 8:00 p.m. in place of supper. All meals were 800 calories. One set of meals contained carbohydrate and fat but no protein. The other set was high in protein. In addition, meals were supplemented with either 2 g tryptophan, 2 g L-leucine, or 2 g placebo. When data were collapsed across amino acid conditions, results indicated that the carbohydrate meals produced significantly greater sleepiness 2 hr after eating than did protein-rich meals.

In order to identify subgroups of the population who might show differential responsivity to nutrients, Spring et al. (151) tested 184 healthy adults between ages

18 and 65 years. In this cross-sectional study, subjects were randomly assigned to eat either a carbohydrate-rich, protein-poor meal, or a protein-rich, carbohydrate-poor meal for breakfast or for lunch. Protein and carbohydrate meals were isocaloric. The high-protein meal was 227 g trimmed turkey breast (containing approximately 57 g protein, 4 g fat, and 1 g carbohydrate). The high-carbohydrate meal was 304 g nondairy sherbet (containing no protein, approximately 4 g fat, and 57 g carbohydrate, of which 47 g was sucrose and 10 g was corn starch). Subjects assigned to eat the test meal for breakfast maintained an overnight fast and consumed the food between 7:15 and 8:30 a.m. Subjects assigned to the lunch groups ate a standard breakfast consisting of black coffee and a pastry (3 g protein, 33 g carbohydrate, and 7 g fat) and consumed the test meal between 11:00 a.m. and 1:00 p.m. Mood was assessed 2 hr after meals were eaten.

Females who ate the carbohydrate meal reported greater sleepiness than did females who ate the protein meal. Males who ate the carbohydrate meal described themselves as feeling calmer than males who ate protein. Both effects, although significant with this sample size, were subtle. The findings raised a question about whether females might be more sensitive than males to the drowsiness following an unbalanced carbohydrate meal. One alternative interpretation was that males might be more reluctant to report frank sleepiness in the work setting where testing was done. Another possible interpretation was that the effects of the standard size carbohydrate meal might be blunted for males because of their larger body size. Both alternative explanations for the sex difference were examined in a subsequent study described below.

Another interesting finding was that older individuals ($\geqslant 40$ years) who ate the carbohydrate meal for breakfast reported feeling more calm and less tense than those who ate protein.

In the absence of a crossover phase or baseline measures, and given the limitation that subjects knew what they were eating, results of the study should be interpreted tentatively. Findings suggest that the effects of foods may differ depending on the time of day the meal is eaten and the age and sex of the consumer. Results indicated that the mood that follows a carbohydrate-rich meal, in comparison to a meal that is protein rich, may be either sleepiness or calmness. Results may indicate that females are more sensitive than males to the drowsiness that follows a carbohydrate meal, although other interpretations are possible. In addition, older individuals may be more sensitive than younger ones to a possible calming effect of a carbohydrate breakfast.

The next study was undertaken to see whether males would also show sleepiness when fed a meal that contained more carbohydrate and when a more powerful within-subjects design was used. A second objective was to determine whether a meal consisting chiefly of starch would produce effects similar to those seen after a sucrose-rich meal. This study of 40 males aged 18 to 28 years was conducted by Lieberman et al. (103), and further details are provided by Spring et al. (150).

Subjects fasted overnight, ate a standard breakfast at 7:30 a.m., and returned to eat the test meals at noon. All subjects ate both a carbohydrate-rich and a protein-rich lunch, with order counterbalanced, on 2 different days separated by a 1-week interval. Self-report mood scales were administered prior to the meals and at hourly intervals until 5:00 p.m. The starch lunch was 152 g of a pita-bread-like substance, comprised of 104.5 g carbohydrate, 0.7 g protein, and 27.1 g fat. This meal supplied 661.1 calories. The protein lunch was 275 g turkey breast salad comprised of 0.8 g carbohydrate, 79.3 g protein, and 37.3 g fat. The protein meal supplied 673.7 calories.

A prior study of six adult males had compared the pita-bread and turkey meals used in this study with an isocaloric dose of sucrose to determine the effects of the meals on the plasma tryptophan ratio (103). By 1 hr after lunch, differences between the ratios generated by the protein versus carbohydrate foods were already significant, and the turkey meal had substantially decreased the tryptophan ratio. This difference in comparison with either a sugar or starch persisted 5 hr after the lunch. By 2 hr after lunch, both sugar and starch lunches had elevated the tryptophan ratio. The increase in the tryptophan ratio persisted until 5 hr after the lunch for the starch meal and until 4 hr after lunch for the sugar meal. Consequently, for the first 4 hr after lunch, the tryptophan ratio was affected very similarly by starch or sugar meals.

Mood findings for the 40 subjects in the complete protocol indicated that, on both days of testing, sleepiness increased and subjective vigor declined significantly over the course of the demanding 5-hr test battery. Visual inspection of the data suggests that a postprandial upswing in sleepiness occurred following both the starch and protein meals in the 3 hr immediately after lunch. Although sleepiness was somewhat greater following the starch meal at 1 and 2 hr after lunch, these differences were not significant.

The patterning of means for the mood data suggests that the males in this study responded to carbohydrate in a qualitatively similar way to the response of female subjects in the Spring et al. (151) study. That is, males became slightly although not significantly sleepier after a carbohydrate than a protein meal. The absence of a statistically significant mood response of males even to a fairly large quantity of carbohydrate may mean that males are not very sensitive to carbohydrate-induced changes in self-reported moods. Before a true gender difference in mood responsivity to carbohydrate can be inferred, however, it is necessary to replicate the finding that carbohydrate-induced drowsiness is a reliable and more pronounced finding in females than in males.

E. Performance

Despite the consistent evidence that tryptophan induces drowsiness, there is a lack of evidence that it impairs performance (149). When given acutely, tryptophan has not been found to slow reaction time or tapping speed in human subjects (72,102). In monkeys as well, learning and social behavior remain unaffected by a high-tryptophan diet, even when animals appear to become very lethargic (23).

1. Studies of Children

Some of the studies reviewed earlier concerning children's activity levels also included tests of performance. Behar et al. (7) detected no effects of sucrose or glucose on vigilance performance or memory. Similarly, Wolraich et al. (171) failed to find effects of sucrose on vigilance, paired associate learning, nonsense-word spelling, the Matching Familiar Figures Test (96), or drawing.

In contrast, Conners et al. (33) found opposite effects of carbohydrates in two studies of children's performance. In a first study, 13 children hospitalized as psychiatric inpatients ate a breakfast of their own choosing at 8:00 a.m. and received 1.25-g/kg challenges of relatively low-dose sucrose, fructose, or aspartame in counterbalanced order at 9:00 a.m. Performance was tested 30 min and 3 hr following challenges. As compared to aspartame, sucrose reduced errors of omission on the CPT of vigilance when the test was administered 30 min but not 3 hr after challenge. The sucrose challenge also speeded reaction time for the earlier but not the later test. Conners et al. (33) suggest that results may indicate a facilitative effect of small dosages of sugar on performance, at least against the background of a normal breakfast that probably contained mixed nutrients. Sample sizes were too small to estimate the effects of self-selected breakfast nutrients compared to challenge nutrients by hierarchical multiple regression.

In evaluating why the Conners et al. (33) findings on the behavioral effects of a sugar challenge differ from those of Behar et al. (7) and Wolraich et al. (171), there are several possible explanations. First, since breakfast meals were not controlled in the Conners et al. study, it is possible that the variability in performance was explained by differences in nutrient intake for breakfast. Second, sample differences may also be involved, since the Conners et al. subjects were psychiatric inpatients. It should also be noted that the sucrose-induced facilitation is in comparison to aspartame. The effects of aspartame on the performance of normal subjects remain unknown. Finally, results are at variance with those from a more carefully controlled study conducted by the Conners et al. group.

In what is apparently the first study to compare the effects of carbohydrate and protein meals on children's behavior, Conners and associates found that a high-carbohydrate breakfast produced detrimental effects on performance, as compared to a protein breakfast or no breakfast. Normal and hyperactive children ($n = 50$) were randomly assigned to fasting, high-carbohydrate breakfast (two slices of buttered toast), or high-protein breakfast (two eggs cooked in butter) eaten at 8:15 a.m. A high-dose 1.75-g/kg sucrose challenge or a 10-mg/kg aspartame challenge was given at 8:30 a.m. The CPT and a warned reaction time test were administered at 8:45 a.m., 10:00 a.m., and 12:15 p.m. At all three intervals, the carbohydrate breakfast, as compared to fasting or the protein breakfast, yielded worse performance on all aspects of vigilance test performance (omissions, commissions, and reaction time). However, the carbohydrate breakfast did not significantly affect warned reaction time. In addition, the sucrose challenge at this high dosage produced a detrimental effect on evoked potential measures of attentiveness when ingested after the carbohydrate breakfast or under fasting conditions but not after protein. The effects of the sugar challenge on performance were apparently similar but not reported in detail.

Results of the second, more carefully controlled Conners et al. (33) study suggest that a carbohydrate breakfast can produce adverse effects on children's attention. A sugar challenge taken immediately after the meal can augment the adverse effect or can be without additional effects. There was no evidence to suggest a facilitating effect of a sugar challenge on performance. The differing results of this study and the previous one demonstrate the utility of controlling and experimentally varying test meals in sugar challenge studies. It is noteworthy that the adverse effects of the carbohydrate breakfast were evident 30 min after eating and were sustained for 4 hr after the meal. It will be informative to plot the relationship between performance, plasma glucose, insulin, and the tryptophan ratio to determine the mechanisms responsible for behavioral differences. The difference between these findings and those of the previous study by Conners et al. (32,33) may also be due in part to dosage differences and to the fact that children in the second study were normal volunteers or outpatients with attention deficit disorders. It remains to be determined whether these two population subgroups responded similarly or differently to carbohydrates.

2. Studies of Adults

In an early study, Simonson et al. (142) found no differences between the effects of a normal lunch and no lunch on a vigilance test similar to the CPT. However, vigilance performance was impaired following a high-carbohydrate meal. Contrary to these results, King et al. (97) found that visual blind spot was less and motor speed fastest after a high-carbohydrate lunch than after no lunch. Tests were conducted as part of a study of altitude tolerance, and three of four sessions occurred after ascent to 17,000 feet. As Craig (38) points out, the protocol incorporates two unusual features: One is that a majority of assessments were made at high altitude; a second is that subjects had been fasting for 6½ to 7½ hr prior to lunch.

Spring et al. (151) examined performance on the dichotic shadowing test of sustained selective attention 2 hr after subjects ate carbohydrate or protein meals. This task requires subjects to repeat back (shadow), syllable by syllable, words presented to one ear over stereo earphones and to ignore distractors sometimes presented to the other ear. Shadowing was significantly less accurate after carbohydrate than protein meals, but this difference was significant only for older subjects who consumed the test meals for lunch. Older (≥40 years) people performed especially poorly after the carbohydrate as compared to the protein lunch. Older people who ate the carbohydrate lunch omitted more syllables than those who ate protein. However, they did not interject more distractor syllables or perform less accurately when distraction was present than when it was absent (149). Results are consistent with a hypothesis that a carbohydrate meal eaten for lunch may, for an older person, promote lapses of sustained attention without enhancing distractibility. A test of simple reaction time did not in this study detect differences attributable to foods.

In a study comparing the effects of starch and protein lunches on the performance of young male adults, Lieberman et al. (103) administered an extensive battery of performance tests from 1 to 5 hr after test meals. The dichotic listening test, administered 3 hr after lunch, did not detect performance deficits in this population, as it had not in the previous sample of younger subjects. However, a simple reaction time test, when administered 1¾ but not 2¾ or 3¾ hr after lunch, revealed significantly slower responses after the starch than the protein lunch. This task involved four times as many trials and waiting intervals half as long as the reaction time test used by Spring et al. (151) and may have yielded more reliable scores. Digit symbol substitution, a test of motor copying and concentration administered 3½ hr after lunch, revealed slightly but significantly worse performance after the carbohydrate than the protein meal. Two tests of vigilance, four-choice reaction time, card sorting, and a tapping test detected no other performance differences following the two meals.

Consistent with the second group of findings for children by Conners et al. (33) results of these two studies suggest adverse effects of carbohydrates on performances involving sustained attention and speed. Many tests did not detect differences, however, and except in the case of older individuals after a carbohydrate lunch, obtained differences were subtle. Further research on the elderly and on children, who might be especially sensitive to nutrient effects, is warranted to evaluate whether adverse effects of carbohydrates on attention represent a reliable finding.

Some have proposed that the behavioral changes observed after carbohydrate intake could be caused by hypoglycemia. In functional reactive hypoglycemia (80), blood glucose levels fall to abnormally low levels (30–40 mg/100 ml) 2½ to 5 hr after a carbohydrate-rich meal (124). At this time, affected individuals experience trembling, sweating, heart palpitations, hunger, and weakness. Prinz and Riddle (125) proposed that hypoglycemia associated with increased production of epinephrine could produce restlessness in hyperactive children who eat sugar. As supporting evidence, the authors cite the finding by Langseth and Dowd (100) that 76% of 261 hyperactive 7- to 9-year-old children had abnormal glucose tolerance curves. Few norms are available for judging whether children's glucose tolerance curves are abnormal, however, and the Langseth and Dowd study (100) lacked a normal control group. Virkkunen (161,162) has suggested that hypoglycemia following sugar consumption might lead to aggressive behavior in adults. This is based on findings of abnormal glucose tolerance test scores in violent offenders (162), as well as enhanced insulin secretion in aggressive individuals with antisocial personalities (161).

Although this is an intriguing suggestion, it must be noted that the majority of well-controlled studies using experimental rather than correlational methods have failed to find evidence that sugar increases activity levels or aggressiveness. In fact, some results suggest that carbohydrate foods may reduce these behaviors, perhaps by enhancing the uptake of tryptophan into the brain.

The relationship between low blood glucose and performance would be of interest to study. For various reasons, however, it appears unlikely that fluctuations in plasma glucose will be sufficient to explain the behavioral changes observed in normal individuals after carbohydrate consumption. First, reactively hypoglycemic individuals constitute only a small minority of the population, and known cases are explicitly excluded from most studies of carbohydrate effects on behavior. Second, plasma glucose levels after glucose challenge fall to similarly low levels in many individuals who do not report symptoms of physiological or psychological distress (M. L. Wolraich and R. Milich, *unpublished manuscript*, 1984). Third, in patients who do report symptoms, their timing is not clearly related to the rate of descent of the glucose level or to the level of glucose at the time of the symptoms (95). Fourth, in studies of the post-lunch dip, subjects who skip lunch presumably have lowered levels of plasma glucose; yet these individuals perform better on psychological tests than those who have higher levels of plasma glucose as a result of eating lunch. Fifth, it does not appear that plasma glucose fluctuations affect the brain under ordinary circumstances. Hence a mechanism by which plasma glucose could affect performance and mood has not been established.

Nonetheless, it would be of interest for study designs to disentangle the effects of plasma glucose and tryptophan. The small segment of the population that is reactively hypoglycemic would represent an interesting homogenous subgroup to study. To determine whether behavioral changes are better explained by fluctuations in plasma glucose or the plasma tryptophan ratio, the two might be independently varied. If alterations in mood and performance most closely parallel the tryptophan ratio, then they would be expected to appear even following a low-carbohydrate diet that is supplemented by tryptophan. Moreover, symptoms would not be expected following a glucose load that is supplemented by valine, which blocks the brain influx of tryptophan.

V. STUDIES OF OTHER NUTRIENTS

A. Tyrosine and Protein

1. Rationale

In the brains of humans or other mammals, the catecholamine neurotransmitters NE and DA are synthesized from the amino acid tyrosine. The rate-limiting initial step in this synthetic pathway is the hydroxylation of tyrosine by tyrosine hydroxylase (TOH) to form the intermediate product DOPA, which is then decarboxylated to form DA. In neurons containing the enzyme dopamine-β-hydroxylase, DA is converted to NE.

In rats, brain tyrosine is increased by a single meal in proportion to its protein content (63). The elevation in brain tyrosine after a meal containing 18 or 40% protein is evident 2 hr after the meal.

In fasted human subjects given a single oral dose of L-tyrosine (100 mg/kg), plasma tyrosine is maximally (twofold) increased 2 hr after ingestion and remains elevated for 8 hr (64). Giving the same amount of tyrosine together with a protein-containing meal causes an even greater elevation of plasma tyrosine. The ratio of plasma tyrosine to competing large neutral amino acids is also elevated. However, the rise in the tyrosine ratio is somewhat less than that following tyrosine alone (64,109) because of the competing large neutral amino acids found in protein.

Despite its effects on the plasma tyrosine ratio, it was initially believed that tyrosine administration would not enhance brain catecholamine synthesis because TOH appeared to be fully saturated. However, subsequent studies demonstrated that TOH is only 75% saturated (21). Moreover, when catecholamine neurons are rapidly firing, TOH becomes activated. The activation of TOH increases the affinity of the enzyme for its cofactor, tetrahydrobiopterin (which is rate limiting under basal conditions) and decreases the susceptibility of the enzyme to end-product inhibition (105,173).

In rats, the rate of catecholamine synthesis is increased by intraperitoneal injection of tyrosine (175) or by consumption of a protein meal (61), as evidenced by heightened accumulation of DOPA following inhibition of its decarboxylation. In animals subjected to cold stress (which increases turnover of brain NE) or probenecid (which blocks the exit of metabolites from CSF), increased brain tyrosine also leads to increased release of NE, as indexed by the accumulation of its metabolite, 3-methoxy-4-hydroxyphenylethylene glycol sulfate (MHPG-SO$_4$).

Tyrosine administration does not ordinarily increase the release of DA. The DA metabolite homovanillic acid (HVA) is not increased after tyrosine intake, even in rats receiving probenecid. However, under conditions that markedly increase the firing rates of DA neurons (e.g., DA-depleting lesions, DA receptor blockade by haloperidol, Parkinson's disease), DA release does appear to be enhanced by tyrosine intake, as evidenced by elevated levels of HVA (74,136).

2. Mood

Several findings have suggested that the metabolism and brain uptake of tyrosine may be altered when individuals are depressed. During the depressed phase of an affective illness, the usual 11:00 a.m. peak in plasma tyrosine is absent (8). Moreover, plasma tyrosine levels are significantly decreased in depressed patients compared to controls, and plasma tyrosine levels rise as patients recover from depression (99). Additional evidence suggests that less tyrosine may be transported into the brains of depressed patients (56). Moreover, a reduced ratio of plasma tyrosine to other large neutral amino acids may correlate with responsiveness to imipramine (115). These findings have been well reviewed by Gelenberg et al. (57).

An early study of tyrosine failed to find it beneficial in the treatment of depression (22). However, a later single-case study did find encouraging results in a 30-year-old unipolar depressed woman. The patient's symptoms improved markedly after

2 weeks of non-blind treatment with tyrosine (100 mg/kg/day) and returned when placebo was substituted. When tyrosine was reinstituted blindly, marked improvement again occurred (58). A subsequent report of two patients who had previously responded to amphetamine also found improvement after non-blind administration of tyrosine (66).

In a pilot study, Gelenberg et al. (57) assigned six depressed patients to tyrosine (100 mg/kg/day) and eight to placebo in a double-blind study lasting 4 weeks. Marked improvement was observed in 67% of tyrosine-treated patients, as compared to 38% of placebo-treated subjects. Moreover, the urinary excretion of MHPG, the major metabolite of NE, was increased 24% in tyrosine-treated patients, suggesting that NE turnover was increased. Analyses of the data from a more extensive comparison of tyrosine, imipramine, and placebo are now in progress.

Although tyrosine may lead to an improvement of mood in some depressed patients, there is a lack of evidence that tyrosine possesses mood-altering properties for normal human subjects. Lieberman et al. (102) administered tyrosine (100 mg/kg) and placebo to 20 healthy males in a double-blind crossover design at 6:15 to 7:15 a.m. No significant differences in mood or performance between tyrosine and placebo were detected.

3. Motor Activity, Aggression, and Behavioral Responses to Stress

There is some evidence to suggest that in mice, 1 week of dietary supplementation with tyrosine and phenylalanine can increase aggression and locomotor activity in an open field (154). In a follow-up to their original study, Thurmond et al. (155) found that the addition of 4% L-tyrosine for 1 week to a usual 12% casein diet led to an increase in the aggressive attacks that the mouse directed toward an intruder into its territory. However, tolerance to this effect developed after 5 weeks of supplementation. Aggressive behavior returned to normal even in the absence of tolerance to increased concentrations of brain catecholamines. Locomotor activity, measured by grid crossings, was also increased after 1 week by either tyrosine or phenylalanine supplementation. Unlike the change in aggression, the elevation in motor activity was sustained after 5 weeks of supplementation. Brady et al. (12) also found that 1 week of supplementation of a 12% casein diet with 4% tyrosine increased aggression in young mice (aged 3 months); however, this effect was not observed in older mice (aged 21 months). Unlike Thurmond et al. (154), Brady et al. (12) failed to find significant changes in locomotor activity following 1 week of tyrosine supplementation.

Acute unavoidable stress results in behavioral deficits, including reductions in spontaneous movement, aggression, and swimming (12,168,169). These behavioral changes, described as learned helplessness (107), have been attributed by some to the hypothalamic and brainstem locus ceruleus depletions in NE, with which they covary (169). An additional finding has been that TOH activity is decreased in the septal area of tree shrews exposed to a chronic social stressor (the visual presence of a dominant animal that subjugated them). These stressed animals died within 4 to 12 days of subjugation. In contrast, animals who were able to avoid the visual presence of the victor were able to survive for at least 50 days. These animals showed increased activity of TOH in the limbic septum and the adrenals (128).

An important question has been whether tyrosine is able to reverse both the behavioral depression and the NE depletion that follow an uncontrollable stressor. Brady et al. (12) found that a 12% casein diet supplemented for 1 week with 4% L-tyrosine prevented the usual diminution in aggression induced in both young and aged mice by cold-swim stress. Tyrosine also prevented the reduction in motor activity ordinarily observed in both stressed and nonstressed aged mice on a second test session. Although stress decreased brain NE and DA in both young and aged mice, and although tyrosine supplementation increased brain tyrosine and DA in both age cohorts, tyrosine did not produce significant changes in brain NE.

In a study of rats, Lehnert et al. (101) administered tail-shock stress or no stress to animals maintained on a 20% protein diet or on diets supplemented with tyrosine alone or tyrosine plus valine. Exposure to stress reduced spontaneous motor activity and decreased exploration of a new environment (measured by hole-poking and standing on hind legs). Stress also caused an increase in NE turnover, increasing MHPG-SO_4 and decreasing NE in the locus ceruleus, hypothalamus, and hippocampus. There were no significant changes in serotonin levels or turnover. Tyrosine supplementation prevented both the behavioral depression and the depletion of NE produced in control animals by stress. Tyrosine supplementation in the absence of stress did not produce changes in behavior or NE turnover. Moreover, coadministration of valine, which competes with tyrosine for brain uptake, eliminated the ability of tyrosine to prevent stress-induced NE depletion and behavioral depression.

Unlike Thurmond et al. (155) and Brady et al. (12), Lehnert et al. (101) found no significant behavioral changes following tyrosine supplementation to unstressed animals. Moreover, Lehnert et al.'s (101) results differ from those of Brady et al. (12) in finding changes in brain NE following tyrosine supplementation. Species differences between mice and rats may have a bearing on these discrepancies.

As Lehnert et al. (101) point out, their results raise an important question about whether tyrosine supplementation might prove beneficial to human subjects exposed to severe uncontrollable stressors. Under such circumstances, noradrenergic neurons, because of their enhanced activity, may become deficient in brain tyrosine and NE. If so, tyrosine might help to reverse these alterations in brain biochemistry and any accompanying psychological effects.

B. Choline and Lecithin

Evidence suggesting an important role for the central cholinergic system in human learning and memory has been well reviewed in an earlier volume in this series (45,47). With great consistency, in normal people, cholinergic antagonists, such as the muscarinic cholinergic blocking agent scopolamine, produce deficits in memory resembling those observed among elderly individuals. Memory disturbances are reversed by physostigmine, a cholinesterase inhibitor that prevents the degradation of acetylcholine within the synapse.

The cognitive performance that is most sensitive to anticholinergic effects involves the learning of new verbal material that exceeds memory span. Memory has been found to be disrupted by anticholinergic agents on tests involving recall of lists of words (113,121,144,158) or digits (135). Tests of immediate memory span (e.g., digit span) do not appear to be disrupted by anticholinergics (46,113). Moreover, retrieval of material learned prior to drug administration is less disrupted than is recall of new material learned afterward (20,46,59).

Much interest has focused on the question of whether consumption of choline (precursor to acetylcholine) or lecithin (phosphatidylcholine; a phospholipid that is the major dietary source of choline) can bring about improvements (or alleviate deficits) in memory. In rats, the administration of choline by injection or via the diet elevates brain acetylcholine levels, especially in the dorsal hippocampus (26,27,89). In humans, consumption of choline, or, more effectively, lecithin, raises choline levels in plasma and CSF (73,174). However, it remains unclear whether the administration of choline increases the synthesis and release of acetylcholine in the human brain.

In mice, the usual age-related decline in retention of a learned passive-avoidance behavior is reduced when animals chronically consume a choline-enriched diet (5). Moreover, in one study of normal young people, choline produced an improvement in memory performance (143). In contrast, among elderly individuals for whom memory disturbance may represent a significant clinical problem, acetylcholine precursors have produced disappointing results. In a recent review of 17 studies using choline or lecithin, Bartus et al. (6) commented that only one study found improvement in a majority (60%) of patients tested, and 10 failed to find evidence of facilitative effects.

It may be that a combination of lecithin and physostigmine will be more beneficial in enhancing memory among the elderly (120). However, in a recent open drug trial, patients with Alzheimer's disease showed temporary improvement in recall memory with physostigmine, regardless of whether or not lecithin was a concomitant aspect of treatment (153a).

In trying to understand why choline and lecithin produce so little benefit for the memory function of elderly individuals, in contrast to their results with animals or younger subjects, Bartus et al. (6) offer several suggestions. First, the muscarinic receptor may be functionally disturbed, such that increasing the synthesis of acetylcholine has little effect. Second, it remains possible that peripherally administered precursors, in the dosages studied, do not produce dramatic changes in the synthesis and release of brain acetylcholine in humans. Third, in the aged brain, deficiencies in choline uptake, CAT activity, oxidative metabolism, or the loss of cholinergic neurons projecting to the cortex may prevent choline from being easily synthesized into acetylcholine.

In summary, although results are presently discouraging, much remains to be learned about the effects of acetylcholine precursors on the human brain. In light of the adverse side effects, narrow effective dosage range, and short duration of benefit from drugs such as physostigmine or arecoline, which represent alternative treatments for memory loss in the elderly, the need for safe and effective treatments remains.

VI. CONCLUSIONS

The study of diet–behavior relationships is still in its infancy. Nonetheless, some intriguing results have emerged from research examining the acute behavioral consequences of administering meals, particular foods, or neurotransmitter precursors to normal individuals. Results of several studies suggest that a lunchtime meal may induce a drop in performance efficiency that occurs approximately 1 hr after the meal. Some positive behavioral aftereffects of eating mixed-nutrient breakfasts have been reported, especially when testing occurs late in the morning. However, the one study to examine changes occurring 30 min to 4 hr after eating a high-carbohydrate breakfast detected consistently negative effects on performance.

An extensive literature has developed concerning the effects of sugar on children's activity levels. A majority of well-controlled experimental studies have detected no change or a slight decrease in activity after sugar consumption. In healthy adults, preliminary evidence suggests that the effects of a carbohydrate-rich meal are similar but subtler than those produced by pure tryptophan. These effects include the induction of drowsiness or calmness and impairments in performance. Problems in concentration have also been found in the one study of children's performance after a carbohydrate meal. Animal research on the effects of tyrosine suggests that it might prove efficacious in alleviating behavioral deficits induced by uncontrollable stress, although studies of human subjects remain to be performed. Finally, despite numerous attempts to ameliorate memory deficits in the elderly, the benefits of choline or lecithin therapy remain elusive.

Many methodologic issues warrant consideration in studies of diet–behavior relationships. These include questions concerning research design, effect sizes, dose-response relationships, the timing of nutrient-related changes and their underlying mechanisms, individual differences, and the choice of the most sensitive behavioral tests. The potential background influences of circadian rhythms, fasting duration, usual dietary habits, and the intake of multiple nutrients all remain to be clearly unraveled.

Food selection represents an intervention that human beings self-administer repeatedly on a daily basis. A knowledge of the actual consequences of consuming particular foods alone or in combination may ultimately facilitate a choice of diets that can enhance the likelihood of desired behavioral consequences. At least, research on diet–behavior relationships can help to evaluate the validity of popular wisdoms about the effects of foods on psychological well-being.

ACKNOWLEDGMENTS

The author is grateful to Sherry Crowell and Donna Isaacson for technical assistance, and to Harris Lieberman and Judith Wurtman for comments on an earlier draft of this manuscript. Preparation of this chapter was supported in part by grants from the Institute of Nutritional Sciences and the Graduate School of Arts and Sciences, Texas Tech University.

REFERENCES

1. Adam, K. (1980): Dietary habits and sleep after bedtime food drinks. *Sleep*, 3:47–58.
2. Adam, K., and Oswald, I. (1979): One gram of tryptophan fails to alter the time taken to fall asleep. *Neuropharmacology*, 18:1025–1027.
3. Anderson, G. H. (1985): Approaches to assessing the dietary component of the diet-behavior connection. *Nutr. Rev. (Suppl.) (in press)*.
4. Asberg, M., Traskman, L., and Thoren, P. (1976): 5-HIAA in the cerebrospinal fluid: A biochemical suicide predictor. *Arch. Gen. Psychiatry*, 33:1193–1197.
5. Bartus, D., Dean, R. L., Goas, J. A., and Lippa, A. S. (1980): Age-related changes in passive avoidance retention: Modulation with dietary choline. *Science*, 209:301–303.
6. Bartus, R. T., Dean, R. L., Beer, B., and Lippa, A. S. (1982): The cholinergic hypothesis of geriatric memory dysfunction. *Science*, 216:408–417.
7. Behar, D., Rapoport, J. L., Adams, A. J., Berg, C. J., and Cornblath, M. (1984): Sugar challenge testing with children considered behaviorally "sugar reactive." *Nutr. Behav.*, 1:277–288.
8. Benkert, O., Renz, A., Marano, C., and Matussek, N. (1971): Daytime plasma levels in endogenous depressive patients. *Arch. Gen. Psychiatry*, 25:359–363.
9. Bierkamper, G. C., and Goldberg, A. M. (1979): Effect of choline on the release of acetylcholine from the neuromuscular junction. In: *Nutrition and the Brain Vol. 5: Choline and Lecithin in Brain Disorders*, edited by A. Barbeau, J. H. Growdon, and R. J. Wurtman, pp. 243–251. Raven Press, New York.
10. Blake, M. J. K. (1971): Temperament and time of day. In: *Biological Rhythms and Human Performance*, edited by W. P. Colquhoun, pp. 39–107. Academic Press, New York.
11. Bowen, D. M., Smith, C. B., White, P., and Davison, A. N. (1976): Neurotransmitter related enzymes and indices of hypoxia in senile dementia and other abiotrophies. *Brain*, 99:459–496.
12. Brady, K., Brown, J. W., and Thurmond, J. B. (1980): Behavioral and neurochemical effects of dietary tyrosine and neurochemical effects in young and aged mice following cold-swim stress. *Pharmacol. Biochem. Behav.*, 12:667–674.
13. Brown, C. C., Horrom, N. J., and Wagman, A. M. I. (1979): Effects of L-tryptophan on sleep onset insomniacs. *Waking Sleeping*, 3:101–108.
14. Brown, C. L., Goodwin, F. K., Ballenger, J. C., Goyer, P. F., and Major, L. F. (1979): Aggression in humans correlated with cerebrospinal fluid amine metabolites. *Psychiatry Res.*, 1:131–139.
15. Brown, G. G., and Nixon, R. K. (1979): Exposure to polybrominated biphenyl: Some effects on personality and cognitive functioning. *JAMA*, 242:523–527.
16. Brown, G. G., Preisman, R. C., Anderson, M. D., Nixon, R. K., Isbister, J. L., and Price, H. A. (1981): Memory performance of chemical workers exposed to polybrominated biphenyls. *Science*, 212:1413–1415.
17. Buckalew, L. W., and Hickey, R. S. (1983): Diet and activity level: An analysis of sucrose effects. *Res. Commun. Psychol. Psychiatry Behav.*, 8:349–352.
18. Bugge, J. F., Opstad, P. K., and Magnus, D. M. (1979): Changes in the circadian rhythm of performance and mood in healthy young men exposed to prolonged, heavy physical work, sleep deprivation, and caloric deficit. *Aviat. Space Environ. Med.*, 50:663–668.
19. Buss, A. H. (1961): *The Psychology of Aggression*. Wiley, New York.
20. Caine, E. D., Weingartner, H., Ludlow, C. L., Cudahy, E. A., and Wehry, S. (1981): Qualitative analysis of scopolamine-induced amnesia. *Psychopharmacology (Berlin)*, 74:74–80.
21. Carlsson, A., and Lindquist, M. (1978): Dependence of 5-HT and catecholamine synthesis on concentrations of precursor amino acids in rat brain. *Naunyn Schmiedebergs Arch. Pharmacol.*, 303:157–164.

22. Carroll, T. J. (1972): Monoamine precursors in the treatment of depression. *Clin. Pharmacol. Ther.*, 12:743–761.
23. Chamove, A. S. (1983): Dietary effects on rhesus social behavior: Altered amino acid diets. *Dev. Psychobiol.*, 16:505–509.
24. Chiel, H. J., and Wurtman, R. J. (1981): Short-term variations in diet composition change the pattern of spontaneous motor activity in rats. *Science*, 213:676–678.
25. Christie, J. J., and McBrearty, E. M. T. (1979): Psychophysiological investigations of post lunch state in male and female subjects. *Ergonomics*, 22:307–323.
26. Cohen, E. L., and Wurtman, R. J. (1975): Brain acetylcholine: Increase after systemic choline administration. *Life Sci.*, 16:1095–1102.
27. Cohen, E. L., and Wurtman, R. J. (1976): Brain acetylcholine: Control by dietary choline. *Science*, 191:561–562.
28. Cohen, J. (1977): *Statistical Power Analysis for the Behavioral Sciences*, revised ed. Academic Press, New York.
29. Cole, J., Hartmann, E., and Brigham, P. (1980): L-tryptophan: Clinical studies. *McLean Hosp. J.*, 5:37–71.
30. Coleman, M. (1971): Serotonin concentrations in whole blood of hyperactive children. *J. Pediatr.*, 78:985–990.
31. Colquhoun, W. P., ed. (1971): Circadian variation in mental efficiency. In: *Biological Rhythms and Human Performance*, pp. 39–107. Academic Press, New York.
32. Conners, C. K., and Blouin, A. G. (1983): Nutritional effects on behavior of children. *J. Psychiatr. Res.*, 17:193–201.
33. Conners, C. K., Caldwell, J., Caldwell, L., Schwab, E., Kronsberg, S., Wells, K. C., Leong, N., and Blouin, A. G. (1985): Experimental studies of sugar and aspartame on autonomic, cortical and behavioral responses to sugar. *Nutr. Rev. (Suppl.) (in press)*.
34. Cooper, A. J. (1979): Tryptophan antidepressant "physiological sedative:" Fact or fancy? *Psychopharmacology (Berlin)*, 61:97–102.
35. Coppen, A., and Wood, K. (1978): Tryptophan and depressive illness. *Psychol. Med.*, 8:49–57.
36. Costello, C. G., and Selby, M. M. (1965): The relationship between sleep patterns and reactive and endogenous depression. *Br. J. Psychiatry*, 111:497–501.
37. Deleted in proof.
38. Craig, A. (1985): Acute effects of meals on perceptual and cognitive functioning. *Nutr. Rev. (Suppl.) (in press)*.
39. Craig, A., Baer, K., and Diekmann, A. (1981): The effects of lunch on sensory-perceptual functioning in man. *Int. Arch. Occup. Environ. Health*, 49:105–114.
40. Crisp, A. H., and Stonehill, E. (1976): *Sleep, Nutrition and Mood*. Wiley, New York.
41. Dalton, K. (1980): *Depression After Childbirth*. Oxford University Press, Oxford, England.
42. Davies, P., and Maloney, A. J. F. (1976): Selective loss of central cholinergic neurons in Alzheimer's disease. *Lancet*, 2:1403.
43. Davis, M., Astrachan, D. I., and Kass, E. (1980): Excitatory and inhibitory effects of serotonin on sensorimotor reactivity measured with acoustic startle. *Science*, 209:521–523.
44. Davis, M., and Sheard, M. H. (1974): Habituation and sensitization of the rat startle response: Effects of raphe lesions. *Physiol. Behav.*, 12:425–431.
45. Deutsch, J. A. (1979): Physiology of acetylcholine in learning and memory. In: *Nutrition and the Brain, Vol. 5*, edited by A. Barbeau, J. H. Growdon, and R. J. Wurtman, pp. 343–350. Raven Press, New York.
46. Drachman, D. A., and Leavitt, J. (1974): Human memory and the cholinergic system: A relationship to aging? *Arch. Neurol.*, 30:113–121.
47. Drachman, D. A., and Sahakian, B. J. (1979): Effects of cholinergic agents on human learning and memory. In: *Nutrition and the Brain, Vol. 5*, edited by A. Barbeau, J. H. Growdon, and R. J. Wurtman, pp. 351–366. Raven Press, New York.
47a. Eckerman, D. A. (1984): Cognitive effects of neurotoxic agents. Paper presented at the workshop on Cognitive Testing Methodology, Committee on Military Nutrition Research, National Academy of Sciences.
48. Eysenck, H. J., and Eysenck, S. B. J. (1963): *Eysenck Personality Inventory*. Educational and Industrial Testing Service, San Diego, California.
49. Feingold, B. F. (1976): *Why Your Child Is Hyperactive*. Random House, New York.

50. Ferguson, B. (1985): Two studies examining the effects of sucrose in comparison to aspartame. *Nutr. Rev. (Suppl.) (in press)*.
51. Fernstrom, J. D., and Wurtman, R. J. (1971): Brain serotonin content: Increase following ingestion of carbohydrate diet. *Science*, 174:1023–1025.
52. Fernstrom, J. D., and Wurtman, R. J. (1972): Brain serotonin content: Physiological regulation by plasma neutral amino acids. *Science*, 178:414–416.
53. Folkard, S. (1983): Diurnal variation. In: *Stress and Fatigue in Human Performance*, edited by G. R. J. Hockey, pp. 245–272. Wiley, New York.
54. Folkard, S., Hume, K. E., Minors, D. S., Waterhouse, J. M., and Watson, F. L. (1985): Independence of the circadian rhythm in alertness from the sleep/wake cycle. *Nature*, 313:678–679.
55. Folstein, M. F., and Luria, R. (1973): Reliability, validity and clinical application of the visual analogue mood scale. *Psychol. Med.*, 3:479–486.
56. Gaillard, J. M., and Tissot, R. (1979): Blood-brain movements of tryptophan and tyrosine in manic-depressive illness and schizophrenia. *J. Neural Transm.*, 15(S):189–196.
57. Gelenberg, A. J., Wojcik, J. D., Gibson, C. J., and Wurtman, R. J. (1983): Tyrosine for the treatment of depression. *J. Psychiatr. Res.*, 17:175–180.
58. Gelenberg, A. J., Wojcik, J. D., Growdon, J. H., Sved, A. F., and Wurtman, R. J. (1980): Tyrosine for the treatment of depression. *Am. J. Psychiatry*, 137:622–623.
59. Ghoneim, M. A., and Mewaldt, S. P. (1975): Effects of diazepam and scopolamine on storage, retrieval and organizational processes in memory. *Psychopharmacologia (Berlin)*, 44:257–262.
60. Gibbons, J. L., Barr, G. A., Bridger, W. H., and Leibowitz, S. F. (1979): Manipulations of dietary tryptophan: Effects on mouse killing and brain serotonin in the rat. *Brain Res.*, 169:139–153.
61. Gibson, C. J., and Wurtman, R. J. (1977): Physiological control of brain catechol synthesis by brain tyrosine concentrations. *Biochem. Pharmacol.*, 26:1137–1142.
62. Gibson, C. J., and Wurtman, R. J. (1978): Physiological control of brain norepinephrine synthesis by brain tyrosine concentration. *Life Sci.*, 22:1399–1406.
63. Glaeser, B. S., Maher, T. J., and Wurtman, R. J. (1983): Changes in brain levels of acidic, basic, and neutral amino acids after consumption of single meals containing various proportions of protein. *J. Neurochem.*, 41:1016–1021.
64. Glaeser, B. S., Melamed, E., Growdon, J. H., and Wurtman, R. J. (1979): Elevation of plasma tyrosine after a single dose of L-tyrosine. *Life Sci.*, 25:265–272.
65. Glenville, M., and Broughton, R. (1980): Reliability of the Stanford Sleepiness Scale compared to short duration performance tests and the Wilkinson auditory vigilance task. In: *Pharmacology of the States of Alertness*, edited by P. Passouant and I. Oswald, pp. 235–244. Pergamon Press, New York.
66. Goldberg, I. K. (1980): L-tyrosine in depression. *Lancet*, 2:364.
67. Goodrich, C. I., and Choy, M. (1978): Body temperature and 5-hydroxytryptamine during early postnatal maturation in mice. *Dev. Psychobiol.*, 11:531–540.
68. Goodrich, C., and Wilk, C. (1981): Temperature preferences and the effect of changes in serotonin in maturing mice. *Physiol. Behav.*, 26:1041–1047.
69. Grahame-Smith, D. G. (1971): Studies in vivo on the relationship between brain tryptophan, brain 5-HTP synthesis and hyperactivity in rats treated with a monoamine oxidase inhibitor and L-tryptophan. *J. Neurochem.*, 18:1053–1066.
70. Grant, L. D., Coscina, D. V., Grossman, S. P., and Freedman, D. K. (1973): Muricide after serotonin depleting lesions of midbrain raphe nuclei. *Pharmacol. Biochem. Behav.*, 1:205–210.
71. Green, D. M., and Swets, J. A. (1966): *Signal Detection Theory and Psychophysics*. Wiley, New York.
72. Greenwood, M. H., Lader, M. H., Kantameneni, B. D., and Curzon, G. (1975): The acute effects of oral (−)-tryptophan in normal subjects. *Br. J. Clin. Pharmacol.*, 2:165–172.
73. Growdon, J., Cohen, E. L., and Wurtman, R. J. (1977): Effects of oral choline administration on serum and C.S.F. choline levels in patients with Huntington's disease. *J. Neurochem.*, 28:229–231.
74. Growdon, J. H., Melamed, E., Logue, M., Hefti, F., and Wurtman, R. J. (1982): Effects of oral L-tyrosine administration on CSF tyrosine and homovanillic acid levels in patients with Parkinson's disease. *Life Sci.*, 38:827–832.
75. Growdon, J. H., Young, R. R., and Shahani, B. T. (1976): L-5-hydroxytryptophan in treatment of several different syndromes in which myoclonus is predominant. *Neurology*, 26:1135–1140.

76. Grunberg, N. (1983): The effects of nicotine and cigarette smoking on food consumption and taste preferences. *Addict. Behav.*, 7:317–331.
77. Grunberg, N. E., Bowen, D. J., and Morse, D. E. (1984): Effects of nicotine on body weight and food consumption in rats. *Psychopharmacology (Berlin)*, 83:93–98.
78. Hagen, J. W. (1967): The effect of distraction on selective attention. *Child Dev.*, 38:685–694.
79. Hare, E. H. (1955): Comparative efficacy of hypnotics: A self-controlled, self-recorded clinical trial in neurotic patients. *Br. J. Prevent. Soc. Med.*, 9:140–141.
80. Harris, S. (1924): Hyperinsulinism and dysinsulin. *JAMA*, 83:729–733.
81. Hartmann, E. (1981): Tryptophan and sleep: Who responds to L-tryptophan? In: *Biological Psychiatry*, edited by C. Perris, G. Struwe, and B. Janssen, pp. 613–621. Elsevier Biomedical, Amsterdam.
82. Hartmann, E., and Greenwald, D. (1984): Tryptophan and human sleep: An analysis of 43 studies. In: *Progress in Tryptophan and Serotonin Research*, edited by H. G. Schlossberger, W. Kochen, B. Linzen, and H. Steinhart, pp. 297–304. Walter de Gruyter, New York.
83. Hartmann, E., Lindsley, J. G., and Spinweber, C. (1983): Chronic insomnia: Effects of tryptophan, flurazepam, secobarbital, and placebo. *Psychopharmacology (Berlin)*, 80:138–142.
84. Hartmann, E., Spinweber, C., and Fernstrom, J. (1977): Diet, amino acids and sleep. *Sleep Res.*, 6:61.
85. Hartmann, E., Spinweber, C. L., and Ware, C. (1976): L-tryptophan, L-leucine, and placebo: Effects on subjective alertness. *Sleep Res.*, 5:57.
86. Hasher, L., and Zacks, R. T. (1979): Automatic and effortful processes in memory. *J. Exp. Psychol. [Gen.]*, 108:356–388.
87. Haubrich, D. R., Wang, P. F. L., Clody, D. E., and Wedeking, P. W. (1975): Increase in rat brain acetylcholine concentration induced by choline or deanol. *Life Sci.*, 17:975–980.
88. Herrington, R. N., Bruce, A., Johnston, E. C., and Lader, M. H. (1976): Comparative trial of L-tryptophan and amitriptyline in depressive illness. *Psychol. Med.*, 6:673–678.
89. Hirsch, M. J., Growdon, J. H., and Wurtman, R. J. (1977): Increase in hippocampal acetylcholine after choline administration. *Brain Res.*, 125:383–385.
90. Hirsch, M. J., and Wurtman, R. J. (1978): Lecithin consumption elevates acetylcholine concentrations in rat brain and adrenal gland. *Science*, 202:223–225.
91. Deleted in proof.
92. Hopkinson, G. (1981): A neurochemical theory of appetite and weight changes in depressive states. *Acta Psychiatr. Scand.*, 64:217–225.
93. Hopkinson, G., and Bland, R. C. (1982): Depressive syndromes in grossly obese women. *Can. J. Psychiatry*, 27:213–215.
94. Irwin, M., Belendiuk, K., McCloskey, K., and Freedman, D. X. (1981): Tryptophan metabolism in children with attentional deficit disorder. *Am. J. Psychiatry*, 138:1082–1085.
95. Johnson, D. D., Dorr, K. E., Swenson, W. M., and Service, F. J. (1980): Reactive hypoglycemia. *JAMA*, 243:1151–1155.
96. Kagan, J., Rosman, B. L., Day, D., Albert, J., and Phillips, W. (1964): Information processing in the child: Significance of analytic and reflective attitudes. *Psych. Monogr.*, 78:578–615.
97. King, C. B., Bickerman, H. A., Bouvet, W., Harrer, C. J., Oyler, J. R., and Seitz, C. P. (1945): Effects of pre-flight and in-flight meals of varying composition with respect to carbohydrate, protein or fat. *J. Aviat. Med.*, 16:69–84.
98. King, R. B. (1980): Pain and tryptophan. *J. Neurosurg.*, 53:44–52.
99. Kishimoto, H., and Hama, Y. (1976): The level and circadian rhythm of plasma tryptophan and tyrosine in manic-depressive patients. *Yokohama Med. Bull.*, 27:89–97.
100. Langseth, L., and Dowd, J. (1978): Glucose tolerance and hyperkinesis. *Food Cosmet. Toxicol.*, 16:129–133.
101. Lehnert, H., Reinstein, D. K., Strowbridge, B. W., and Wurtman, R. J. (1984): Neurochemical and behavioral consequences of acute, uncontrollable stress: Effects of dietary tyrosine. *Brain Res.*, 303:215–223.
102. Lieberman, H., Corkin, S., Spring, B., Growdon, J. H., and Wurtman, R. J. (1983): Mood, performance and sensitivity: Changes induced by food constituents. *J. Psychiatr. Res.*, 17:135–145.
103. Lieberman, H. R., Spring, B. J., and Garfield, G. S. (1985): The behavioral effects of food constituents: Strategies used in studies of amino acids, protein, carbohydrate and caffeine. *Nutr. Rev. (Suppl.) (in press)*.

104. Lindberg, D., Ahlfors, U. G., Dencker, S. J., Fruensgaard, K., Hansten, S., Tensen, K., Ose, E., and Kinkanen, T. A. (1979): Symptom reduction in depression after treatment with L-tryptophan or imipramine. *Acta Psychiatr. Scand.*, 60:287–294.
105. Lovenberg, W., Ames, M. M., and Lerner, D. (1978): Mechanisms of acute regulation of tyrosine hydroxylase. In: *Psychopharmacology: A Generation of Progress*, edited by M. A. Lipton, A. DiMascio, and K. F. Killam, pp. 247–259. Raven Press, New York.
106. Lytle, L. D., Messing, R. B., Fisher, L., and Phebus, L. (1975): Effect of chronic corn consumption on brain serotonin and the response to electric shock. *Science*, 190:692–694.
107. Maier, S. F., and Seligman, M. E. P. (1976): Learned helplessness: Theory and evidence. *J. Exp. Psychol. [Gen.]*, 105:3–46.
108. McNair, P. M., Lorr, M., and Dropplemen, L. F. (1971): *Profile of Mood States Manual.* Educational and Industrial Testing Service, San Diego, California.
109. Melamed, E., Glaeser, B., Growdon, J. H., and Wurtman, R. J. (1980): Plasma tyrosine in normal humans: Effects of oral tyrosine and protein-containing meals. *J. Neural Transm.*, 47:299–306.
110. Menzies, I. C. (1984): Disturbed children: The role of food and chemical sensitivities. *Nutr. Health*, 3:39–54.
111. Modigh, K. (1972): Central and peripheral effects of 5-hydroxytryptophan on motor activity in mice. *Psychopharmacologia (Berlin)*, 23:48–54.
112. Modigh, K. (1973): Effects of chlorimipramine and protriptyline on the hyperactivity induced by 5-hydroxytryptophan after peripheral decarboxylase inhibition in mice. *J. Neural Transm.*, 34:101–109.
113. Mohs, R. C., Davis, K. L., and Levy, M. L. (1981): Partial reversal of anticholinergic amnesia by choline chloride. *Life Sci.*, 29:1317–1323.
114. Møller, S. E., Kirk, L., and Femming, K. H. (1976): Plasma amino acids as an index for subgroups in manic depressive psychosis, correlation to effect of tryptophan. *Psychopharmacology (Berlin)*, 49:205–213.
115. Møller, S. E., Reisby, N., Ortmann, J., Elley, J., and Krautwald, O. (1981): Relevance of tryptophan and tyrosine availability in endogenous and "non-endogenous" depressives treated with imipramine or clomipramine. *J. Affective Disord.*, 3:231–244.
116. Morand, C., Young, S. N., and Ervin, F. R. (1983): Clinical response of aggressive schizophrenics to oral tryptophan. *Biol. Psychiatry*, 18:575–578.
117. Nicholson, A. N., and Stone, B. M. (1979): L-tryptophan and sleep in healthy man. *Electroencephalogr. Clin. Neurophysiol.*, 47:539–545.
118. Deleted in proof.
119. Oswald, I., Ashcroft, G. W., Berger, R. J., Eccleston, D., Evans, J. I., and Thacore, V. R. (1966): Some experiments in the chemistry of normal sleep. *Br. J. Psychiatry*, 112:391–399.
120. Peters, B. H., and Levin, H. S. (1979): Effects of physostigmine and lecithin on memory in Alzheimer's disease. *Ann. Neurol.*, 6:219–221.
121. Peterson, R. C. (1977): Scopolamine induced learning failures in man. *Psychopharmacology (Berlin)*, 52:283–289.
122. Pollitt, E., Leibel, K. L., and Greenfield, D. (1981): Brief fasting, stress and cognition in children. *Am. J. Clin. Nutr.*, 34:1526–1533.
123. Pollitt, E., Lewis, N. L., Garza, C., and Shulman, R. J. (1983): Fasting and cognitive function. *J. Psychiatr. Res.*, 17:169–174.
124. Porte, D., and Halter, J. B. (1981): The endocrine pancreas and diabetes mellitus. In: *Textbook of Endocrinology*, 6th ed., edited by R. H. Williams, pp. 716–843. W. B. Saunders, Philadelphia.
125. Prinz, R. J., and Riddle, D. B. (1985): Associations between nutrition and behavior in five-year-old children. *Nutr. Rev. (Suppl.) (in press)*.
126. Prinz, R. J., Roberts, W. A., and Hantman, E. (1980): Dietary correlates of hyperactive behavior in children. *J. Consult. Clin. Psychol.*, 48:760–769.
127. Puhringe, W., Wirz-Justice, A., Graw, P., et al. (1976): Intravenous L-5-hydroxytryptophan in normal subjects: An interdisciplinary precursor loading study. I. Implication of reproducible mood elevation. *Pharmacopsychiatria*, 9:260–268.
128. Raab, A., and Oswald, R. (1980): Coping with social conflict: Impact on the activity of tyrosine hydroxylase in the limbic system and in the adrenals. *Physiol. Behav.*, 24:387–394.
129. Rapoport, J. L. Diet and hyperactivity. *Nutr. Rev. (Suppl.) (in press)*.

130. Rapoport, J. L., Berg, C. J., Ismond, D. R., Zahn, T. P., and Neims, A. (1984): Behavioral effects of caffeine in children. *Arch. Gen. Psychiatry*, 41:1073–1079.
131. Rapoport, J. L., Quinn, P., Scribanu, N., et al. (1974): Platelet serotonin of hyperactive school age boys. *Br. J. Psychiatry*, 125:138–140.
132. Rippere, V. (1983): Food additives and hyperactive children: A critique of Conners. *Br. J. Clin. Psychol.*, 22:19–32.
133. Rosenthal, N. E., Davenport, Y., Gillin, C., Goodwin, F. K., Lewy, A., Mueller, P. S., and Sack, D. A. (1984): Seasonal affective disorder. *Arch. Gen. Psychiatry*, 41:72–80.
134. Rosenthal, R., and Jacobson, L. (1968): *Pygmalion in the Classroom: Teacher Expectation and Pupils' Intellectual Development.* Holt, Rinehart & Winston, New York.
135. Safer, D. J., and Allen, R. P. (1971): The central effects of scopolamine in man. *Biol. Psychiatry*, 3:347–355.
136. Scally, M. D., Ulus, I. H., and Wurtman, R. J. (1979): Brain tyrosine level controls striatal dopamine synthesis in haloperidol-treated rats. *J. Neural Transm.*, 41:1–6.
136a. Schneider-Helmert, D., and Spinweber, C. L. (1984): Evaluation of L-tryptophan for treatment of insomnia: A review. Naval Health Research Center Report #84-4, San Diego.
137. Seltzer, S., Dewart, D., Pollack, R. L., and Jackson, E. (1983): The effects of dietary tryptophan on chronic maxillofacial pain and experimental pain tolerance. *J. Psychiatr. Res.*, 17:181–186.
138. Seltzer, S., Stoch, R., Marcus, R., and Jackson, E. (1982): Alteration of human pain thresholds by nutritional manipulation and L-tryptophan supplementation. *Pain*, 13:385–393.
139. Sheard, M. (1969): The effect of p-chlorophenylalanine on behavior in rats: Relation to brain serotonin and 5-hydroxyacetic acid. *Brain Res.*, 15:524–528.
140. Sheard, M. (1975): Lithium in the treatment of aggression. *J. Nerv. Ment. Dis.*, 100:108–117.
141. Shiffron, R. M., and Schneider, W. (1977): Controlled and automatic human information processing: II. Perceptual learning, automatic attending and a general theory. *Psychol. Rev.*, 84:127–190.
142. Simonson, E., Brozek, J., and Keys, A. (1948): Effects of meals on visual performance and fatigue. *J. Appl. Psychol.*, 1:270–278.
143. Sitaram, N., Weingartner, H., Caine, E. D., and Gillin, J. C. (1978): Choline: Selective enhancement of serial learning and encoding of low imagery words in man. *Life Sci.*, 22:1555–1560.
144. Sitaram, N., Weingartner, H., and Gillin, J. C. (1978): Human serial learning: Enhancement with arecoline and impairment with scopolamine correlated with performance on placebo. *Science*, 201:274–276.
145. Slesinger, D. P., McDivitt, M., and O'Donnell, F. M. (1980): Food patterns in an urban population: Age and sociodemographic correlates. *J. Gerontol.*, 35:432–441.
146. Sloviter, R. S., Drust, E. G., and Conner, J. D. (1978): Evidence that serotonin mediates some behavioral effects of amphetamine. *J. Pharmacol. Exp. Ther.*, 206:348–352.
147. Smith, B., and Prockop, D. J. (1962): CNS effects of ingestion of L-tryptophan by normal subjects. *N. Engl. J. Med.*, 267:1338–1341.
148. Spinweber, C. L., Ursin, R., Hilbert, R. P., and Hilderbrand, R. L. (1983): L-tryptophan: Effects on daytime sleep latency and on the waking EEG. *Electroencephalogr. Clin. Neurophysiol.*, 55:652–661.
149. Spring, B. (1984): Recent research on the behavioral effects of tryptophan and carbohydrate. *Nutr. Health*, 3:55–68.
150. Spring, B., Lieberman, H., Swope, G., and Garfield, G. (1985): Effects of carbohydrates on mood and behavior. *Nutr. Rev. (Suppl.) (in press).*
151. Spring, B., Maller, O., Wurtman, J., Digman, L., and Cozolino, L. (1983): Effects of protein and carbohydrate meals on mood and performance: Interactions with sex and age. *J. Psychiatr. Res.*, 17:155–167.
152. Sternbach, R. A., Janowsky, D. S., Huey, L. Y., and Segal, D. S. (1976): Effects of altering brain serotonin activity on human chronic pain. In: *Advances in Pain Research and Theory, Vol. 1,* edited by J. J. Bonica and D. Albe-Fessard, pp. 601–606. Raven Press, New York.
153. Taylor, M. (1976): Effects of L-tryptophan and L-methionine on activity in the rat. *Br. J. Pharmacol.*, 58:117–119.
153a. Thal, L. J., Masur, M. S., Sharpless, N. S., Fuld, P. A., and Davies, P. (1984): Acute and chronic effects of oral physostigmine and lecithin in Alzheimer's disease. In: *Alzheimer's Disease: Advances in Basic Research and Therapies*, edited by R. J. Wurtman, S. H. Corkin, and J. H.

Growdon, pp. 333–348. Proceedings of the Third Meeting of the International Study Group on the Treatment of Memory Disorders Associated with Aging. Zurich, Switzerland.

154. Thurmond, J. B., Lasley, S. M., Conkin, A. L., and Brown, J. W. (1977): Effects of dietary tyrosine, phenylalanine, and tryptophan on aggression in mice. *Pharmacol. Biochem. Behav.*, 6:475–478.

155. Thurmond, J. B., Lasley, S. M., Kramercy, N. R., and Brown, J. W. (1979): Differential tolerance to dietary amino acid-induced changes in aggressive behavior and locomotor activity in mice. *Psychopharmacology (Berlin)*, 66:301–308.

156. Treiser, S. L., Cascio, C. S., O'Donohue, T. L., Thoa, N. B., Jacobowitz, D. M., and Kellae, K. J. (1981): Lithium increases serotonin release and decreases serotonin receptors in the hippocampus. *Science*, 213:1529–1531.

157. Trimble, M., Chadwick, D., Reynolds, E., et al. (1975): L-5-hydroxytryptophan and mood. *Lancet*, 1:583.

158. Tune, L. E., Strauss, M. E., Lew, M. F., Breitlinger, E., and Coyle, J. T. (1982): Serum levels of anticholinergic drugs and impaired recent memory in chronic schizophrenic patients. *Am. J. Psychiatry*, 139:1460–1462.

159. Valcuikas, J. A., Lilis, R., Wolff, M. S., and Anderson, H. A. (1978): Comparative neurobehavioral study of a polybrominated biphenyl-exposed population in Michigan and a nonexposed group in Wisconsin. *Environ. Health Perspect.*, 23:199–210.

160. Van Praag, H. M. (1980): Central monoamine metabolism in depressions. I. Serotonin and related compounds. *Compr. Psychiatry*, 21:30–43.

161. Virkkunen, M. (1983): Insulin secretion during the glucose tolerance test in antisocial personality. *Br. J. Psychiatry*, 142:598–604.

162. Virkkunen, M., and Huttunen, M. O. (1982): Evidence for abnormal glucose tolerance test among violent offenders. *Neuropsychology*, 8:30–34.

163. Van Woert, M. H., Rosenbaum, D., Howieston, J., and Bowers, M. B. (1976): Serotonin and myoclonus. *Monogr. Neural Sci.*, 3:71–80.

164. Walinder, J., Skott, A., Carlsson, A., Nagy, A., and Roos, B. E. (1976): Potentiation of the antidepressant action of clomipramine by tryptophan. *Arch. Gen. Psychol.*, 33:1384–1389.

165. Walters, J. K., Davis, M., and Sheard, M. H. (1979): Tryptophan-free diet: Effects on the acoustic startle reflex in rats. *Psychopharmacology (Berlin)*, 62:103–109.

166. Warbritton, J. D., Stewart, R. M., and Baldessarini, R. J. (1978): Decreased locomotor activity and attenuation of amphetamine hyperactivity with intraventricular infusion of serotonin in the rat. *Brain Res.*, 143:373–382.

167. Weiss, B. (1983): Behavioral toxicology and environmental health science: Opportunity and challenge for psychology. *Am. Psychol.*, 38:1174–1187.

168. Weiss, J. M. (1971): Effects of coping behavior in different warning conditions on stress pathology in rats. *J. Comp. Physiol. Psychol.*, 77:1–13.

168a.Weiss, B., Williams, J. H., Margen, S., Citron, L. J., Cox, C., McKibben, J., Ogar, D., and Schultz, S. (1980): Behavioral responses to artificial food colors. *Science*, 207:1487–1489.

169. Weiss, J. M., Goodman, P. A., Losito, B. G., Corrigan, S., Carry, J. M., and Bailey, W. H. (1981): Behavioral depression produced by an uncontrollable stressor: Relationship to norepinephrine, dopamine and serotonin levels in various regions of rat brain. *Brain Res. Rev.*, 3:167–205.

170. Wender, P. H. (1969): Platelet serotonin level in children with minimal brain dysfunction. *Lancet*, 2:1021.

171. Wolraich, M. L., Milich, R., Stumbo, P., and Schultz, F. (1985): The effects of sucrose ingestion on the behavior of hyperactive boys. *J. Pediatr.*, 106:675–682.

172. Wurtman, R. J. (1982): Nutrients that modify brain function. *Sci. Am.*, 246:50–59.

173. Wurtman, R. J., Hefti, F., and Melamed, E. (1981): Precursor control of neurotransmitter synthesis. *Pharmacol. Rev.*, 32:315–335.

174. Wurtman, R. J., Hirsch, M. J., and Growdon, J. H. (1977): Lecithin consumption raises serum free choline levels. *Lancet*, 2:68–69.

175. Wurtman, R. J., Larin, F., Mostafapour, S., and Fernstrom, J. D. (1974): Brain catechol synthesis: Control by brain tyrosine concentrations. *Science*, 185:183–184.

176. Yensen, R. (1959): Some factors affecting taste sensitivity in man. I: Food intake and time of day. *Q. J. Exp. Psychol.*, 11:221–229.

177. Yogman, M. W., and Zeisel, S. (1983): Diet and sleep patterns in newborn infants. *N. Engl. J. Med.*, 309:1147–1149.

178. Yogman, M. W., Zeisel, S. H., and Roberts, C. (1983): Dietary precursors of serotonin and newborn behavior. *J. Psychiatr. Res.*, 17:123–133.
179. Yokogoshi, H., Roberts, C. H., Caballero, B., and Wurtman, R. (1984): Effects of aspartame and glucose administration on brain and plasma levels of large neutral amino acids and brain 5-hydroxyindoles. *Am. J. Clin. Nutr.*, 40(1):1–7.
180. Young, S. (1985): The effect of altering tryptophan levels on aggression. *Nutr. Rev. (Suppl.) (in press)*.
181. Yuwiler, A., Brammer, G. L., Morley, J. E., Raleigh, M. J., Flannery, J. W., and Geller, E. (1981): Short-term and repetitive administration of oral tryptophan in normal men. *Arch. Gen. Psychiatry*, 38:619–626.

Nutrition and the Brain, Vol. 7, edited by
R. J. Wurtman and J. J. Wurtman. Raven Press,
New York © 1986.

The Clinical Psychopharmacology
of Tryptophan

S. N. Young

Department of Psychiatry, McGill University, Montreal, Quebec, Canada H3A 1A1

I. INTRODUCTION

The behavioral effects of tryptophan have been studied for more than 25 years. Lauer et al. (112), who published the first report on this topic in 1958, gave L-tryptophan (0.2 mg/kg/day for 6 weeks) to seven schizophrenic patients who were also receiving the monoamine oxidase inhibitor (MAOI) iproniazid. The authors found that "the patients exhibited an increase in energy level and motor activity and improvement in the ability to accept interpersonal relationships, and displayed more affect." The rationale given by the authors for the use of tryptophan is clearly stated. They discussed the fact, then newly discovered, that iproniazid increases brain levels of serotonin (5-hydroxytryptamine, 5-HT), and that the immediate precursor of serotonin, 5-hydroxytryptophan (5-HTP), could cross the blood-brain barrier. They went on to state that 5-HTP

> has many undesirable side effects, but the dietary precursor of serotonin, L-tryptophan, which can be converted to 5-hydroxytryptophan, does not have these deleterious properties in physiological amounts. Thus it was thought that if the degradation of serotonin could be impeded by a monoamine oxidase inhibitor, and its synthesis simultaneously accelerated by giving the precursor from which it is formed, effects might be obtained which were more pronounced.

It was not until 3 years later that Hess and Doepfner (90) actually demonstrated that tryptophan increased the brain 5-HT content of rats pretreated with a MAOI. In 1965, Ashcroft et al. (6) demonstrated the same effect in the absence of MAO inhibition. However, it was not until 1970 that the assumption made by Lauer et al. (112), that tryptophan increases 5-HT synthesis in the central nervous system (CNS) of humans, was finally confirmed by Eccleston et al. (54). These authors demonstrated that oral ingestion of tryptophan in humans caused a significant increase in the level of the 5-HT metabolite, 5-hydroxyindoleacetic acid (5-HIAA), in the lumbar cerebrospinal fluid (CSF), indicating an increased turnover of 5-HT in the CNS.

Tryptophan has been used extensively without a MAOI in clinical biochemical studies. In one such study in 1960, Olson et al. (147) gave 10 g DL-tryptophan to normal subjects and mentioned that they invariably experienced some mental symptoms, "mainly euphoria and lightheadedness, but including dizziness, headache and rarely nausea, which lasted for one or two hours." The first study to look specifically at CNS effects of tryptophan given alone in humans was by Smith and Prockop in 1962 (169). They gave normal subjects single doses of L-tryptophan, up to 90 mg/kg, and noted alternating drowsiness and euphoria. The majority of the subsequent studies on the clinical psychopharmacology of tryptophan have followed up on the original observations of Lauer et al. (112) and Smith and Prockop (169), that tryptophan tends to cause euphoria and sedation, and have been concerned with the antidepressant and hypnotic properties of tryptophan. There are some studies, however, that are based not on these early clinical observations but on animal studies. There is a large body of literature on the behavioral effects of 5-HT in rodents. The relatively small literature on the action of tryptophan in conditions such as pain, pathological aggression, and eating disorders is based on the conclusion from animal studies that 5-HT is involved in, among other things, the regulation of pain perception, aggression, and food intake.

The rationale given by Lauer et al. (112) for the clinical use of tryptophan is still valid today. Tryptophan increases synthesis of 5-HT in the brain and therefore may stimulate 5-HT release and function. Because it is a natural constituent of the diet, tryptophan should have low toxicity and produce few side effects. The assumption that tryptophan will necessarily produce an increase in 5-HT release is questionable and is discussed in more detail in Section II.C. Tryptophan does indeed have low toxicity and few side effects, but, as discussed in Section III, it is not without its potential dangers. Besides low toxicity, another advantage in the use of a dietary component, such as tryptophan, is acceptability to patients. Dietary components, even at pharmacological doses, are considered more "natural" than compounds that are unambiguously drugs. Of course, it is not natural to give an amino acid in purified form at several times the normal daily dietary intake. Furthermore, there is no evidence that tryptophan is correcting a deficiency of tryptophan in most of the situations in which it is used clinically. Thus it cannot be considered a "natural" treatment. The term *drug* would seem appropriate in a situation in which tryptophan has no nutritive value and is given for the sole purpose of manipulating metabolism of a neurotransmitter.

Although there are certainly advantages in the use of dietary components as drugs, there is one disadvantage that is not always adequately appreciated. Regulatory mechanisms in the body will often work to overcome the desired effect on administration of a natural product. As discussed in Section II.B, plasma tryptophan is normally metabolized fairly rapidly; hence tryptophan ingested in purified form has a much shorter half-life than most drugs. In addition, the increase in 5-HT release occurring when 5-HT synthesis is increased is limited (see Section II.C). Despite these problems, however, there is good evidence that tryptophan can influence 5-HT-medicated neurotransmission in some circumstances. Because an understanding of the biochemistry and physiology of tryptophan is important in interpreting data on its clinical effects, this background material is discussed in Section II. Section III discusses background information relevant to the choice of appropriate dosage of tryptophan for clinical use; and Section IV deals with the toxicity and side effects of tryptophan. The clinical studies described in Section V concern both experimental studies on normal subjects and clinical trials in patients. The experimental studies include those in which tryptophan levels were lowered, as well as those involving tryptophan administration, as the former type of study should help provide a better overall picture on the role and importance of tryptophan availability. The final sections summarize available information and propose future directions of research.

II. BACKGROUND

A. Tryptophan and Diet

An adult male needs 0.25 g tryptophan to maintain nitrogen balance (2), while a normal diet contains 1 to 1.5 g tryptophan per day (38,143). Although dietary deficiencies, such as pellagra (180) and protein-energy malnutrition (4), are known to cause large decreases in plasma tryptophan levels, little is known about how chronic ingestion of qualities or quantities of protein within the nutritionally adequate range affects tryptophan availability and thus 5-HT synthesis. On the other hand, the acute effects of food ingestion are reasonably well understood with respect to the different influences of the macronutrients.

One regulatory system of crucial importance for the control of brain tryptophan occurs at the level of the blood-brain barrier. All the large neutral amino acids, including tryptophan, are transported into the brain across the blood-brain barrier by the same transport system. Because there is competition among the various amino acids for the carrier (146), protein and carbohydrate have different effects on brain tryptophan; and the effects are not in the direction that would be expected. Thus ingestion of protein, which contains tryptophan, will lower brain tryptophan and 5-HT (58). This is because tryptophan is the least abundant amino acid in protein. Therefore, the rise in plasma tryptophan is less than the rise in the plasma levels of the amino acids that compete with tryptophan for transport into brain. On the other hand, carbohydrate, which of course contains no tryptophan, raises brain tryptophan and 5-HT (59). Carbohydrate ingestion causes release of insulin, which stimulates the uptake of the branched chain amino acids leucine, isoleucine, and valine into muscle. Therefore, their plasma levels fall, competition for the transport of tryptophan decreases, and brain levels of tryptophan and 5-HT increase. These mechanisms have been elucidated primarily in experimental animals. There is only one published study on the acute effects of food ingestion in humans. When humans ingested a balanced meal, there was a significant decline in the CSF levels of tryptophan and 5-HIAA (152). This suggests that in humans, as in rats (58), when both protein and carbohydrate are ingested in proportions that would occur in a balanced meal, the effect of protein will predominate.

B. Effect of Peripheral Tryptophan Metabolism on Brain Levels

Competition among all the large neutral amino acids for entry into brain is an important factor controlling brain tryptophan levels, as is peripheral tryptophan metabolism because of the effect it has on plasma tryptophan. There are two quantitatively important pathways of tryptophan metabolism in the periphery: protein synthesis, which is reversible, and the irreversible catabolic pathway, which is initiated by L-tryptophan-2,3-dioxygenase (tryptophan pyrrolase). When tryptophan is ingested as a part of protein in a meal, peripheral protein metabolism will determine its net effect on the plasma tryptophan (36,142). After a protein meal, there is rapid uptake of amino acids by liver and other tissues. The liver disposes of some of these amino acids (for example, the aromatic compounds) fairly rapidly, both by catabolism and by protein synthesis. However, in other tissues that lack the necessary catabolic enzymes for tryptophan, such as muscle, its only metabolic pathway is into protein. This rapid protein synthesis after a meal limits the rise of plasma amino acids. In the rat, the whole-body stores of free tryptophan are equivalent to only about 2% of the rat's daily requirement. In the postabsorptive state, release of amino acids from these labile protein stores by protein catabolism prevents a large decline in plasma amino acid levels (142). Thus tryptophan is released from the liver into the blood as early as 2 hr after food is removed from rats (16). Protein synthesis obviously will not play any role in regulating plasma tryptophan after ingestion of purified tryptophan.

The enhancement of protein synthesis by exogenous amino acids provides a convenient and simple way to lower brain 5-HT for experimental purposes. When rats are given a day's supply of amino acids in a single dose, but devoid of tryptophan, there is a sharp and long-lasting (24 hr) decline in plasma and brain tryptophan and in brain 5-HT (13). An amino acid mixture lacking only the one essential amino acid will induce protein synthesis, and the free tryptophan in blood and tissues is incorporated into protein. This results in a decline in plasma tryptophan. Competition by the other amino acids for entry into brain will play a role in regulating brain tryptophan in these circumstances, but this effect is relatively small compared with that of the decrease in plasma tryptophan caused by its utilization for protein synthesis (64).

This technique can by applied to humans to investigate the acute mental changes that might accompany a lowering of brain 5-HT. When humans ingest an amino acid mixture devoid of tryptophan but containing all the other essential and most nonessential amino acids in the same proportion that they occur in milk, plasma tryptophan falls. One hundred grams of such a mixture (containing the amount of amino acids in about 500 g steak) caused a steady decline in plasma tryptophan, which reached its lowest point (24% of the original value) at 5 hr after the mixture was ingested (201). In rats, a decline in plasma tryptophan of this magnitude caused a 50% decline in brain 5-HT levels (13). In the human experiment, control subjects received a nutritionally balanced amino acid mixture of the same composition but containing the appropriate amount of tryptophan. Thus the only neurochemical difference between control and treated subjects should have been that brain tryptophan and 5-HT were lower in the treated subjects. However, as the balanced mixture would have tended to lower brain tryptophan and 5-HT, due to competition at the blood-brain barrier, the control is a conservative one. The effects of this type of 5-HT manipulation on mental function are described in Section V.

When tryptophan is ingested by itself, protein metabolism will play no role in regulating its availability. As a neglible amount is excreted in the urine (133), irreversible catabolic pathways are the main factor controlling its level, and by far the most quantitatively significant of these is initiated by tryptophan pyrrolase. Tryptophan pyrrolase is induced by glucocorticoids and by tryptophan itself. Plasma glucocorticoids can be markedly elevated in depressed patients (161), and studies on rats have shown that induction of tryptophan pyrrolase by glucocorticoids (106) or by tryptophan (200) can greatly diminish the increase in brain tryptophan and 5-HT that occurs after a tryptophan load. However, the increased plasma glucocorticoid levels characteristic of depressed patients do not seem to be sufficient to influence plasma tryptophan in clinical use: two studies have shown that tryptophan absorption, distribution, and elimination after a tryptophan load, as indicated by plasma tryptophan levels, are not significantly different in depressed patients and controls (92,138). Also, the increase in CSF 5-HIAA is not significantly different in depressed patients and neurological controls when both receive a single oral dose of tryptophan (5).

On the other hand, clinical data suggest that tryptophan pyrrolase may have a powerful effect on tryptophan availability after tryptophan ingestion. Thus the duration of the increase of plasma tryptophan after a load is relatively small. Also, larger tryptophan loads, which probably induce tryptophan pyrrolase more than small loads, do not increase plasma tryptophan in direct proportion to their size. In neurological patients who received 50 mg/kg tryptophan, an amount often given as a single dose in clinical studies, CSF tryptophan and 5-HIAA remained elevated for only 12 hr (54). Increasing doses shorten the plasma half-life of tryptophan in normal subjects (72) and lead to only slightly higher peak values. Thus 50 mg/kg tryptophan caused a peak ninefold increase in plasma tryptophan, but 100 mg/kg increased the value only 12-fold (204). However, a study on neurological patients showed that higher doses are capable of prolonging the rise of CSF 5-HIAA (199).

Clinical data suggest that chronic treatment with very large doses of tryptophan may lead to a progressive induction of tryptophan pyrrolase. In normal subjects who received either a single or a double dose of tryptophan every day for 7 days, the rise of plasma tryptophan after the last dose was less than that seen after an acute dose (72,205). In schizophrenic subjects receiving a constant 6 g/day, the rise in plasma tryptophan was less at 6 weeks than at 3 weeks (30). However, although tryptophan pyrrolase may limit the rise of brain tryptophan in subjects receiving high tryptophan doses, there is sufficient evidence from studies in which CSF 5-HIAA was measured in patients receiving tryptophan chronically to show that tryptophan will increase brain 5-HT synthesis when used therapeutically (17,28,100,115,143).

One consequence of the relatively rapid metabolism of tryptophan might be wide fluctuations in brain tryptophan levels. If studies on CSF tryptophan levels in neurological patients receiving an acute dose of tryptophan (54,199) provide any insights as to brain tryptophan, levels may vary over a 10-fold range in patients receiving two daily doses of 3 g tryptophan. Variability in the increase of plasma tryptophan from day to day can also be very great for any individual receiving a constant daily dose of tryptophan (31), although the reason for this is not understood.

The fluctuations in plasma and brain tryptophan that occur after chronic high-dose tryptophan loading could theoretically be minimized and the dose of tryptophan reduced, if tryptophan pyrrolase were inhibited. Studies on rats have been interpreted as showing that allopurinol (8) or nicotinamide (202) would be suitable inhibitors. However, clinical studies have failed to show that these compounds, when given at clinically acceptable doses, influence plasma tryptophan levels after a tryptophan load (73,133,135). The hypothesis that inhibiting tryptophan pyrrolase potentiates exogenous tryptophan will have to await testing until development of an effective and nontoxic tryptophan pyrrolase inhibitor.

C. Influence of Tryptophan on 5-HT Synthesis, Release, and Function

Tryptophan increases the synthesis of 5-HT because the rate-limiting enzyme in 5-HT synthesis, tryptophan hydroxylase, is not fully saturated with tryptophan. Studies on the accumulation of 5-HT in rat brain after inhibition of MAO (70), and on the accumulation of 5-HTP after inhibition of aromatic amino acid decarboxylase (24), suggest that tryptophan hydroxylase is normally about half saturated. Thus tryptophan loading can double the rate of 5-HT synthesis in rat brain. The same may be true in humans. In neurological patients, a 3-g tryptophan load approximately doubled CSF 5-HIAA, while a 6-g load caused no further increase (199). When neurosurgical patients received an infusion of tryptophan, which produced plasma concentrations comparable to those found when treating depression or insomnia with tryptophan, excised brain tissue revealed sixfold elevations in cortical tryptophan levels (67). An increase of this magnitude would be enough to maximize 5-HT synthesis. Although it is possible that tryptophan hydroxylase has different properties in different types of patients, this is unlikely; the small amount of evidence available shows similar tryptophan responses in different diagnostić groups. Thus when unipolar depressed patients, bipolar depressed patients, bipolar manic patients, and neurological patients were given a tryptophan load, the increases in CSF 5-HIAA were similar in all groups (5).

One important question is whether a twofold or smaller increase in 5-HT synthesis is enough to affect 5-HT release and function. Animal studies show that a rise in the rate of 5-HT synthesis is usually accompanied by an increase in 5-HT levels, but nothing is known about the subcellular distribution of the additional 5-HT. Specifically, it is not known whether a rise in 5-HT levels will result in a greater density of 5-HT within "releasable" pools, if such distinct pools actually exist. An increase in 5-HT release in response to tryptophan loading would imply either an increase in 5-HT release each time a neuron fires, an increase in the rate of firing of 5-HT neurons, or additional release of the neurotransmitter independent of neuronal firing. Although animal studies have not yet shown which possibility actually occurs, there are data relevant to this choice.

The cell bodies of 5-HT neurons are situated in the raphe nuclei of the brainstem. Single unit recordings of cells in the raphe nuclei of rats show that they have a slow rhythmic discharge rate (60). Experimental manipulations of neuronal firing in cat brain (89) indicate that the release of labeled 5-HT (formed endogenously from isotopically labeled tryptophan) is dependent on nerve activity. This relationship between 5-HT release and raphe cell firing rates may be physiological inasmuch as both are reduced by sleep in the cat (156). When rats are given tryptophan or 5-HTP, there is a dose-related decline in raphe unit activity, which is seen at quite low doses (178) and is dependent on an increase in local (raphe) 5-HT concentrations (60). The data available from experiments on rats suggest that the combination of increased brain 5-HT and decreased raphe firing after tryptophan loading may result in either a moderate or a negligible increase in 5-HT release. The effect of tryptophan and 5-HTP on release of 5-HT into the perfused ventricles was studied in the rat (175). Acute ingestion of 5-HTP caused an immediate, important, and long-lasting increase of 5-HT release, while a tryptophan load, given intraperitoneally, or a long-lasting tryptophan infusion gave a transient and moderate elevation of 5-HT release. The elevation of brain 5-HT levels outlasted by several hours the increase in 5-HT release.

Two techniques that may eventually supply important information on 5-HT release in specific brain areas of freely moving animals are *in vivo* voltammetry and *in vivo* dialysis. In a study using voltammetric analysis of the rat striatum, tryptophan caused no increase in the signal, which was thought to be due to 5-HT, while the combination of tryptophan and a MAOI caused a small but steady increase in the signal (124). However, because more recent data suggest that part of the signal may have been attributable to uric acid, as well as to 5-HT and 5-HIAA (148), these results should be interpreted with caution.

The consequences of giving tryptophan alone may be different from those when it is given along with a MAOI. Thus in rodents, tryptophan tends to inhibit locomotor activity (130), while the combination of tryptophan with a MAOI (70) or 5-HTP (129) tend to increase locomotor activity. The increase in brain 5-HT can be much larger after 5-HTP or with the combination of tryptophan and a MAOI than after tryptophan alone. The larger increases may cause diffusion of 5-HT out of the raphe neuron. Thus 5-HT may affect synaptic and neuronal functions in ways not dependent on neuronal firing (74). In this situation, 5-HT release will be influenced less by the decline in the rate of neuronal firing that can accompany elevated 5-HT levels.

Experimental data on the acute effects of tryptophan in rodents provide no more than a framework for speculating about changes that might occur in raphe neuron firing rates or 5-HT release when patients receive tryptophan chronically. Ultimately, it is the clinical data that are most important. If tryptophan influences a behavior thought to be modulated by 5-HT, this can be taken as an indication that it has altered 5-HT-mediated neurotransmission. However, some of the clinical data are consistent with animal results. Thus, as discussed in Section V, the combination of tryptophan and a MAOI produces a much clearer antidepressant effect than tryptophan by itself, while the same could be said of the two treatments in relation to 5-HT release in the rat.

If 5-HT release after tryptophan (given without a MAOI) is affected in part by the rate of raphe firing, then it is pertinent to ask what other factors influence firing rates. In the cat, there is a strong positive correlation between single unit discharge rates in the raphe and the level of behavior arousal (179). Higher discharge rates might potentiate the enhancement of 5-HT release after tryptophan. Thus tryptophan might be more effective in the treatment of clinical conditions with high arousal (e.g., mania, pathological aggression) than in those associated with low arousal (e.g., depression). The available clinical data (discussed in Section V) may point slightly in this direction, but much more evidence is required before this assertion can be made with any confidence.

D. Other Influences of Tryptophan on Brain Metabolism

It is often assumed that any change in brain function that accompanies altered tryptophan levels must be mediated by altered 5-HT function. However, there are many other tryptophan metabolites besides 5-HT in brain, including tryptamine, the pineal indoles, products of the action of indoleamine-2,3-dioxygenase, and condensation products, such as tetrahydro-β-carboline (196). The role of tryptophan availability in controlling the levels of most of these compounds in brain is not known, but tryptophan administration can increase pineal 5-hydroxytryptophol and melatonin contents in the rat (198).

The only other compound besides 5-HT whose metabolism and function in the brain has been studied in detail is tryptamine. Studies on the relative amounts of the acid metabolites of 5-HT and tryptamine in human CSF suggest that the rate of tryptamine metabolism in human CNS may be about 15% of that of 5-HT. Unlike 5-HT metabolism, which will not increase more than twofold in response to tryptophan loading, levels of tryptamine metabolites increase in proportion to the size of a tryptophan load, with 6 g producing a fourfold increase (199). Animal data indicate that release of tryptamine, unlike that of 5-HT, is not dependent on neuronal firing (89). Tryptamine can modulate, at low levels, the influence of iontophoretically applied 5-HT on the firing rates of single neurons in rat cortex (104). It can also modify the responses of rat cortical neurons evoked by stimulating the raphe nucleus medianus (103) and, in animals, the actions of 5-HT on various behaviors (102).

Thus it is possible that endogenous tryptamine, formed after tryptophan administration, also affects the 5-HT-mediated behavioral effects of tryptophan in people. The most likely situation in which this might occur is after the use of tryptophan in combination with a MAOI. In the rat, this combination produces very large increases in brain tryptamine (185). Moreover, animal behavioral studies implicate both 5-HT and tryptamine in the etiology of the characteristic syndrome that occurs with tryptophan and a MAOI (125). The only relevant clinical evidence on this question comes from a 1964 study by Hodge et al. (91), who showed that high doses (1.5 g) of a decarboxylase inhibitor (Ro4–4602) almost completely abolished the acute central effects of administering tryptophan with a MAOI. The decarboxylase inhibitor could have diminished the syntheses of both 5-HT and tryptamine.

Tryptophan is capable of influencing brain levels of more than just its own metabolites. Because of the competition between the large neutral amino acids for entry into brain, it is pertinent to ask whether tryptophan administration would lower the brain level of phenylalanine, tyrosine, or histidine. In rats, a tryptophan dose of 50 mg/kg i.p. depressed brain tyrosine levels significantly by 19% (190). In psychiatric patients, a single 5-g tryptophan dose failed to lower CSF tyrosine levels (182). As this dose is larger than that usually given at a single time therapeutically, it seems unlikely that exogenous tryptophan affects brain tyrosine (or catecholamine) levels in patients.

Tryptophan has at least one other effect on brain metabolism that is not related to monoamine synthesis: Its administration to rats reportedly enhances brain protein synthesis, as it does in other tissues (105). The clinical implications of this effect are obscure.

III. APPROPRIATE DOSAGE SCHEDULES FOR TRYPTOPHAN

To readers inexperienced in the therapeutic use of amino acids, tryptophan dosage levels may initially seem large. However, even the normal daily dietary intake of tryptophan (1–1.5 g) is large compared with dosages of many drugs, and this is a useful reference point in considering tryptophan dosages. The manner in which tryptophan is to be given will depend on the desired effect. For example, if tryptophan is given as a hypnotic, the aim would presumably be to maximize brain 5-HT synthesis for a relatively short period, so that sleep latency could be reduced without influencing sleep architecture. In this situation, a single small dose taken before bedtime is appropriate, and one dose-response study suggests about 1 g is all that is needed (82). Giving the tryptophan with carbohydrate in order to enhance tryptophan uptake into the brain may be helpful in this situation (190), but protein, as in a glass of milk, would be counterproductive, because of the inhibition of tryptophan uptake into the brain by the other amino acids. If the dose of tryptophan were large enough, concomitant ingestion of protein would probably not matter much, but carbohydrate might lessen the dose of tryptophan needed. The action of carbohydrate would be relatively short lived, which would be appropriate when tryptophan is given as a hypnotic. Similar arguments would apply for administering tryptophan with a small amount of a carbohydrate for short-term appetite suppression or pain relief (117,189).

When tryptophan is given in psychiatric disorders, such as depression, mania, or aggression, the objective would be to ensure continuous maximization of 5-HT synthesis. Because of the relatively fast metabolism of tryptophan, and because very high doses might conceivably induce tryptophan pyrrolase (Section II.B), a divided dosage schedule would be preferable to a single daily dose. After a single 6-g dose of tryptophan, plasma tryptophan has almost returned to normal after 12 hr (199). When tryptophan was given in three doses of 2 g spaced throughout the day in depressed patients, however, morning fasting plasma tryptophan values were elevated (33), suggesting that they also were elevated throughout the day. This discussion is based on the assumption that a continuous elevation of brain 5-HT synthesis would be more likely to have a therapeutic effect than an episodic elevation. Although this assumption is intuitively reasonable, it is admittedly without experimental foundation.

The actual dosage of tryptophan to use during chronic tryptophan administration is difficult to assess. Amounts in the range of 6 to 8 g/day, given in divided doses, would probably keep tryptophan hydroxylase reasonably close to saturation throughout most of the day. Higher doses presumably would only increase synthesis of tryptamine, induction of tryptophan pyrrolase, and the possibility of side effects, without having an appreciably greater effect on brain 5-HT.

Several years ago, I suggested that there might be a therapeutic window in the dosage of tryptophan needed for treatment of depression, with doses above 6 g being less effective than those of 6 g or less (203). This conclusion was based on an analysis of the dose and efficacy of tryptophan in studies published up to that time.

Studies published since then have not maintained the same pattern, and I now suggest that it is unlikely that the efficacy of tryptophan is reduced at higher doses.

Although concomitant ingestion of carbohydrate with tryptophan may be useful when it is given as a hypnotic, this would not necessarily be the case when it is given chronically for the treatment of psychiatric disorders. For example, if tryptophan were given in three daily doses of 2 g, the tryptophan level in the brain immediately after ingestion of a single dose would likely be more than enough to saturate tryptophan hydroxylase. Thus no further benefit would be obtained from carbohydrate. Eight hours later, just before the next dose, tryptophan hydroxylase might not be fully saturated. However, it is unlikely that the effect on brain tryptophan of carbohydrate, given with the tryptophan dose, would have persisted for that length of time. (Indeed, if tryptophan were given with protein, it might help to minimize the fluctuations of brain tryptophan by attenuating the initial large rise of brain tryptophan.) Thus, based on the information currently available, it would seem reasonable to give tryptophan at mealtimes. This would have the additional benefit of tending to reduce any nausea produced by tryptophan ingestion.

In this chapter, tryptophan refers exclusively to the L isomer unless the DL mixture is specified. In some of the earlier studies, before L-tryptophan was freely available, DL-tryptophan was used. As humans probably cannot use the D isomer (196), the dose of DL-tryptophan used in such studies should be halved to obtain the effective tryptophan dose.

IV. TOXICITY AND SIDE EFFECTS OF TRYPTOPHAN

The LD_{50} for L-tryptophan in the rat is 1.6 g/kg (76). At this dose, symptoms of toxicity appeared between 10 min and 2 hr after ingestion; death, which was probably due to the accumulation of breakdown products, such as urea and ammonia, occurred between 5 hr and 3 days. The equivalent dose for a human would be 80 g or more, and considerably lower doses ingested orally would be expected to cause vomiting. Autopsies performed on animals 10 days after surviving an LD_{50} dose showed no evidence of pathology, either gross or microscopic. Thus tryptophan is unlikely to cause long-term detrimental effects through overdose in humans. Lower doses added to the diet of weanling rats causes depression of food intake and growth. This does not seem to be related specifically to tryptophan and occurs with any diet containing amino acid imbalances. The adverse effects of amino acid imbalance are exacerbated by diets low in protein and diminished by high-protein diets (77).

One of the concerns about the clinical use of tryptophan is the possibility that it might cause or promote bladder cancer. This line of research was started by the discovery that addition of DL-tryptophan to the diet enhanced the carcinogenicity of 2-fluorenylacetamide for the rat bladder (53). Subsequently, it was shown that when pellets that contained any of seven tryptophan metabolites formed by tryptophan pyrrolase were implanted in the bladder, the incidence of bladder cancer increased (22). Active metabolites included kynurenine, 3-hydroxykynurenine, 3-

hydroxyanthranillic acid, and xanthurenic acid, but not tryptophan itself. This effect is seen only when implants provide a source of irritation in the bladder. In a large study carried out by the National Cancer Institute, tryptophan was not found to produce cancer in either rats or mice (144), although tryptophan has been reported to either promote or inhibit the carcinogenic action of a variety of known carcinogens. Related observations have recently been reviewed by Sourkes (174).

Elevated levels of tryptophan metabolites in the urine have been reported both in bladder cancer patients relative to controls, and in patients who had a recurrence of cancer relative to those who did not (195). While this association does not necessarily imply cause, it does imply that urinary levels of such metabolites should be kept as low as possible during tryptophan treatment. Elevated levels of urinary tryptophan metabolites are seen not only after tryptophan ingestion but also in functional vitamin B6 deficiency (187). Chronic tryptophan treatment in humans may also cause an increased requirement for vitamin B6, as supplements of this vitamin were found in one study to attenuate the increase in urinary tryptophan metabolites that occurred when normal human subjects are given very large doses of tryptophan every day for a week (71). As long as vitamin B6 supplements are given, bladder cancer probably need not be a concern, except perhaps when susceptible populations receive very large doses. The vitamin supplement may or may not influence the actions of tryptophan on the brain (e.g., by accelerating the metabolism of tryptophan in the periphery). In one small study on depressed patients, the therapeutic efficacy of tryptophan was not modified by giving it with vitamins (41).

Other detrimental effects of tryptophan that have been reported in animals are mainly of concern to special groups. Xanthurenic acid, which is increased on tryptophan loading (187), has a diabetogenic action in animals, possibly due to its ability to bind insulin (84,101), suggesting caution in the use of tryptophan in patients with a family history of diabetes. Supplementation of tryptophan (to 1.8% in the diet) in pregnant hamsters caused significant reductions in embryo and neonate survival and in neonatal weight of the pups, an effect possibly mediated by an increase in 5-HT levels in the periphery (126). In ruminants, oral tryptophan causes marked pulmonary edema and emphysema. This effect seems to be mediated by bacterial conversion of tryptophan to skatole (3-methylindole), which causes the same type of lung lesions (23). This would not normally be of concern in humans except where bacteria exist high in the gastrointestinal tract due to conditions such as achlorhydria, or where tryptophan reaches the bacterial populations lower in the gastrointestinal tract due to malabsorption.

Finally, animal data suggest that photooxidation of tryptophan and some of its metabolites, such as kynurenine, may be involved in cataract formation (206). Although there is no evidence that this occurs in humans, tryptophan administration is likely to raise lenticular tryptophan and kynurenine concentrations, and this might make subjects more susceptible to cataract formation, particularly if exposed to ultraviolet light.

In reports of clinical trials of tryptophan, side effects are often not mentioned and, when discussed, have usually been mild. In two reports of studies using high doses of tryptophan, 9.6 g/day in patients with affective disorders (143) and 20 g/day in schizophrenic patients (66), no indication was given of any undesirable side effects. When 24 acutely manic patients were given 12 g tryptophan per day for 1 week, there were seven cases of nausea (six mild, one severe), two of anorexia (moderate), one of dizziness (mild), and one of headache (mild). During the second week, half the patients were switched to placebo under double-blind conditions; the only side effects seen were one case of mild drowsiness in the tryptophan group and one in the placebo group of mild nausea and moderate anorexia (32). The most important report that considered side effects, both because of its size (115 patients) and duration (12 weeks), compared the effects of tryptophan, amitriptyline, their combination, and a placebo when given by general practitioners to depressed patients (177). Tryptophan (3 g/day) produced significantly less dry mouth and drowsiness than either amitriptyline or the combination. The increase in heart rate seen with amitriptyline was much less marked in the combined treatment group, and it is possible that tryptophan antagonizes some of the peripheral effects of amitriptyline. The side effects seen in the tryptophan and placebo groups were not significantly different. In other studies where side effects were noted, they were generally mild; the most common were nausea and lightheadedness (19,26,33).

As tryptophan is on the market in Britain as an antidepressant, the conclusion, drawn from the above clinical trials, that it has few side effects is strengthened by the almost complete lack of such problems in normal clinical use. The only side effect noted in this way is sexual disinhibition, which has been reported several times. In the original study, three of four male chronic schizophrenics showed sexual disinhibition when treated with tryptophan along with phenothiazines; in addition, one male manic-depressive patient showed the same symptom when given tryptophan alone (55). In other reports, two depressed male patients treated with tryptophan and a MAOI (141) and one depressed female patient treated with tryptophan and electroconvulsive therapy (ECT) also showed sexual disinhibition (99). In a research report, five of seven chronic schizophrenic women showed "compulsive sexual excitatory behavior" during combined treatment with tryptophan and a MAOI. All five patients were also on neuroleptics, while the other two, who did not show sexual disinhibition, had been withdrawn from neuroleptics before treatment with tryptophan was started (52). The picture that emerges from these reports is not consistent, but it seems that tryptophan alone is not sufficient to produce this side effect. Seven of the 12 patients exhibiting sexual disinhibition were on MAOIs, while eight of them were on neuroleptics known to be capable of blocking 5-HT receptors. It is not known what the net effect on 5-HT-mediated neurotransmission would be of increasing 5-HT synthesis and partially blocking 5-HT receptors. However, a large amount of data from experiments on animals indicate that 5-HT has an inhibitory effect on sexual activity, and there are two clinical reports in which tryptophan, given alone, decreased sexual function in males (168).

Although tryptophan seems to be relatively free of side effects when given alone, the literature reveals a consistent increase in side effects when tryptophan is given concurrently with a MAOI. In studies comparing the antidepressant action of a MAOI with that of a MAOI plus tryptophan, the most common side effects seen with the combination were dizziness, nausea, and headache (7,43,68). Other symptoms resembled those described in an early study in which single doses of 20 to 50 mg/kg tryptophan were given to hypertensive patients on MAOIs. The effects included ethanol-like intoxication, drowsiness, hyperreflexia, and clonus (145). Single case reports of adverse reactions to the drug combination include hypomanic behavior, ocular oscillation, ataxia, and myoclonus (10,20,176). Some of these reactions resemble the "serotonin syndrome" seen in experimental animals, which consists of tremor, hypertonus, myoclonus, and hyperreactivity (20,176). These adverse effects limit the utility of tryptophan–MAOI combinations, but the symptoms disappear soon after cessation of tryptophan, and no detrimental long-term effects have been seen.

Studies on the toxicity of tryptophan in experimental animals and clinical reports describing possible side effects lead to a number of recommendations concerning its use: (i) to minimize the risk of bladder cancer, it may be wise to give vitamin B6 supplements, if the tryptophan doses are many times in excess of those consumed normally in dietary protein; (ii) tryptophan probably should be withheld from patients with a history of bladder cancer, or with a source of physical irritation in the bladder; (iii) patients chronically taking high doses of tryptophan should not also be protein deprived, lest effects due to amino acid imbalance ensue; (iv) because of the diabetogenic effect of xanthurenic acid, patients with diabetes or a family history of diabetes receiving tryptophan should be monitored for possible changes in glucose tolerance; (v) very high doses of any amino acid, including tryptophan, should not be given to pregnant women; (vi) because of the toxicity to the lung of skatole, tryptophan should not be given to patients with achlorhydria or those not able to absorb it in the upper bowel; (vii) patients on tryptophan should be followed carefully to ensure that they do not develop cataracts; (viii) caution should be used when adding tryptophan to MAOIs, and possible side effects should be monitored carefully; and (ix) possible signs of sexual disinhibition should be noted when tryptophan is added to neuroleptics or MAOIs. Despite these perhaps overly conservative qualifications, tryptophan seems to have few side effects, all of which are usually mild, and it is well tolerated by the majority of patients.

V. CLINICAL EFFECTS OF ALTERED TRYPTOPHAN LEVELS

A. Effect of Raising or Lowering Tryptophan on Food Intake

When considering the control of neurotransmitter synthesis through the availability of precursor amino acids, one constant question is: why should brain neurotransmitter metabolism be vulnerable to dietary intake? There is a logical answer: to regulate food intake. However, the part of food intake regulation that is mediated by 5-HT probably occurs in very specific groups of brain neurons, perhaps in the hypothalamus, while food consumption or tryptophan administration will affect 5-HT not just in these nuclei but throughout the brain. One consequence is that food consumption can, via brain tryptophan and 5-HT, influence a variety of behaviors, albeit for most, with no apparent logical reason for this relationship. Because food intake regulation is the one behavior where a rationale is immediately apparent, it is discussed first.

Protein tends to lower, and carbohydrate to raise, brain tryptophan and 5-HT (Section II.A). A variety of animal data suggest that a decrease in 5-HT-mediated neurotransmission will increase carbohydrate intake relative to that of protein, and, conversely, that increasing 5-HT release increases protein relative to carbohydrate (3,189,191). Thus the composition of one meal can affect macronutrient intake at the next, and the amount of protein and carbohydrate ingested over a period of days should stay within certain limits. Three experiments have looked at aspects of this mechanism in humans. Tryptophan was given over a 2-week period to obese subjects with a craving for carbohydrate snacks, at a dose of 2.4 g/day given in three doses per day. It significantly diminished carbohydrate intake in three of the eight treated subjects, and increased it in one subject; it did not significantly modify snacking patterns in the group as a whole (189). Tryptophan was also tested against placebo in a double-blind crossover study in healthy lean men. Tryptophan, in doses from 1 to 3 g, or placebo was given 45 min before subjects selected from a buffet luncheon. Either 3 or 2 g reduced total calorie intake significantly by 13 to 20%; 1 had no effect; and all three doses had no significant effect on relative macronutrient selection (98).

The other study on tryptophan and food intake used a tryptophan-deficient diet to deplete plasma and brain tryptophan, as described in Section II.B. In a double-blind crossover design, normal male subjects received 50 g of either a tryptophan-deficient amino acid mixture or, as a control, a nutritionally balanced amino acid mixture containing tryptophan (204). Five hours later, the subjects selected from a buffet luncheon. Tryptophan depletion caused a significant 13% decline in protein intake. There was a similar but nonsignificant fall in total calorie intake and no effect on carbohydrate selection. These three studies, taken together, suggest that tryptophan availability in the brain can play some role in regulating food intake in humans, that the overall type of effect seen is similar to that elucidated in animal work, but that many details must be worked out. How humans might select for carbohydrate or protein is not known, but it is probably not through cognitive processes. Thus in a double-blind comparison of the effects of tryptophan (0.5 g) and placebo on various measures in a questionnaire, tryptophan had no effect on the subjects' own rating of their hunger or carbohydrate/protein preference, even though they found tryptophan significantly more sedating (113). Also in the study of different dosages and their effect on food intake, described above, visual analogue scale ratings of "hunger" or "urge to eat" were not always related to actual changes in food intake (98).

B. Effect of Tryptophan on Arousal and Sleep

In 1962, Smith and Prockop (169) reported on the CNS effects of ingestion of tryptophan by normal subjects. Among the symptoms they found were drowsiness, a finding that has repeatedly been confirmed in other studies (29,75,113,117). The first study to look at the effect of tryptophan on sleep was that of Oswald et al. (149) published in 1966. They found that tryptophan (5–10 g orally) could shorten the time before onset of rapid eye movement (REM) sleep, and that this effect was prevented by prior administration of the 5-HT blocker methysergide. Since then more than 40 studies have been published on the effect of tryptophan on sleep. These studies have been reviewed in detail by Cole et al. (38) and by Hartmann and Greenwald (80), so this review is selective rather than exhaustive. Many of the earlier studies dealt with changes in sleep stages. For example, in one study, normal subjects given 7.5 g tryptophan showed a decrease in REM sleep and an increase in non-REM sleep (192). Other studies have not reported changes in sleep stages, a discrepancy that may be related in part to use of different dosages of tryptophan. In a dose-response study, tryptophan doses of 1 to 15 g decreased sleep latency, but only doses above 5 g produced any alteration in sleep stages—in this case, a decrease in desynchronized sleep and an increase in slow-wave sleep (79).

Decreased sleep latency appears to be the most common and most consistent effect of tryptophan on sleep. Although this effect has not been observed universally, Hartmann and Greenwald (80) have identified some factors that might affect its appearance. Dose is important. While doses above 1 g seem to decrease sleep latency with equal efficiency (79), doses of 0.25 and 0.5 g showed a trend toward decreased latency, but the effect was not statistically significant (82).

Another important variable is time of administration. Subjects given 4 g tryptophan were asked to fill out the Stanford Sleepiness Scale every 15 min. Tryptophan had a definite effect in producing sleepiness, but its effect became significantly different from that of placebo only starting at 45 min after administration (83). (Perhaps it took this long for brain 5-HT to rise sufficiently to influence arousal.) The type of subject tested for sleep latency can also affect responses (80). Tryptophan, given at an adequate dose, was invariably found to decrease sleep latency in subjects with mild insomnia or in subjects with a long sleep latency who did not complain of insomnia. In studies on normal subjects or in patients with chronic or severe insomnia, however, positive results occurred only sometimes. In normal subjects who fall asleep easily, there is diminished scope for reduced latency, which may explain some of the negative results. The negative results with chronic and severe insomniacs may suggest that tryptophan is less effective in this type of patient than in mild insomniacs.

The idea that tryptophan is relatively ineffective in severe insomnia is supported by the results of a study comparing 1 g tryptophan with secobarbital, flurazepam, and placebo in 96 serious insomniacs (81). Flurazepam produced significant improvement on several sleep measures compared to placebo, whereas tryptophan and secobarbital did not. Thus tryptophan was not as effective as a standard hypnotic agent. The same conclusion came from a study comparing tryptophan, chloral hydrate, and placebo in geriatric patients (121). In the former study, an analysis of those who did and did not respond to tryptophan indicated that responders tended to have shorter sleep latencies but broken sleep, while nonresponders had longer sleep latencies (119). Thus it may be possible to select specific types of severe insomniacs who show a good response to tryptophan.

In several studies, ingestion of tryptophan at bedtime for several nights was followed by ingestion of placebo for several nights, with continuing improvement during the placebo period (i.e., relative to the pre-tryptophan baseline) (69,81,162, 192). This has led to suggestions that interval therapy might be useful. When eight severe chronic insomniacs were given 2 g tryptophan for three nights, followed by a four-night placebo period, there were highly significant sleep improvements in the placebo period relative to baseline (162). However, further studies will be needed to confirm the tentative finding that tryptophan may be a more effective hypnotic when given intermittently than when given continuously.

The mechanism mediating the success of interval therapy is unknown. However, in rats, single tryptophan loads can increase pineal melatonin (198), while animal studies show that melatonin, given at the same time every day, is capable of entraining free-running rhythms (159). Thus tryptophan may be working through a melatonin-mediated entrainment of the diurnal sleep rhythm.

In summary, single doses of tryptophan decrease arousal, and this can decrease sleep latency in subjects with mild insomnia. For this purpose, 1 g tryptophan given 45 min before bedtime seems to be suitable. If further research confirms the utility of intermittent use of tryptophan, this approach may make tryptophan suitable for use in severe or chronic insomnia.

C. Effect of Tryptophan on Pain

A large body of literature derived from animal experiments indicates that 5-HT is one of the many neurotransmitters involved in modulating pain perception. In addition, 5-HT may be involved in the analgesia produced by morphine and other opiates. Thus it is surprising that tryptophan has been tested for the treatment of clinical pain in only a few studies, most of them on a small number of patients.

The effect of tryptophan on pain perception in normal subjects has been tested in two studies. Pain perception and tolerance thresholds were measured in 30 normal subjects by electrical stimulation of dental pulps before and after receiving either placebo or 2 g tryptophan per day in three divided doses for 7 days (164). Perception threshold levels were similar in tryptophan and placebo subjects; however, pain tolerance levels were significantly higher in the group receiving tryptophan. In a second study, eight healthy men were given tryptophan (50 mg/kg), tyrosine (100 mg/kg), or placebo in a double-blind crossover experiment. The subjects rated heat stimuli. Tryptophan but not tyrosine significantly reduced pain discriminability (117).

The use of tryptophan alone in the treatment of clinical pain has been tested in three studies. In a double-blind study, 30 patients with chronic maxillofacial pain were assigned to placebo or tryptophan (3 g/day in six divided doses). After 4 weeks, there was a greater reduction in reported clinical pain and a greater increase in pain tolerance in the tryptophan group than in the placebo group (163). Another study found negative results in a comparison of tryptophan (a single 5-g dose given at bedtime) and chlorpromazine in patients with fibrositis syndrome (131). Chlorpromazine but not tryptophan was associated with increased slow-wave sleep and amelioration of pain and mood. In an open study, 9 g tryptophan per day, given in three daily doses for 10 days, prevented migraine altogether in three of five patients and reduced the incidence of headache in a fourth (154).

Tryptophan has been found useful in reversing tolerance to three different analgesic treatments. Five patients were given tryptophan when they developed tolerance to the ability of electrical stimulation of periaqueductal and periventricular gray matter to ameliorate severe intractable pain. Tryptophan was given orally for 2-month periods at a dose of 3 g/day in four divided doses, interspersed by 2-month placebo periods. One patient stopped taking tryptophan because of acute gastric pain. In the other four, tryptophan reversed tolerance to the electrical stimulation (94). In three patients, tryptophan administration was shown to restore the release of β-endorphin immunoreactivity into the ventricular CSF on electrical stimulation; such release had stopped concurrent with the development of tolerance to the analgesic effect of electrical stimulation (96). Tryptophan (4 g/day for 2–9 weeks) also reversed tolerance to opiates in five patients who had been given opiates chronically to treat low back and leg pain. Tryptophan enabled the patients to lead more active lives and to reduce their daily opiate intake (95). Finally, tryptophan (2 g/day) was given to five rhizotomy and cordotomy patients in whom pain had resumed and sensory deficits had diminished. Their sensory deficits for both touch and pinprick reexpanded to the maximum extent initially recorded after surgery (107).

The results so far with tryptophan and pain are encouraging and suggest that tryptophan may not only be an analgesic when given by itself, but also may be useful in reversing tolerance to other treatments. Because of these preliminary results and the few side effects that occur with tryptophan treatment, it now seems appropriate that large-scale studies be done to test the clinical utility of tryptophan in the treatment of a variety of types of pain.

D. Effect of Raising or Lowering Tryptophan Levels on Aggression

Among the psychiatric disorders, pathological aggression is of interest because of the availability of abundant data from animal studies on its neurochemical basis. However, this information has not been applied to clinical situations to any appreciable extent. Animal studies suggest that 5-HT has an inhibitory effect on aggression. Recently, Brown et al. (21) reviewed the clinical evidence from CSF studies that low 5-HT is associated both with aggression directed toward others and the self-directed aggression of suicide. Only one study has so far applied this information by testing the use of tryptophan in pathological aggression (140). The subjects were 12 male schizophrenics at a hospital for mentally ill offenders. All of them had been convicted of murder or other person-related crimes. They continued to show episodes of threatening aggression and responded poorly to neuroleptics. In a double-blind placebo crossover design, tryptophan (4 or 8 g/day) and placebo were each given for 4 weeks. A 17-item ward checklist was filled in daily on each patient to record physical assault, verbal abuse, and other uncontrolled behaviors. This checklist showed a significant (30%) decline in incidents while the patients were on tryptophan relative to placebo.

In addition to this study on pathologically aggressive patients, one study has looked at the acute effects of manipulating tryptophan levels on performance in a laboratory test of aggression in normal subjects (172). Thirty-six normal males were assigned to treatment with tryptophan-deficient, nutritionally balanced, or tryptophan-supplemented amino acid mixtures, as described in Section II.B. These treatments were designed to lower or raise brain tryptophan and 5-HT, with the nutritionally balanced mixture serving as a control. The test of aggression was a modified Buss paradigm in which the subjects give electric shocks to a (nonexistent) partner. The intensity and duration of shock administered is the measure of aggression. In this study, there was no significant difference between the mean shock duration or intensity administered by the three groups.

Much more clinical work is needed on how tryptophan availability can influence aggression. The preliminary indication that tryptophan may be useful needs testing in a variety of different types of pathological aggression. As far as studies on normal subjects are concerned, it remains to be seen whether the negative results are due to differences between normals and the pathologically aggressive. For example, if 5-HT were one of many inhibitory systems modulating aggression in normal subjects, it may be that altering 5-HT would not affect aggression appreciably, but that in the pathologically aggressive, whose inhibitory systems are inadequate, manipulating even one of them, 5-HT, might produce clinically significant results. Alternatively, the laboratory test used in the normal subjects may not have been an adequate measure of the types of aggression actually exhibited by normal subjects in the real world.

E. Tryptophan and Mood

1. The Use of Tryptophan with Other Antidepressant Treatments

The first test of the use of tryptophan as an antidepressant was published by Coppen et al. in 1963 (43). In a double-blind study, DL-tryptophan (10–17 g) or placebo was added to the MAOI tranylcypromine during the second week of treatment. Improvement in the tryptophan group was significantly more rapid than in the placebo group, starting with the second week of treatment. In the same year, Pare (150) published results of a study in which tryptophan (7.5–15 g/day) had been given to patients who had responded to various MAOIs and tricyclic antidepressants but who had relapsed on reduced dosages. While only one in 10 of the patients on tricyclic antidepressants responded, six of the 14 patients on MAOIs showed a striking improvement 2 or 3 days after starting tryptophan. Substitution of placebo for the tryptophan caused relapse within 2 to 7 days.

Two other controlled studies have looked at the ability of tryptophan to potentiate the action of MAOIs. In 20 patients given either phenelzine and placebo or phenelzine and tryptophan (12–18 g/day) under double-blind conditions, response was significantly better in the tryptophan group (68). When 30 depressed patients receiving nialamide were given DL-tryptophan (6 g/day) or placebo in a double-blind study, the tryptophan group showed faster and greater improvement (7). In a study investigating the effect of adding the MAOI tranylcypromine to DL-tryptophan (5–7 g/day), there was a trend for the patients treated with the combination to show a greater improvement than those treated by tryptophan alone, but this effect was not statistically significant (44).

As mentioned above, in 1963, Pare (150) found no potentiation of the action of imipramine or amitriptyline by tryptophan, and several other studies have come to similar conclusions. These include studies using 6 g tryptophan per day with clomipramine or desipramine (165), an incremental dosage schedule of up to 6 g tryptophan per day in patients receiving imipramine (33), and 0.1 g/kg DL-tryptophan with zimelidine (183). This last study is of interest because CSF 5-HIAA measurements were made. Zimelidine, as expected with all 5-HT uptake inhibitors, lowered CSF 5-HIAA, but the decline was even greater in patients receiving tryptophan with zimelidine. Thus there was no evidence that tryptophan was increasing 5-HT synthesis in the zimelidine-treated patients. This is a surprising finding, especially as the same dose of tryptophan did increase 5-HT synthesis in clomipramine-treated patients in another study (184). Tryptophan reversed the clomipramine-mediated decline in CSF 5-HIAA.

The combination of tryptophan and clomipramine also resulted in a more rapid and greater improvement in depression and anxiety than a tryptophan–placebo combination. Tryptophan (3 g/day) improved depression more effectively than placebo in patients receiving amitriptyline, but the difference was not statistically significant (122). The most important study on the combined treatment, because it contained the largest number of patients and was of 12 weeks' duration, compared the action of tryptophan (3 g/day in 29 patients), amitriptyline (31 patients), their combination (27 patients), and placebo (28 patients) (177). The treatments were given by general practitioners, and the patients were less depressed [mean Hamilton Depression Scale (HDS) scores of less than 20] than in most of the other studies, which were hospital based. The HDS total showed no significant difference between the effects of tryptophan, amitriptyline, and their combination, although the HDS item *Depressed Mood* showed significantly better improvement for the combination than for either active treatment alone. A visual analogue scale filled in by the patients suggested that both amitriptyline and the combination were better than tryptophan alone.

The three studies that found a potentiation of the action of tricyclic antidepressants used relatively small doses of tryptophan. It is obvious, therefore, to ask whether variation in tryptophan availability within the physiological range influences response to tricyclic antidepressants. The results on this question are mixed. Patients who responded to unspecified tricyclics had significantly higher plasma tryptophan levels than nonresponders (160). However, this finding was not confirmed in three other studies (46,134,139), two of which found that the plasma ratio of tryptophan to the amino acids that compete with it for uptake into brain was inversely related to response to imipramine or amitripytline (134,139).

The ability of tryptophan to potentiate the action of ECT has been tested in two studies. Tryptophan was no better than placebo when infused intravenously at a dose of 10 mg/kg 5 min before each ECT (108). A negative result might have been expected from this study, as the patients can have received no more than 2 g tryptophan each week, considerably less than dietary intake. Oral tryptophan (6 g/day) was tested against placebo, with treatment being initiated 1 day before the first ECT and terminated 4 days after the last ECT (50). Tryptophan caused a significant potentiation of the antiretardation effect of ECT, but this effect was considered of little importance clinically.

The combination of tryptophan with lithium has also been used in depressed patients. Thirty-one bipolar depressed patients received either 6 g tryptophan per day or the same dose of tryptophan plus lithium in a double-blind 3-week trial (188). The combination was significantly better than tryptophan alone from the second week on. Tryptophan was also given in a single daily dose of 100 mg/kg together with lithium in a 4-week open study on 43 depressed patients, with amitriptyline as the control medication (93). There was no difference in the antidepressive efficacy of the two treatments. The two studies show some promise, but what is needed now is a controlled trial of the addition of tryptophan or placebo to patients receiving lithium.

A rather different approach to the use of combinations is described in a double-blind study of tryptophan, a combination of tryptophan and 5-HTP, and a low dose of nomifensine as control (157). Tryptophan was given at a maximum dose of 3 g/day when given alone. The patients receiving the combination received 2.85 g tryptophan and 0.15 g 5-HTP. The combination was significantly better than nomifensine, while tryptophan alone was not. The combination showed a trend toward being significantly better than tryptophan on several measures. These results are impressive, as there were only eight patients per group. In this study, 5-HTP was given because of indications that it could attenuate the rise of tryptophan pyrrolase in tryptophan-treated animals (37); it may also have been acting as a 5-HT precursor or, as discussed elsewhere in this volume, to release catecholamines. This intriguing finding requires follow-up.

Overall, the studies described above suggest that tryptophan can bring about a clear-cut improvement when added to a MAOI. However, because side effects also tend to be potentiated, this combination is not generally useful. Tryptophan may also cause a clinically significant improvement when added to tricyclic antidepressants. This effect has been seen most clearly at low doses of tryptophan and in mildly depressed patients. More work will be needed to determine whether this potentiation of clinical efficacy is confined to these conditions. The use of tryptophan with other therapies, such as ECT, lithium, and 5-HTP, needs further assessment.

2. The Use of Tryptophan by Itself in Depression

There are a large number of published studies on the efficacy of tryptophan given alone as an antidepressant, and the many excellent reviews of this area of research (9,25,35,38,39,49,63,181,186,197), like the studies themselves, show no consensus on the efficacy of tryptophan. This is both because the studies come to different conclusions and because they use very different designs, dosages, and types of patients. Often a distinction, such as differential response in unipolar and bipolar patients, which is stressed in one study, will be ignored in another, which will not even mention the numbers of unipolar or bipolar patients tested. A further problem is the small sample size used in most of the studies. In general, studies belong to one or more of three types: (i) those with no adequate control group, (ii) those which compared tryptophan to a standard antidepressant, and (iii) the most rigorous test of all, those which compared tryptophan to placebo.

The majority of studies with no control group found little therapeutic effect. Four studies were almost entirely negative (17,61,127,188), whereas two found almost no response in unipolar patients but improvement in approximately 50% of a small group of bipolar patients (57,143). A further three studies found a good response in approximately 75% of the depressed patients given tryptophan (19,34,167). In these studies, the positive results are obviously easier to explain, by the placebo effect, than are the negative results.

The majority of the studies on tryptophan have compared it with standard antidepressant treatments. In five double-blind studies (33,45,109,118,158) and in one that was not double blind (19), tryptophan, at doses in the range of 3 to 9 g/day, was found not to be significantly different in antidepressive efficacy from imipramine. A similar conclusion was reached with respect to amitriptyline (87) and mianserin (12) in double-blind studies using tryptophan in the same dosage range. Tryptophan was significantly less effective than both clomipramine and doxepin, but in this study, tryptophan was used as an active placebo at a very low dose (1.5 g/day) (120). In the largest and longest lasting (12 weeks) study, tryptophan (3 g/day) was not significantly different from amitriptyline on the HDS and a Global Rating Scale, but tryptophan was less effective than amitriptyline on a visual analogue scale filled in by the patients (177). As the visual analogue scale went from "most depressed ever" to "happiest ever," while the other scales had euthymia as their end point, this might indicate that amitriptyline but not tryptophan was causing euphoria in the patients.

The comparison of tryptophan with a standard antidepressant drug is not a particularly demanding one unless the sample size used is larger than that in the studies described above. Because the margin of efficacy between placebo and any antidepressant drug is relatively small, the finding that tryptophan is not significantly different from a standard antidepressant does not imply that tryptophan is better than placebo, except with a large sample. Tryptophan has also been put to the more demanding test of a comparison with ECT. These studies did not employ dummy ECTs and thus were not double blind. In two studies employing 7 g (26) and 6 to 8 g (86) tryptophan per day, tryptophan was inferior to ECT. In a study using 0.1 g/kg DL-tryptophan, the two treatments were not significantly different (44), whereas in one study using 3 g tryptophan per day, tryptophan was found to be superior to unilateral ECT administered twice weekly (123). There does not seem to be any simple way of reconciling these discrepancies, although it is interesting that in the studies that found positive results relative to ECT, the initial levels of depression were lower than in those studies that found ECT better than tryptophan.

The best test of any antidepressant medication is against placebo, and tryptophan has been put to this test in several studies. In a double-blind crossover study, patients received an average of 9.6 g/tryptophan per day. Of 16 unipolar patients, only one responded to tryptophan, and this patient failed to relapse on placebo. Five of eight bipolar patients responded to tryptophan, and three of the five relapsed on placebo (143). Using an incremental dosage schedule from 3 to 16 g/day, only one of six patients responded to tryptophan, whereas none of the three patients on placebo did (127). In somewhat larger studies, 4 g tryptophan was no more effective than placebo in unipolar patients (12 per group), while 8 g/day was no more effective than placebo in bipolar patients (nine per group) (35). Two placebo-controlled studies have tested the action of tryptophan in special categories of depressed patients. A daily dose of 3 g tryptophan was no better than placebo in the treatment of "maternity blues" (78). In 40 geriatric patients with mild to moderate depression of mixed etiology (including endogenous and reactive depression and depression secondary to organic disease), 6 g tryptophan per day produced significant improvement after 4 weeks, while placebo did so after 6 weeks. However, there was no significant difference between the efficacies of placebo and drug (40). The only positive result with tryptophan against placebo occurred in the study mentioned above, in which 3 g tryptophan per day was compared with amitriptyline, the combination of tryptophan and amitriptyline, and placebo (177). Using the HDS and a Global Rating Scale, tryptophan was significantly better than placebo and was comparable in efficacy to amitriptyline.

The results from the study that found tryptophan more effective than placebo must be given more weight than any other individual study, because this study was both larger and longer lasting than the others. Thus the group sizes were from 27 to 31 patients, compared with a maximum of 20 patients in other studies, while the duration of the study was 12 weeks, compared with a norm of 3 or 4 weeks for the other studies. However, all the other placebo-controlled studies, as well as some of the open studies, suggest that tryptophan was not effective as an antidepressant drug. For reasons given above, the studies comparing tryptophan with other antidepressant drugs do not provide convincing evidence of the efficacy of tryptophan. These discrepant results make it difficult to say whether or not tryptophan is an antidepressant, but there may be differences related to the type of patients. In the study that found tryptophan significantly better than placebo, the medication was prescribed by general practitioners. All the other studies were hospital based; many were carried out on inpatients, and the initial levels of depression were, in general, much higher. Thus the mean HDS scores in the groups treated by the general practitioners started at less than 20. If it is assumed that the results of all the placebo-controlled studies are correct, then the tentative conclusion must be that tryptophan is more effective in mild or moderately depressed subjects than in severely depressed patients.

With a therapy such as tryptophan, which acts relatively specifically on a particular neurochemical system, it is obvious to ask whether responses would be better in a biochemically distinct subgroup of patients. In this case, a better response might be expected in subjects with low 5-HT, with or without low brain tryptophan, particularly if the low 5-HT were involved in the etiology of the depression. Determination of CSF tryptophan and 5-HIAA would be a useful method for selecting such a group, but this has not been done. Pretreatment plasma tryptophan levels do not predict clinical responses to tryptophan (33,34,136), but the plasma ratio of tryptophan to the amino acids which compete with it for entry into brain may provide a better measure than plasma tryptophan alone (132,137). In patients with a pretreatment ratio less than the 15th percentile, a good clinical response occurred in 80% within 2 weeks. In patients with a ratio above the 30th percentile, a good response was seen in only 7%. When the ratio was measured in 87 depressed patients, the calculated response rate, from the previous data, was 28%, comparable to a placebo effect. However, the original study involved a single daily tryptophan dose of 100 mg/kg, which is probably not an ideal dosage schedule (see Section III). A low plasma ratio may be related to increased severity of depression (51). If this is so, the suggestion that the best response to tryptophan is seen in patients with a low ratio and the alternative suggestion that the best response is seen in mildly depressed patients are not compatible. Obviously, more work will be needed to identify the types of depressed patients who show a good response to tryptophan.

3. Tryptophan as an Antimanic Agent

There are several reasons to test the antimanic efficacy of tryptophan. In experimental animals, brain 5-HT levels seem to have an inverse relationship to responses to various stimuli, while enhanced responsivity to their environment is a characteristic of manic patients. Clinical data indicate that tryptophan has a sedative effect (Section V.B), while low 5-HT has been suggested as one factor involved in the etiology of mania (155). The effect of tryptophan in mania has been tested in four studies. When 10 acutely manic or hypomanic patients were given an average dose of 9.6 g tryptophan per day, seven improved. Three of the seven relapsed when placebo was substituted for tryptophan under double-blind conditions (143). A daily dose of 6 g tryptophan was compared with moderate doses of chlorpromazine in a double-blind crossover study on 10 patients, in which each treatment was given first in half the patients (155). Tryptophan was slightly superior to chlorpromazine in all respects. The same dose of tryptophan was used in a double-blind, placebo-controlled, 2-week trial on 10 acutely manic patients (27). In view of the fact that there were only five patients per group and that nitrazepam and chlorpromazine were also given to the patients, it is hardly surprising that there was no significant difference between tryptophan and placebo. In a modified double-blind placebo crossover design, 12 g tryptophan per day was given to 24 acutely manic patients for 1 week (32). During the second week, half the patients were substituted onto placebo. A good therapeutic response was seen in the first week, and the continued response during the second week was better in the tryptophan group than in the placebo group. Overall, these studies suggest that tryptophan has a clinically useful therapeutic effect in acute mania.

One obvious area in which to extend research on tryptophan in the affective disorders is to determine whether tryptophan can potentiate the action of lithium, and to determine if it has a prophylactic action in bipolar patients. A small amount of information is already available on these matters. A group of 16 patients receiving lithium (nine bipolar in the manic phase and seven schizoaffective) were given either 9 g tryptophan per day or placebo for 3 weeks (18). Significant improvement on tryptophan relative to placebo was seen on a Manic State Rating Scale and the Brief Psychiatric Rating Scale for both diagnostic subgroups. Three single case studies indicate that tryptophan may have a prophylactic action in bipolar subjects who did not respond adequately to lithium, when given either alone (11,88) or with lithium (31). This is a promising area which needs further study.

4. The Effects of Raising or Lowering Tryptophan on Mood in Normal Subjects

The studies on the acute mood-elevating effects of tryptophan in normal subjects, like the studies on the chronic mood-elevating effect of tryptophan in depressed patients, have given variable results. Some have found that tryptophan produces euphoria (29,169), while others have not (75,113,117,201). There are no apparent reasons for these discrepancies in the literature.

The effect of lowering tryptophan on mood in normal subjects has been tested using the tryptophan-deficient amino acid mixture described in Section II.B. The experiment was carried out on 36 normal males who were divided into three groups. Each received, under double-blind conditions, a tryptophan-deficient (T −) amino acid mixture to lower tryptophan, a nutritionally balanced (B) amino acid mixture to serve as a control, and a mixture containing excess tryptophan (T +) to raise tryptophan levels (201). Two measures of mood were used. One was the depression scale of the Multiple Affect Adjective Checklist (MAACL). The other, a measure of dysphoria, was based on distractability during attentional proofreading tasks. The subjects performed proofreading tasks as quickly as possible while listening to tapes of varying emotional content over headphones. Low and high distractors served as controls for a dysphoric distractor, which contained themes of hopelessness and helplessness. Cognitive theories predict that individuals who are depressed will be more distracted by dysphoric themes than people who are not depressed. Both measures indicated that the group who received the T− mixture had significantly lower mood than the groups receiving the B and T+ mixtures at 5 hr after mixture ingestion. Plasma tryptophan was at its lowest at this time.

In the experiment described above, subjects remained in a sparsely furnished room and spent most of their time filling in various paper and pencil tests. To test whether this relatively negative environment might have made the subjects in the T− group more susceptible to a mood-lowering effect, a second experiment was performed with subjects in either positive or negative environments (171). In the negative environment, the subjects were kept in a sparsely furnished room and forbidden to do anything other than work on the tests provided. In the positive environment, the subjects were kept in a comfortable room with a supportive atmosphere and were entertained during the time between amino acid ingestion and testing 5 hr later. These manipulations were sufficient to influence the B group in the expected way, as indicated by changes in MAACL scores. However, in the T− group, the increase in MAACL depression scale scores was not significantly different in the positive and negative environments. This replicated the original finding and showed that the decline in mood induced by tryptophan depletion was robust with respect to an environmental manipulation.

The mood-lowering effect of tryptophan depletion produces a state within the normal range rather than clinical depression. Indeed, anything else would be surprising over a period of a few hours. Nonetheless, these data do suggest that, in some patients, low 5-HT might contribute to clinical depression. The tests used in the studies do not provide much information on the type of mental state produced by tryptophan depletion, and it remains to be seen whether it is more somatic or related more to mental state, and, if the latter, to exactly what components of mental state.

F. Effect of Tryptophan in Schizophrenia

The early studies on the action of tryptophan in schizophrenia were on patients treated with MAOIs. In general, there was an elevation of mood and motor activity, but this was also sometimes accompanied by increased anxiety and hallucinatory activity (1,112,153). When tryptophan was given at 2 to 4 g/day to six schizophrenics not on MAOIs, there was a slight decrease in anxiety and tension but less than that subsequently produced by neuroleptics. In a double-blind crossover study, eight chronic schizophrenic patients were given placebo or tryptophan at daily doses up to 20 g (66). Tryptophan had no therapeutic effect. Tryptophan was also given to chronic schizophrenics using an incremental dosage schedule up to 6 g/day over 6 weeks in a two-group comparison with chlorpromazine (300–900 mg/day) (30). The patients (16 per group) had previously been withdrawn from neuroleptics. Brief Psychiatric Rating Scale measures showed that chlorpromazine was clearly superior to tryptophan. Tryptophan (8 g/day) was also inferior to the combination of tryptophan and chlorpromazine when the two were compared in a double-blind

4-week study in chronic schizophrenics (28). The group treated with tryptophan alone showed exacerbation of psychotic symptoms, while the group given tryptophan and chlorpromazine showed no change.

In schizoaffective patients, tryptophan may have a beneficial mood-stabilizing effect. In a double-blind comparison of lithium plus tryptophan (9 g/day) and lithium plus placebo in seven manic schizoaffective patients, tryptophan was significantly better than placebo (18). In 12 depressed schizoaffective patients treated daily with 8 g tryptophan for 4 weeks, there was an improvement in affective symptoms (28).

Overall, these results suggest that tryptophan is of little use in schizophrenia, although it may be of some use as a mood stabilizer in schizoaffective patients.

G. Use of Tryptophan in the Treatment of L-DOPA-Induced Side Effects

In parkinsonian patients treated with DOPA, psychiatric side effects, including psychotic episodes and depression, are quite common. In a postmortem study, tryptophan was measured in brain areas of parkinsonian patients who had been on DOPA. In patients who had developed psychoses, tryptophan levels were lower than in those who did not become psychotic (14). Because DOPA is a large neutral amino acid, it will compete with tryptophan both for absorption in the intestine and for entry into the brain. Administration of tryptophan can normalize the low brain 5-HT found in DOPA-treated rats (56), providing a rationale for the testing of tryptophan in the treatment of psychosis produced by DOPA. In the four clinical studies performed so far, tryptophan was successful in alleviating the mental symptoms that develop during DOPA therapy (15,62,114,128). In addition, the effect of tryptophan has been tested on the depression found in parkinsonian patients that is not related to DOPA intake. The combination of tryptophan with DOPA, but not DOPA alone, caused a significant improvement in mood when comparing pre- and posttreatment scores, but the between-group comparison did not reveal any significant differences (42).

Tryptophan seems to be effective in relieving DOPA-induced side effects in parkinsonian patients. However, it is not clear to what extent this is due to tryptophan restoring brain 5-HT levels or inhibiting DOPA uptake by brain and thus reducing its effective dosage.

H. Other Psychopharmacological Uses of Tryptophan

Tryptophan has been tested in a variety of clinical conditions in addition to those described above. Obviously, the conditions most likely to respond to tryptophan are those in which low brain tryptophan or 5-HT are thought to have etiological significance. This is so in two types of epilepsy. Progressive myoclonus epilepsy is a distinct clinical entity of unknown etiology that occurs in Finland. Because there is deficient intestinal absorption of tryptophan (110) and low CSF 5-HIAA (115) in this condition, tryptophan has been tested in two studies. The first was a double-blind crossover trial with 2 g tryptophan or placebo carried out in seven patients

(111). The 8-week trial was followed by a 3-month open study of the same dose of tryptophan. In six of seven patients, tryptophan improved ambulation, myoclonic jerks, and general condition. However, the effect disappeared in three of the patients after 3 to 4 weeks of treatment. The second study used a higher dose of tryptophan (100 mg/kg/day) in 11 patients over 6 weeks (116). The increase in CSF 5-HIAA caused by the tryptophan was accompanied by an improvement in activities of daily living, a decrease of active myoclonus, and a decreased frequency of seizures. Tryptophan has also been tested in postanoxic myoclonus, a condition with low CSF 5-HIAA which responds to 5-HTP administration. In two such patients, treatment with 10 g tryptophan in five daily doses caused a moderate improvement, which was reversed by substitution of placebo (48). The only other study on epileptic subjects was a controlled trial of tryptophan in the hyperactive child syndrome associated with epilepsy (65). In a crossover study, 11 children received 5 weeks of treatment with tryptophan (40 mg/kg/day) or placebo. No therapeutic effect was seen, which could indicate that either 5-HT does not inhibit the hyperactivity associated with epilepsy or that the dose was too low.

Another neurological condition in which low CSF 5-HIAA is known to occur, at least in severe cases, is multiple sclerosis. The action of tryptophan has been tested in this condition (100). When tryptophan was given to 12 patients for 30 days in an open study, there was a modest improvement in mood and neurological symptoms. Because of the variable course of this disease, however, these findings must be accepted with caution.

Among the psychiatric disorders in which low 5-HT has been suggested are phobias and obsessive–compulsive disorders. In a 10-week double-blind study comparing the action of clomipramine plus tryptophan (increasing to 8 g/day) with clomipramine plus placebo in 24 agoraphobics and 16 social phobics, tryptophan did not potentiate the beneficial effect of clomipramine on phobic avoidance, phobic fears, or the incidence of panic attacks (151). In an open study on seven obsessive–compulsive patients, a daily dose of 3 to 9 g tryptophan caused considerable improvement after 1 month of therapy (193). After 6 to 12 months of therapy, the patients' conditions were stabilized.

Tryptophan has been tested in demented gerontopsychiatric patients (170). Twenty-eight patients received either tryptophan (3 g given as a single dose in the evening) or casein (as a placebo) for 1 month each, using a double-blind crossover design. Tryptophan failed to have a significant effect on the mental condition of the patients as a whole.

Case reports suggest that tryptophan may have some action in various miscellaneous states. Thus tryptophan was found to diminish sexual desire in two male subjects, in keeping with the animal data suggesting that 5-HT has an inhibitory effect on sexual function (168). This was the desired effect of tryptophan administration in one of the subjects, but in the other, it was an undesired side effect. Tryptophan has also been reported to have a beneficial effect in three cases of isolated sleep paralysis (173). In 12 children treated for anxiety, which manifested as difficulties in school or a disturbed relationship with parents, tryptophan was claimed to have a beneficial effect (97).

Two effects of tryptophan, which are not related to its therapeutic actions, are of interest. First, tryptophan, at a dose of 2 g/day, caused a significant decrease in frontal voltages in 18 normal subjects and 10 nonpsychotic psychiatric patients in an electrophysiological study (47). This is in keeping with the sedative action of tryptophan. Surprisingly, the same treatment in 30 schizophrenic subjects had an opposite voltage-increasing effect. Second, when tryptophan was given to eight depressed patients, it significantly improved the subjects' impaired performance on serial and free recall verbal learning tasks, even though it had no effect on depression in these subjects (85). This might suggest that 5-HT has an effect on learning independent of its effect on mood.

VI. CLINICAL PROFILE OF TRYPTOPHAN

From the clinical data, tryptophan seems to have varied actions: it is a hypnotic, at least in mild insomniacs; it may be an antidepressant, although perhaps not in severely depressed subjects; it has a calming effect in acute mania; it may have analgesic effects and potentiate the action of other analgesic treatments; it seems to be therapeutic in some types of myoclonus; and it can attenuate DOPA-induced side effects in parkinsonian patients. In addition, there are preliminary indications that it influences food intake and is therapeutic in pathological aggression, while case reports indicate still other uses, such as for the prophylaxis of acute episodes in bipolar depressed patients and in the treatment of hypersexuality, isolated sleep paralysis, and obsessive–compulsive conditions. Indeed, there is a reasonably sound theoretical framework for believing that tryptophan might have useful actions in many conditions.

In view of the multiplicity of the actions of tryptophan, it is perhaps surprising that side effects are not seen more often. For example, drowsiness and anorexia have not been reported to any appreciable extent in depressed patients on tryptophan. It has been noted that tryptophan does not seem to influence sleep in depressed patients, except insofar as would be expected from the change in clinical condition (33,45). Part of the reason for this might depend on the fact that the actions of tryptophan depend on the state of the subject being treated. The currently available evidence suggests that tryptophan is an antidepressant in mildly depressed patients but not in severe depression, that it is a better hypnotic in mild insomnia than in severe insomnia, and that altering tryptophan levels can influence aggression in pathologically aggressive subjects but not in normal people. Similarly, the efficacy of tryptophan will be influenced greatly by the circumstances under which it is given. A single dose given 1 hr before bedtime would not be expected to have an antidepressant effect or to influence food intake, nor would three daily doses taken at mealtimes be expected to have a hypnotic effect. Rather than trying to answer the question of whether or not tryptophan is, for example, an antidepressant, it is more meaningful to question under what particular circumstances tryptophan might be seen to have an antidepressant action. There is not necessarily any discrepancy in the fact that tryptophan may be therapeutically effective in pathological aggression and yet not influence aggression in normal subjects.

The idea that the psychopharmacological effects of tryptophan may depend to a large extent on the circumstances in which it is given can be reconciled with our present fragmentary knowledge of the neural systems controlling complex brain functions, such as mood, aggression, or pain perception. The functions are controlled in a complex manner by a multiplicity of systems, of which 5-HT neurons are only one. It is reasonable to suggest that the effect of 5-HT on a complex function will depend largely on the state of the other systems controlling that function and on how 5-HT interacts with those systems. Furthermore, as discussed in Section II.C, the effects of tryptophan on 5-HT release may depend on the rate of firing of 5-HT neurons, which in turn is controlled in part through other unknown mechanisms related to the level of behavioral arousal and possibly other factors. The practical implication of this is that the type of patient used in clinical studies should be defined as closely as possible.

Although the list of possible indications for the use of tryptophan is long, there are precedents for drugs influencing more than one clinical condition. One example of special interest in relation to tryptophan is lithium. Lithium is not generally thought to be an effective antidepressant, although some studies have suggested that it may have antidepressant properties. Lithium is effective in the treatment of acute mania and also in prophylaxis in bipolar patients. In addition, lithium is effective in the treatment of pathological aggression (166). This pattern is similar to some of the effects of tryptophan, which is not generally thought to be an effective antidepressant, although one good study does suggest it has an action in mild depression. Tryptophan is effective in the treatment of acute mania, and case reports, still to be confirmed in controlled trials, suggest that it may be useful for prophylaxis in bipolar patients. In addition, there is a preliminary indication that tryptophan is useful in the treatment of pathological aggression. If the similarity between the clinical profiles of tryptophan and lithium is confirmed, this would have important implications for our understanding of the mechanism of action of both compounds. Lithium has complex actions on 5-HT, but a discussion of these actions is beyond the scope of this chapter.

VII. WILL DIET ALTER BRAIN FUNCTION THROUGH CHANGES IN BRAIN TRYPTOPHAN?

Experimental manipulations of tryptophan alter brain functions in some circumstances. It is obvious, therefore, to ask whether acute dietary intake, which also affects brain tryptophan, will influence brain 5-HT function. There is no direct experimental evidence on this, but experimental manipulations of tryptophan have been done in situations with a close resemblance to normal feeding. Babies 2 to 3 days old were given a feeding of tryptophan in 10% glucose, valine in 5% glucose, or normal infant formula (194). The amount of tryptophan was approximately the amount in the infant formula, while the valine was approximately half that in the infant formula. The infants fed tryptophan entered sleep 14 min sooner than they did after the formula, while those fed valine entered sleep 16 min later than they did after the formula. These results are consistent with what is known about the effect of tryptophan on sleep in adults. However, while the tryptophan would be expected to have a reasonably specific effect on brain tryptophan and 5-HT, the valine would have inhibited uptake into brain not only of tryptophan but also of phenylalanine, tyrosine, and histidine and therefore may have influenced the catecholamines and histamine. The infant formula, on the other hand, would have influenced not only the aromatic amino acids but also possibly choline, the precursor of acetylcholine.

While food intake will influence tryptophan, and therefore almost certainly in some circumstances will influence 5-HT function, there could be several other effects of food intake on brain function. The overall effect on the brain will depend on all these changes. In addition, psychological factors, social factors, and expectancy may play an important role in influencing mood and behavior after food ingestion. Therefore, it would not be surprising if the effects of food were different from the effects expected when considering only tryptophan and 5-HT changes. As the behavioral effects of food ingestion are not yet well delineated, it is not possible to give hard data in this area. Nonetheless, ingestion of a balanced meal is known to lower brain 5-HT metabolism in humans (152). An experimentally induced lowering of 5-HT in normal subjects lowers mood (Section V.E.4), while most people would agree that a lowering of mood is not a normal concomitant of meal ingestion. Obviously, much work will be needed in order to determine the relative importance of altered brain tryptophan and other factors in controlling the mood and behavioral changes that occur after eating different foods.

VIII. CONCLUSIONS AND PROSPECTS FOR THE FUTURE

The number of studies on the clinical psychopharmacology of tryptophan is large, and yet the number of definitive statements that can be made about its actions is small. One recurring problem has been that many studies have been performed on relatively small numbers of subjects and have not given conclusive results. Part of the reason for this is probably related to funding of studies. The necessary large placebo-controlled studies are expensive to perform. For most psychopharmacological agents, such studies are funded by drug companies. Unfortunately, it is often difficult to interest drug companies in the drug use of natural products, such as tryptophan, because patent laws diminish the chances for profitable marketing.

Most studies on the action of tryptophan have concerned its antidepressant and hypnotic actions. These studies have been following up original clinical observations made more than 20 years ago. There is certainly scope for definite large-scale placebo-controlled studies on the action of tryptophan in the affective disorders and on sleep. More information is needed on the action of tryptophan in depression and mania, while controlled studies are needed to determine whether it has a prophylactic action in bipolar patients. In the area of sleep research, more work is needed on the type of patient who responds best to tryptophan and on the use of interval therapy.

The most intriguing development in the area of tryptophan research is the use of tryptophan in clinical conditions suggested by basic research. Animal data indicate that 5-HT is one of many neurotransmitters involved in control of food intake, aggression, and pain perception. There are already preliminary indications that tryptophan is of use in clinical situations to control food intake, aggression, and pain, but much more work is needed in these areas. If it turns out that a simple nontoxic amino acid with few side effects is useful in the control of obesity, pathological aggression, or chronic pain, this would be an important advance. Because tryptophan is relatively specific for its effects on brain 5-HT, future research may lead not only to improved pharmacotherapy but also to more information on the effects of raising or lowering 5-HT in normal subjects. The data available so far have given clear indications for useful future areas of research on tryptophan, and the tools to carry out this research are available. If these problems are thought to be of sufficient interest, intriguing data should emerge in the future.

REFERENCES

1. Alexander, F., Curtis, G. C., Sprince, H., and Crosley, A. P., Jr. (1963): L-Methionine and L-tryptophan feedings in non-psychotic and schizophrenic patients with and without tranylcypromine. *J. Nerv. Ment. Dis.*, 137:135–142.
2. Altman, P. L., and Dittmer, D. S., eds. (1968): *Metabolism*, pp. 114–115, *Fed. Am. Soc. Exp. Biol.*, Bethesda.
3. Anderson, G. H. (1979): Control of protein and energy intake: Role of plasma amino acids and brain neurotransmitters. *Can. J. Physiol. Pharmacol.*, 57:1043–1057.
4. Antener, I., Tonney, G., Verwilghen, A. M., and Mauron, J. (1981): Biochemical study of malnutrition. IV. Determination of amino acids in the serum, erythrocytes and stool ultrafiltrates. *Int. J. Vitam. Nutr. Res.*, 51:64–78.
5. Ashcroft, G. W., Crawford, T. B. B., Cundall, R. L., Davidson, D. L., Dobson, J., Dow, R. C., Eccleston, D., Loose, R. W., and Pullar, I. A. (1973): 5-Hydroxytryptamine metabolism in affective illness: The effect of tryptophan administration. *Psychol. Med.*, 3:326–332.
6. Ashcroft, G. W., Eccleston, D., and Crawford, T. B. B. (1965): 5-Hydroxyindole metabolism in rat brain: A study of intermediate metabolism using the technique of tryptophan loading; methods. *J. Neurochem.*, 12:483–492.
7. Ayuso Gutierrez, J. L., and Lopez-Ibor Alino, J. J. (1971): Tryptophan and an MAOI (nialamide) in the treatment of depression: A double-blind study. *Int. Pharmacopsychiatry*, 6:92–97.
8. Badawy, A. A. B., and Evans, M. (1973): The mechanism of inhibition of rat liver tryptophan pyrrolase activity by 4-hydroxypyrazolo[3,4-d]pyrimidine (Allopurinol). *Biochem. J.*, 113:585–591.
9. Baldessarini, R. J. (1984): Treatment of depression by altering monoamine metabolism: Precursors and metabolic inhibitor. *Psychopharmacol. Bull.*, 20:224–239.
10. Baloh, R. W., Dietz, J., and Spooner, J. W. (1982): Myoclonus and ocular oscillations induced by L-tryptophan. *Ann. Neurol.*, 11:95–97.
11. Beitman, B. D., and Dunner, D. L. (1982): L-Tryptophan in the maintenance treatment of bipolar II manic-depressive illness. *Am. J. Psychiatry*, 139:1498–1499.
12. Bennie, E. H. (1982): Mianserin hydrochloride and L-tryptophan compared in depressive illness. *Br. J. Clin. Social Psychiatry*, 1:90–91.
13. Biggio, G. Fadda, F., Fanni, P., Tagliamonte, A., and Gessa, G. L. (1974): Rapid depletion of serum tryptophan, brain tryptophan, serotonin and 5-hydroxyindoleacetic acid by a tryptophan-free diet. *Life Sci.*, 14:1321–1329.

14. Birkmayer, W., Danielczyk, W., Neumayer, E., and Riederer, P. (1974): Nucleus ruber and L-dopa psychosis: Biochemical post-mortem findings. *J. Neural Transm.*, 35:93–116.
15. Birkmayer, W., and Neumayer, E. (1972): Die Behandlung der Dopa-Psychosen mit L-Tryptophan. *Nervenarzt*, 43:76–78.
16. Bloxam, D. L., Warren, W. H., and White, P. J. (1974): Involvement of the liver in the regulation of tryptophan availability: Possible role in the responses of liver and brain to starvation. *Life Sci.*, 15:1443–1455.
17. Bowers, M. B. (1970): Cerebrospinal fluid 5-hydroxyindoles and behavior after L-tryptophan and pyridoxine administration to psychiatric patients. *Neuropharmacology*, 9:599–604.
18. Brewerton, T. D., and Reus, V. I. (1983): Lithium carbonate and L-tryptophan in the treatment of bipolar and schizoaffective disorders. *Am. J. Psychiatry*, 140:757–760.
19. Broadhurst, A. D. (1970): L-Tryptophan versus E.C.T. *Lancet*, i:1392–1393.
20. Brotman, A. W., and Rosenbaum, J. F. (1984): MAOIs plus tryptophan: A cause of the serotonin syndrome. *Mass. Gen. Hosp. Newsletter Biol. Ther. Psychiatry*, 7:45–46.
21. Brown, G. L., Ebert, M. H., Goyer, P. F., Jimerson, D. C., Klein, W. J., Bunney, W. E., and Goodwin, F. K. (1982): Aggression, suicide, and serotonin: Relationship to CSF amine metabolites. *Am. J. Psychiatry*, 139:741–746.
22. Bryan, D. J. (1971): The role of urinary tryptophan metabolites in the etiology of bladder cancer. *Am. J. Clin. Nutr.*, 24:841–846.
23. Carlson, J. R., Yokoyama, M. T., and Dickinson, E. O. (1972): Induction of pulmonary edema and emphysema in cattle and goats with 3-methylindole. *Science*, 176:298–299.
24. Carlsson, A., and Lindqvist, M. (1978): Dependence of 5-HT and catecholamine synthesis on concentrations of precursor amino-acids in rat brain. *Naunyn Schmiedebergs Arch. Pharmacol.*, 303:157–164.
25. Carroll, B. J. (1971): Monoamine precursors in the treatment of depression. *Clin. Pharmacol. Ther.*, 12:743–761.
26. Carroll, B. J., Mowbray, R. M., and Davies, B. (1970): Sequential comparison of L-tryptophan with E.C.T. in severe depression. *Lancet*, i:967–969.
27. Chambers, C. A., and Naylor, G. J. (1978): A controlled trial of L-tryptophan in mania. *Br. J. Psychiatry*, 132:555–559.
28. Chandramouli, R., and Subrahmanyam, S. (1981): L-Tryptophan loading in schizoaffective and chronic schizophrenia. *Biomedicine*, 1:37–42.
29. Charney, D. S., Heninger, G. R., Reinhard, J. F., Sternberg, D. E., and Hafstead, K. M. (1982): The effect of IV L-tryptophan on prolactin, growth hormone, and mood in healthy subjects. *Psychopharmacology*, 78:38–43.
30. Chouinard, G., Annable, L., Young, S. N., and Sourkes, T. L. (1978): A controlled study of tryptophan-benserazide in schizophrenia. *Commun. Psychopharmacol.*, 2:21–31.
31. Chouinard, G., Jones, B. D., Young, S. N., and Annable, L. (1979): Potentiation of lithium by tryptophan in a case of bipolar illness. *Am. J. Psychiatry*, 136:719–720.
32. Chouinard, G., Young, S. N., and Annable, L. (1985): A controlled clinical trial of L-tryptophan in acute mania. *Biol. Psychiatry*, 20:546–557.
33. Chouinard, G., Young, S. N., Annable, L., and Sourkes, T. L. (1979): Tryptophan-nicotinamide, imipramine and their combination in depression: A controlled study. *Acta Psychiatr. Scand.*, 59:395–414.
34. Chouinard, G., Young, S. N., Annable, L., Sourkes, T. L., Kiriakos, R. Z. (1978): Tryptophan-nicotinamide combination in the treatment of newly admitted depressed patients. *Commun. Psychopharmacol.*, 2:311–318.
35. Chouinard, G., Young, S. N., Bradwejn, J., and Annable, L. (1983): Tryptophan in the treatment of depression and mania. In: *Management of Depressions with Monoamine Precursors: Advances in Biological Psychiatry, Vol. 10*, edited by H. M. van Praag and J. Mendlewicz, pp. 47–66. Karger, Basel.
36. Christensen, H. N. (1964): Free amino acids and peptides in tissues. In: *Mammalian Protein Metabolism, Vol. 1*, edited by H. N. Munro and J. B. Allison, pp. 105–124. Academic Press, New York.
37. Clark, J. A., Clark, M. S. G., Palfreyman, E. S., and Palfreyman, M. G. (1975): The effect of tryptophan and a tryptophan/5-hydroxytryptophan combination on indoles in the brain of rats fed a tryptophan-deficient diet. *Psychopharmacology*, 45:183–188.
38. Cole, J. O., Hartmann, E., and Brigham, P. (1980): L-Tryptophan: Clinical studies. In: *Psycho-

pharmacology Update, edited by J. O. Cole, pp. 119–148. The Collamore Press, Lexington, Massachusetts.

39. Cooper, A. J. (1979): Tryptophan antidepressant "physiological sedative:" Fact or fancy? *Psychopharmacology*, 61:97–102.
40. Cooper, A. J., and Datta, S. R. (1980): A placebo controlled evaluation of L-tryptophan in depression in the elderly. *Can. J. Psychiatry*, 25:386–390.
41. Coppen, A. (1976): Treatment of unipolar depression. *Lancet*, i:90–91.
42. Coppen, A., Metcalf, M., Carroll, J. D., and Morris, J. G. L. (1972): Levodopa and L-tryptophan therapy in parkinsonism. *Lancet*, i:654–658.
43. Coppen, A., Shaw, D. M., and Farrell, J. P. (1963): Potentiation of the antidepressant effect of a monoamine-oxidase inhibitor by tryptophan. *Lancet*, i:79–81.
44. Coppen, A., Shaw, D. M., Herzberg, B., and Maggs, R. (1967): Tryptophan in the treatment of depression. *Lancet*, ii:1178–1180.
45. Coppen, A., Whybrow, P. C., Noguera, R., Maggs, R., and Prange, A. J. (1972): The comparative antidepressant value of L-tryptophan and imipramine with and without attempted potentiation by liothyronine. *Arch. Gen. Psychiatry*, 26:234–241.
46. Coppen, A., and Wood, K. (1977): Total and non-bound plasma tryptophan in depressive illness. *Lancet*, i:94.
47. Cowen, M. A. (1976): An electrophysiological study on the effects of tryptophan and cortisol on schizophrenic and other mentally ill patient groups and on normal subjects. *Biol. Psychiatry*, 11:389–401.
48. DeLean, J., and Richardson, J. C. (1975): Relief of myoclonus by L-tryptophan. *Lancet*, ii:870–871.
49. d'Elia, G., Hanson, L., and Raotma, H. (1978): L-Tryptophan and 5-hydroxytryptophan in the treatment of depression: A review. *Acta Psychiatr. Scand.*, 57:239–252.
50. d'Elia, G., Lehmann, J., and Raotma, H. (1977): Evaluation of the combination of tryptophan and ECT in the treatment of depression. I. Clinical analysis. *Acta Psychiatr. Scand.*, 56:303–318.
51. DeMyer, M. K., Shea, P. A., Hendrie, H. C., and Yoshimura, N. N. (1981): Plasma tryptophan and five other amino acids in depressed and normal subjects. *Arch. Gen. Psychiatr*, 38:642–646.
52. Doust, J. W. L., and Huszka, L. (1972): Amines and aphrodisiacs in chronic schizophrenia. *J. Nerv. Ment. Dis.*, 155:261–264.
53. Dunning, W. F., Curtis, M. R., and Maun, M. E. (1950): The effect of added dietary tryptophan on the occurrence of 2-acetylaminofluorene induced liver and bladder cancer in rats. *Cancer Res.*, 10:454–459.
54. Eccleston, D., Ashcroft, G. W., Crawford, T. B. B., Stanton, J. B., Wood, D., and McTurk, P. H. (1970): Effect of tryptophan administration on 5HIAA in cerebrospinal fluid in man. *J. Neurol. Neurosurg. Psychiatry*, 33:269–272.
55. Egan, G. P., and Hammad, G. E. M. (1976): Sexual disinhibition with L-tryptophan. *Br. Med. J.*, 2:701.
56. Fahn, S., Snider, S., Prosad, A. L. N., Lane, E., and Madadon, J. (1975): Normalization of brain serotonin by L-tryptophan in levodopa-treated rats. *Neurology*, 25:861–865.
57. Farkas, T., Dunner, D. L., and Fieve, R. R. (1976): L-Tryptophan in depression. *Biol. Psychiatry*, 11:295–302.
58. Fernstrom, J. D., and Faller, D. V. (1978): Neutral amino acids in the brain: Changes in response to food ingestion. *J. Neurochem.*, 30:1513–1538.
59. Fernstrom, J. D., and Wurtman, R. J. (1971): Brain serotonin content: Increase following ingestion of a carbohydrate diet. *Science*, 174:1023–1025.
60. Gallagher, D. W., and Aghajanian, G. K. (1976): Inhibition of firing of raphe neurons by tryptophan and 5-hydroxytryptophan: Blockade by inhibiting serotonin synthesis with Ro-4-4602. *Neuropharmacology*, 15:149–156.
61. Gayford, J. J., Parker, A. L., Phillips, E. M., and Rowsell, A. R. (1973): Whole blood 5-hydroxytryptamine during treatment of endogenous depressive illness. *Br. J. Psychiatry*, 122:597–598.
62. Gehlen, W., and Müller, J. (1974): Zur Therapie der Dopa-Psychosen mit L-Tryptophan. *Dtsch. Med. Wochenschr.*, 99:457–463.
63. Gelenberg, A. S., Gibson, C. J., and Wojcik, J. D. (1982): Neurotransmitter precursors for the treatment of depression. *Psychopharmacol. Bull.*, 18:7–18.
64. Gessa, G. L., Biggio, G., Fadda, F., Corsini, G. V., and Tagliamonte, A. (1974): Effect of the

oral administration of tryptophan-free amino acid mixtures on serum tryptophan, brain tryptophan and serotonin metabolism. *J. Neurochem.*, 22:869–870.

65. Ghose, K. (1983): *L*-Tryptophan in hyperactive child syndrome associated with epilepsy: A controlled study. *Neuropsychobiology*, 10:111–114.
66. Gillin, J. C., Kaplan, J. A., and Wyatt, R. J. (1976): Clinical effects of tryptophan in chronic schizophrenic patients. *Biol. Psychiatry*, 11:635–639.
67. Gillman, P. K., Bartlett, J. R., Bridges, P. K., Hunt, A., Patel, A. J., Kantamaneni, B. D., and Curzon, G. (1981): Indolic substances in plasma, cerebrospinal fluid, and frontal cortex of human subjects infused with saline or tryptophan. *J. Neurochem.*, 37:410–417.
68. Glassman, A. H., and Platman, S. R. (1969): Potentiation of a monoamine oxidase inhibitor by tryptophan. *J. Psychiatr. Res.*, 7:83–88.
69. Gnirss, F., Schneider-Helmert, D., and Schenker, J. (1978): L-Tryptophan + oxprenolol: A new approach to the treatment of insomnia. *Pharmacopsychiatria*, 11:180–185.
70. Grahame-Smith, D. G. (1971): Studies *in vivo* on the relationship between tryptophan, brain 5-HT synthesis and hyperactivity in rats treated with a monoamine oxidase inhibitor and L-tryptophan. *J. Neurochem.*, 18:1053–1066.
71. Green, A. R., and Aronson, J. K. (1980): Metabolism of an oral tryptophan load. III. Effect of a pyridoxine supplement. *Br. J. Clin. Pharmacol.*, 10:617–619.
72. Green, A. R., Aronson, J. K., Curzon, G., and Woods, H. F. (1980): Metabolism of an oral tryptophan load. I. Effects of dose and pretreatment with tryptophan. *Br. J. Clin. Pharmacol.*, 10:603–610.
73. Green, A. R., Aronson, J. K., Curzon, G., and Woods, H. F. (1980): Metabolism of an oral tryptophan load. II. Effect of pretreatment with the putative tryptophan pyrrolase inhibitors nicotinamide or allopurinol. *Br. J. Pharmacol.*, 10:611–615.
74. Green, A. R., and Grahame-Smith, D. G. (1976): Effects of drugs on the processes regulating the functional activity of brain 5-hydroxytryptamine. *Nature*, 260:487–491.
75. Greenwood, M. H., Lader, M. H., Kantameneni, and Curzon, G. (1975): The acute effects of oral (−)-tryptophan in human subjects. *Br. J. Clin. Pharmacol.*, 2:165–172.
76. Gullino, P., Winitz, M., Birnbaum, M, Cornfield, J., Otey, M. C., and Greenstein, J. P. (1956): Studies on the metabolism of amino acids and related compounds *in vivo*. 1. Toxicity of essential amino acids, individually and in mixtures, and the protective effect of L-arginine. *Arch. Biochem. Biophys.*, 64:319–332.
77. Harper, A. E., Benevenga, N. J., and Wohlhueter, R. M. (1970): Effects of ingestion of disproportional amounts of amino acids. *Physiol. Rev.*, 50:428–558.
78. Harris, B. (1980): Prospective trial of L-tryptophan in maternity blues. *Br. J. Psychiatry*, 137:233–235.
79. Hartmann, E., Cravens, J., and List, S. (1974): Hypnotic effects of L-tryptophan. *Arch. Gen. Psychiatry*, 31:394–397.
80. Hartmann, E., and Greenwald, D. (1984): Tryptophan and human sleep: An analysis of 43 studies. In: *Progress in Tryptophan and Serotonin Research*, edited by H. G. Schlossberger, W. Kochen, B. Linzen, and H. Steinhart, pp. 297–304. Walter de Gruyter, Berlin.
81. Hartmann, E., Lindsley, J. G., Spinweber, C. (1983): Chronic insomnia: Effects of tryptophan, flurazepam, secobarbital, and placebo. *Psychopharmacology*, 80:138–142.
82. Hartmann, E., and Spinweber, C. L. (1979): Sleep induced by L-tryptophan: Effect of dosages within the normal dietary intake. *J. Nerv. Ment. Dis.*, 167:497–499.
83. Hartmann, E., Spinweber, C. L., and Ware, C. (1976): L-Tryptophan, L-leucine, and placebo: Effects on subjective alertness. *Sleep Res.*, 5:57.
84. Hattori, M., Kotake, Y., Kotake, Y., Otsuka, H., and Shibata, Y. (1984): Studies on the urinary excretion of xanthurenic acid in diabetics. In: *Progress in Tryptophan and Serotonin Research*, edited by H. G. Schlossberger, W. Kochan, B. Linzen, and H. Steinhart, pp. 347–354. Walter de Gruyter, Berlin.
85. Henry, G. M., Weingartner, H. W., and Murphy, D. L. (1973): Influence of affective states and psychoactive drugs on verbal learning and memory. *Am. J. Psychiatry*, 130:966–971.
86. Herrington, R. N., Bruce, A., Johnstone, E. C., and Lader, M. H. (1974): Comparative trial of L-tryptophan and E.C.T. in severe depressive illness. *Lancet*, ii:731–734.
87. Herrington, R. N., Bruce, A., Johnstone, E. C., and Lader, M. H. (1976): Comparative trial of L-tryptophan and amitriptyline in depressive illness. *Psychol. Med.*, 6:673–678.
88. Hertz, D., and Sulman, F. G. (1968): Preventing depression with tryptophan. *Lancet*, i:531–532.

89. Hery, F., Simonnet, G., Bourgoin, S., Soubrie, P., Artand, F., Hamon, M., and Glowinski, J. (1979): Effect of nerve activity on the in vivo release of (³H) serotonin continuously formed from L-(³H)tryptophan in the caudate nucleus of the cat. *Brain Res.*, 169:317–334.

90. Hess, S. M., and Doepfner, W. (1961): Behavioral effects and brain amine content in rats. *Arch. Int. Pharmacodyn.*, 134:89–99.

91. Hodge, J. V., Oates, J. A., and Sjoerdsma, A. (1964): Reduction of the central effects of tryptophan by a decarboxylase inhibitor. *Clin. Pharmacol. Ther.*, 5:149–155.

92. Hoes, M. J. A. J. M., Loeffen, T., and Vree, T. B. (1981): Kinetics of L-tryptophan in depressive patients: A possible correlation between the plasma concentrations of L-tryptophan and some psychiatric rating scales. *Psychopharmacology*, 75:350–353.

93. Honore, P., Møller, S. E., and Jørgensen, A. (1982): Lithium + L-tryptophan compared with amitriptyline in endogenous depression. *J. Affective Disord.*, 4:79–82.

94. Hosobuchi, Y. (1978): Tryptophan reversal of tolerance to analgesia induced by central grey stimulation. *Lancet*, ii:47.

95. Hosobuchi, Y., Lamb, S., and Baskin, D. (1980): Tryptophan loading may reverse tolerance to opiate analgesics in humans: A preliminary report. *Pain*, 9:161–169.

96. Hosobuchi, Y., Rossier, J., and Bloom, F. E. (1980): Oral loading with L-tryptophan may augment the simultaneous release of ACTH and beta-endorphin that accompanies periaqueductal stimulation in humans. In: *Neural Peptides and Neuronal Communications*, edited by E. Costa and M. Trabucchi, pp. 563–570. Raven Press, New York.

97. Hoyes, S. (1982): Experiences with L-tryptophan in a child and family psychiatric department. *J. Int. Med. Res.*, 10:157–159.

98. Hrboticky, N., Leiter, L. A., and Anderson, G. H. (1985): Effects of L-tryptophan on short term food intake, subjective hunger and mood in healthy lean men. *Nutr. Res.*, 5:595–607.

99. Hullin, R. P., and Jerram, T. (1976): Sexual disinhibition with L-tryptophan. *Br. Med. J.*, 2:1010.

100. Hyyppä, M. T., Jolma, T., Riekkinen, P., and Rhine, U. K. (1975): Effects of L-tryptophan treatment on central indoleamine metabolism and short-lasting neurologic disturbances in multiple sclerosis. *J. Neural Transm.*, 37:297–304.

101. Ikeda, S., and Kotake, Y. (1984): Urinary excretion of xanthurenic acid and zinc in diabetes. In: *Progress in Tryptophan and Serotonin Research*, edited by H. G. Schlossberger, W. Kochen, B. Linzen, and H. Steinhart, pp. 355–358. Walter de Gruyter, Berlin.

102. Jones, R. S. G. (1981): *In vivo* pharmacological studies on the interactions between tryptamine and 5-hydroxytryptamine. *Br. J. Pharmacol.*, 73:485–493.

103. Jones, R. S. G. (1982): Tryptamine modifies cortical neurone responses evoked by stimulation of nucleus raphe medianus. *Brain Res. Bull.*, 8:435–437.

104. Jones, R. S. G., and Boulton, A. A. (1980): Tryptamine and 5-hydroxytryptamine: Actions and interactions on cortical neurones in the rat. *Life Sci.*, 27:1849–1856.

105. Jørgensen, A. J. F., and Majumdar, A. P. N. (1976): Bilateral adrenalectomy: Effect of tryptophan force-feeding on amino acid incorporation into feritin, transferrin, and mixed proteins of liver, brain and kidneys *in vivo*. *Biochem. Med.*, 16:37–46.

106. Joseph, M. H., Young, S. N., and Curzon, G. (1976): The metabolism of a tryptophan load in rat brain and liver: The influence of hydrocortisone and allopurinol. *Biochem. Pharmacol.*, 25:2599–2604.

107. King, R. B. (1980): Pain and tryptophan. *J. Neurosurg.*, 53:44–52.

108. Kirkegaard, C., Møller, S. E., and Bjørum, N. (1978): Addition of L-tryptophan to electroconvulsive treatment in endogenous depression: A double-blind study. *Acta Psychiatr. Scand.*, 58:457–462.

109. Kline, N. S., and Shah, B. K. (1973): Comparable therapeutic efficacy of tryptophan and imipramine: Average therapeutic ratings versus "true" equivalence: An important difference. *Curr. Ther. Res.*, 15:484–487.

110. Koskiniemi, M.-L. (1980): Deficient intestinal absorption of L-tryptophan in progressive myoclonus epilepsy without lafora bodies. *J. Neurol. Sci.*, 47:1–6.

111. Koskiniemi, M.-L., Hyyppä, M., Sainio, K., Salmi, T., Sarna, S., and Uotila, L. (1980): Transient effect of L-tryptophan in progressive myoclonus epilepsy without lafora bodies: Clinical and electrophysiological study. *Epilepsia*, 21:351–357.

112. Lauer, J. W., Inskip, W. M., Bernsohn, J., and Zeller, E. A. (1958): Observations on schizophrenic patients after iproniazid and tryptophan. *AMA Arch. Neurol. Psychiatry*, 80:122–130.

113. Leathwood, P. D., and Pollet, P. (1983): Diet-induced mood changes in normal populations. *J. Psychiatr. Res.*, 17:147–154.
114. Lehmann, J. (1963): Tryptophan metabolism in levodopa-treated Parkinsonian patients. *Acta Med. Scand.*, 194:181–189.
115. Leino, E., MacDonald, E., Airaksinen, M. M., and Riekkinen, P. J. (1980): Homovanillic acid and 5-hydroxyindoleacetic acid levels in cerebrospinal fluid of patients with progressive myoclonus epilepsy. *Acta Neurol. Scand.*, 62:45–54.
116. Leino, E., MacDonald, E., Airaksinen, M. M., Riekkinen, P. J., and Salo, H. (1981): L-Tryptophan-carbidopa trial in patients with long-standing progressive myoclonus epilepsy. *Acta Neurol. Scand.*, 64:132–141.
117. Lieberman, H. R., Corkin, S., Spring, B. J., Growdon, J. H., and Wurtman, R. J. (1983): Mood, performance, and pain sensitivity: Changes induced by food constituents. *J. Psychiatr. Res.*, 17:135–145.
118. Lindberg, D., Ahlfors, U. G., Dencker, S. J., Fruensgaard, K., Hansten, S., Jensen, K., Ose, E., and Pihkanen, T. A. (1979): Symptom reduction in depression after treatment with L-tryptophan or imipramine: Item analysis of Hamilton rating scale for depression. *Acta Psychiatr. Scand.*, 60:287–294.
119. Lindsley, J. G., Hartmann, E. L., and Mitchell, W. (1983): Selectivity in response to L-tryptophan among insomniac subjects: A preliminary report. *Sleep*, 6:247–256.
120. Linnoila, M., Seppala, T., Mattila, M. J., Vihko, R., Pakarinen, A., and Skinner, J. T. (1980): Clomipramine and doxepin in depressive neurosis: Plasma levels and therapeutic response. *Arch. Gen. Psychiatry*, 37:1295–1299.
121. Linnoila, M., Viukari, M., Nummunen, A., and Auvinen, J. (1980): Efficacy and side effects of chloral hydrate and tryptophan as sleeping aids in psychogeriatric patients. *Int. Pharmacopsychiatry*, 15:124–128.
122. Lopez-Ibor Aliño, J. J., Ayuso Gutierrez, J. L., and Montejo Iglesias, M. L. (1973): Tryptophan and amitriptyline in the treatment of depression: A double-blind study. *Int. Pharmacopsychiatry*, 8:145–151.
123. MacSweeney, D. A. (1975): Treatment of unipolar depression. *Lancet*, ii:510–511.
124. Marsden, C. A., Conti, J., Strope, E., Curzon, G., and Adams, R. N. (1979): Monitoring 5-hydroxytryptamine release in the brain of the freely moving unanaesthetized rat using in vivo voltammetry. *Brain Res.*, 171:85–99.
125. Marsden, C. A., and Curzon, G. (1978): The contribution of tryptamine to the behavioural effects of L-tryptophan in tranylcypromine-treated rats. *Psychopharmacology*, 57:71–76.
126. Meier, A. H., and Wilson, J. M. (1983): Tryptophan feeding adversely influences pregnancy. *Life Sci.*, 32:1193–1196.
127. Mendels, J., Stinnett, J. L., Burns, D., and Frazer, A. (1975): Amine precursors and depression. *Arch. Gen. Psychiatry*, 32:22–30.
128. Miller, E. M., and Nieburg, H. A. (1974): L-Tryptophan in the treatment of levodopa-induced psychiatric disorders. *Dis. Nerv. Syst.*, 35:20–23.
129. Modigh, K. (1972): Central and peripheral effects of 5-hydroxytryptophan on motor activity in mice. *Psychopharmacology*, 23:48–54.
130. Modigh, K. (1973): Effects of L-tryptophan on motor activity in mice. *Psychopharmacology*, 30:123–143.
131. Moldofsky, H., and Lue, F. A. (1980): The relationship of alpha and delta EEG frequencies to pain and mood in "fibrositis" patients treated with chlorpromazine and L-tryptophan. *Electroencephalogr. Clin. Neurophysiol.*, 50:71–80.
132. Møller, S. E. (1980): Evaluation of the relative potency of individual competing amino acids to tryptophan transport in endogenously depressed patients. *Psychiatr. Res.*, 3:141–150.
133. Møller, S. E. (1981): Pharmacokinetics of tryptophan, renal handling of kynurenine and the effect of nicotinamide on its appearance in plasma and urine following L-tryptophan loading of healthy subjects. *Eur. J. Clin. Pharmacol.*, 21:137–142.
134. Møller, S. E., Honore, P., and Larsen, O. B. (1983): Tryptophan and tyrosine ratios to neutral amino acids in endogenous depression: Relation to antidepressant response to amitriptyline and lithium + L-tryptophan. *J. Affective Disord.*, 5:67–79.
135. Møller, S. E., and Kirk, L. (1978): The effect of allopurinol on the kynurenine formation in humans following a tryptophan load. *Acta Vitaminol. Enzymol.*, 32:159–162.

136. Møller, S. E., Kirk, L., and Honore, P. (1979): Free and total plasma tryptophan in endogenous depression. *J. Affective Disord.*, 1:69–76.
137. Møller, S. E., Kirk, L., and Honore, P. (1980): Relationship between plasma ratio of tryptophan to competing amino acids and the response to L-tryptophan treatment in endogenously depressed patients. *J. Affective Disord.*, 2:47–49.
138. Møller, S. E., Kirk, L., and Honore, P. (1982): Tryptophan tolerance and metabolism in endogenous depression. *Psychopharmacology*, 76:79–83.
139. Møller, S. E., Reisby, N., Ortmann, J., Elley, J., and Krautwald, O. (1981): Relevance of tryptophan and tyrosine availability in endogenous and "non-endogenous" depressives treated with imipramine and clomipramine. *J. Affective Disord.*, 3:231–244.
140. Morand, C., Young, S. N., and Ervin, F. R. (1983): Clinical response of aggressive schizophrenics to oral tryptophan. *Biol. Psychiatry*, 18:575–578.
141. Morgan, R. (1977): Tryptophan overdosage. *Br. J. Psychiatry*, 131:548–549.
142. Munro, H. N. (1970): Free amino acid pools and their role in regulation. In: *Mammalian Protein Metabolism, Vol. 4*, edited by H. N. Munro, pp. 299–386. Academic Press, New York.
143. Murphy, D. L., Baker, M., Goodwin, F. K., Miller, L., Kotin, J., and Bunney, W. E. (1974): L-Tryptophan in affective disorders: Indoleamine changes and differential clinical effects. *Psychopharmacology*, 34:11–20.
144. National Cancer Institute (1978): *Bioassay of L-Tryptophan for Possible Carcinogenicity, National Cancer Institute Carcinogenesis Technical Report Series No. 71.* DHEW Publication No. (NIH)78–1321.
145. Oates, J. A., and Sjoerdsma, A. (1960): Neurologic effects of tryptophan in patients receiving a monoamine oxidase inhibitor. *Neurology*, 10:1076–1078.
146. Oldendorf, W. H., and Szabo, J. (1976): Amino acid assignment to one of three blood-brain barrier amino acid carriers. *Am. J. Physiol.*, 230:94–98.
147. Olson, R. E., Gursey, D., and Vester, J. W. (1960): Evidence for a defect in tryptophan metabolism in chronic alcoholism. *N. Engl. J. Med.*, 263:1169–1174.
148. O'Neill, R. D., Fillenz, M., Grünewald, R. A., Bloomfield, M. R., Alberg, W. J., Jamieson, C. M., Williams, J. H., and Gray, J. A. (1984): Voltammetric carbon paste electrodes monitor uric acid and not 5HIAA at the 5-hydroxyindole potential in the rat brain. *Neurosci. Lett.*, 45:39–46.
149. Oswald, I., Ashcroft, G. W., Berger, R. J., Eccleston, D., Evans, J. I., and Thacore, V. R. (1966): Some experiments in the chemistry of normal sleep. *Br. J. Psychiatry*, 112:391–399.
150. Pare, C. M. B. (1963): Potentiation of monoamine-oxidase inhibitors by tryptophan. *Lancet*, ii:527–528.
151. Pecknold, J. C., McClure, D. J., Appeltauer, L., Allan, T., and Wrzesinski, L. (1982): Does tryptophan potentiate clomipramine in the treatment of agoraphobic and social phobic patients? *Br. J. Psychiatry*, 140:484–490.
152. Perez-Cruet, J., Chase, T. N., and Murphy, D. L. (1974): Dietary regulation of brain tryptophan metabolism by plasma ratio of free tryptophan and neutral amino acids in humans. *Nature*, 248:693–695.
153. Pollin, W., Cardon, P. V., and Kety, S. S. (1961): Effects of amino acid feedings in schizophrenic patients treated with iproniazid. *Science*, 133:104–105.
154. Poloni, M., Nappi, G., Arringo, A., and Savoldi, F. (1974): Cerebrospinal fluid 5-hydroxyindoleacetic acid level in migrainous patients during spontaneous attacks, during headache-free periods and following treatment with L-tryptophan. *Experientia*, 30:640–641.
155. Prange, A. J, Wilson, I. C., Lynn, C. W., Alltop, L. B., and Strikeleather, R. A. (1974): L-Tryptophan in mania: Contribution to a permissive hypothesis of affective disorders. *Arch. Gen. Psychiatry*, 30:56–62.
156. Puizillout, J. J., Gaudin-Chazal, G., Daszuta, A., Seyfritz, N., and Ternaux, J. P. (1979): Release of endogenous serotonin from "encephale isole" cats. II. Correlations with raphe neuronal activity and sleep and wakefulness. *J. Physiol. (Paris)*, 75:531–537.
157. Quadbeck, H., Lehmann, E., and Tegeler, J. (1984): Comparison of the antidepressant action of tryptophan, tryptophan/5-hydroxytryptophan combination and nomifensine. *Neuropsychobiology*, 11:111–115.
158. Rao, B., and Broadhurst, A. D. (1976): Tryptophan and depression. *Br. Med. J.*, i:460.
159. Redman, J., Armstrong, S., and Ng, K. T. (1983): Free-running activity rhythms in the rat: Entrainment by melatonin. *Science*, 219:1089–1091.

160. Riley, G. J., and Shaw, D. M. (1976): Total and non-bound tryptophan in unipolar illness. *Lancet*, ii:1249.
161. Sachar, E. J., Helman, L., Roffwarg, H., Halpern, F., Fukushima, D., and Gallagher, T. (1973): Disrupted 24-hour patterns of cortisol secretion in psychotic depression. *Arch. Gen. Psychiatry*, 28:19–24.
162. Schneider-Helmert, D. (1981): Interval therapy with *L*-Tryptophan in severe chronic insomniacs: A predictive laboratory study. *Int. Pharmacopsychiatry*, 16:162–173.
163. Seltzer, S., Dewart, D., Pollack, R., and Jackson, E. (1983): The effects of dietary tryptophan on chronic maxillofacial pain and experimental pain tolerance. *J. Psychiatr. Res.*, 17:181–186.
164. Seltzer, S., Stoch, R., Marcus, R., and Jackson, E. (1982): Alteration of human pain thresholds by nutritional manipulation and L-tryptophan supplementation. *Pain*, 13:385–393.
165. Shaw, D. M., MacSweeney, D. A., Hewland, R., and Johnston, A. L. (1975): Tricyclic antidepressants and tryptophan in unipolar depression. *Psycho. Med.*, 5:276–278.
166. Sheard, M. H. (1975): Lithium in the treatment of aggression. *J. Nerv. Ment. Dis.*, 100:108–117.
167. Shopsin, B. (1978): Enhancement of the antidepressant response to L-tryptophan by a liver pyrrolase inhibitor: A rational treatment approach. *Neuropsychobiology*, 4:188–192.
168. Sicuteri, F. (1974): Serotonin and sex in man. *Pharmacol. Res. Commun.*, 6:403–411.
169. Smith, B., and Prockop, D. J. (1962): Central-nervous-system effects of ingestion of L-tryptophan by normal subjects. *N. Engl. J. Med.*, 267:1338–1341.
170. Smith, D. F., Strömgren, E., Petersen, H. N., Williams, D. G., and Sheldon, W. (1984): Lack of effect of tryptophan treatment in demented gerontopsychiatric patients: A double-blind, crossover-controlled study. *Acta Psychiatr. Scand.*, 70:470–477.
171. Smith, S., Pihl, R. O., Young, S. N., and Ervin, F. R. (1985): A test of possible cognitive and environmental influences on the mood lowering effect of tryptophan depletion in normal males. *Psychopharmacology (submitted)*.
172. Smith, S., Pihl, R. O., Young, S. N., and Ervin, F. R. (1985): The elevation and reduction of plasma tryptophan and their effects on aggression and pain sensitivity in normal males. *Aggress. Behav. (in press)*.
173. Snyder, S., and Hams, G. (1982): Serotoninergic agents in the treatment of isolated sleep paralysis. *Am. J. Psychiatry*, 139:1202–1203.
174. Sourkes, T. L. (1983): Toxicology of monoamine precursors. In: *Advances in Biological Psychiatry, Vol. 10*, edited by H. M. van Praag and J. Mendlewicz, pp. 160–175. Karger, Basel.
175. Ternaux, J. P., Boireau, A., Bourgoin, S., Hamon, M., Hery, F., and Glowinski, J. (1976): *In vivo* release of 5-HT in the lateral ventricle of the rat: Effects of 5-hydroxytryptophan and tryptophan. *Brain Res.*, 101:533–548.
176. Thomas, J. M., and Rubin, E. H. (1984): Case report of a toxic reaction from a combination of tryptophan and phenelzine. *Am. J. Psychiatry*, 141:281–283.
177. Thomson, J., Rankin, H., Ashcroft, G. W., Yates, C. M., McQueen, J. K., and Cummings, S. W. (1982): The treatment of depression in general practice: A comparison of L-tryptophan, amitriptyline, and a combination of L-tryptophan and amitriptyline with placebo. *Psychol. Med.*, 12:741–751.
178. Trulson, M. E., and Jacobs, B. L. (1976): Dose-response relationships between systematically administered L-tryptophan or L-5-hydroxytryptophan and raphe unit activity in the rat. *Neuropharmacology*, 15:339–344.
179. Trulson, M. E, and Jacobs, B. L. (1979): Raphe unit activity in freely moving cats: Correlations with level of behavioral arousal. *Brain Res.*, 169:135–150.
180. Truswell, A. S., Hansen, J. D. L., and Wannenberg, P. (1968): Plasma tryptophan and other amino acids in pellagra. *Am. J. Clin. Nutr.*, 21:1314–1320.
181. van Praag, H. M. (1981): Management of depression with serotonin precursors. *Biol. Psychiatry*, 16:291–310.
182. van Praag, H. M., Flentge, F., Korf, J., Dols, L. C. W., and Schut, T. (1973): The influence of probenecid on the metabolism of serotonin, dopamine and their precursors in man. *Psychopharmacology*, 33:141–151.
183. Walinder, J., Carlsson, A., and Persson, R. (1981): 5-HT reuptake inhibitors plus tryptophan in endogenous depression. *Acta Psychiatr. Scand. [Suppl. 290]*, 63:179–190.
184. Walinder, J., Skott, A., Carlsson, A., Nagy, and Roos, B.-E. (1976): Potentiation of the antidepressant action of clomipramine by tryptophan. *Arch. Gen. Psychiatry*, 33:1384–1389.

185. Warsh, J. J., Coscina, D. V., Godge, D. D., and Chan, P. W. (1979): Dependence of brain trypta-mine formation on tryptophan availability. *J. Neurochem.*, 32:1191–1196.
186. Wirz-Justice, A. (1977): Theoretical and therapeutic potential of indoleamine precursors. *Neuropsychobiology*, 3:199–233.
187. Wolf, H. (1974): Studies on tryptophan metabolism in man. *Scand. J. Clin. Lab. Invest. [Suppl.]*, 136:1–186.
188. Worrall, E. P., Moody, J. P., Peet, M., Dick, P., Smith, A., Chambers, C., Adams, M., and Naylor, G. J. (1979): Controlled studies of the acute antidepressant effects of lithium. *Br. J. Psychiatry*, 135:255–262.
189. Wurtman, J. J., Wurtman, R. J., Growdon, J. H., Henry, P., Lipscomb, A., and Zeisel, S. H. (1981): Carbohydrate craving in obese people: Suppression by treatments affecting serotoninergic transmission. *Int. J. Eating Disord.*, 1:2–15.
190. Wurtman, R. J., Hefti, F., and Melamed, E. (1981): Precursor control of neurotransmitter synthesis. *Pharmacol. Rev.*, 32:315–335.
190a. Wurtman, R. J., Larin, F., Mostafapour, S., and Fernstrom, J. D. (1974): Brain catechol synthesis: Control by brain tyrosine concentration. *Science*, 185:183–184.
191. Wurtman, R. J., and Wurtman, J. J. (1984): Nutrients, neurotransmitter synthesis, and the control of food intake. In: *Eating and Its Disorders*, edited by A. J. Stunkard and E. Stellar, pp. 77–86. Raven Press, New York.
192. Wyatt, R. J., Engelman, K., Kupfer, D. J., Fram, D. H., Sjoerdsma, A., and Snyder, F. (1970): Effects of L-tryptophan (a natural sedative) on human sleep. *Lancet*, ii:842–846.
193. Yaryura-Tobias, J. A., and Bhagavan, H. M. (1977): L-Tryptophan in obsessive-compulsive disorders. *Am. J. Psychiatry*, 134:1298–1299.
194. Yogman, M. W., and Zeisel, S. H. (1983): Diet and sleep patterns in newborn infants. *N. Engl. J. Med.*, 309:1147–1149.
195. Yoshida, O., Brown, R. R., and Bryan, G. T. (1971): A possible role of urinary metabolites of tryptophan in the heterotopic recurrence of bladder cancer in man. *Am. J. Clin. Nutr.*, 24:848–851.
196. Young, S. N. (1983): The significance of tryptophan, phenylalanine, tyrosine and their metabolites in the nervous system. In: *Handbook of Neurochemistry, Vol. 3*, edited by A. Lajtha, pp. 559–581. Plenum, New York.
197. Young, S. N. (1984): Monoamine precursors in the affective disorders. In: *Advances in Human Psychopharmacology, Vol. 3*, edited by G. D. Burrows and J. S. Werry, pp. 251–285. JAI Press, Greenwich, Connecticut.
198. Young, S. N., and Anderson, G. M. (1982): Factors influencing melatonin, 5-hydroxytryptophol, 5-hydroxyindoleacetic acid, 5-hydroxytryptamine and tryptophan in rat pineal glands. *Neuroendocrinology*, 35:464–468.
199. Young, S. N., and Gauthier, S. (1981): Effect of tryptophan administration on tryptophan, 5-hydroxyindoleacetic acid and indoleacetic acid in human lumbar and cisternal cerebrospinal fluid. *J. Neurol. Neurosurg. Psychiatry*, 44:323–328.
200. Young, S. N., and Oravec, M. (1979): The effect of growth hormone on the metabolism of a tryptophan load in liver and brain of hypophysectomized rats. *Can. J. Biochem.*, 57:517–522.
201. Young, S. N., Smith, S., Pihl, R. O., and Ervin, F. R. (1985): Tryptophan depletion causes a rapid lowering of mood in normal males. *Psychopharmacology (in press)*.
202. Young, S. N., and Sourkes, T. L. (1974): The antidepressant action of tryptophan. *Lancet*, ii:897–898.
203. Young, S. N., and Sourkes, T. L. (1977): Tryptophan in the central nervous system: Regulation and significance. In: *Advances in Neurochemistry, Vol. 2*, edited by B. W. Agranoff and M. H. Aprison, pp. 133–191. Plenum, New York.
204. Young, S. N., Tourjman, S. V., Teff, K., Pihl, R. O., Ervin, F. R., and Anderson, G. H. (1985): The effect of lowering plasma tryptophan levels on food selection in normal males. *(Manuscript in preparation.)*
205. Yuwiler, A., Brammer, G. L., Morley, J. E., Raleigh, M. J., Flannery, J. W., and Geller, E. (1981): Short-term and repetitive administration of oral tryptophan in normal men. *Arch. Gen. Psychiatry*, 38:619–626.
206. Zigman, S. (1984): The role of tryptophan oxidation in ocular tissue damage. In: *Progress in Tryptophan and Serotonin Research*, edited by H. G. Schlossberger, W. Kochen, B. Linzen, and H. Steinhart, pp. 449–467. Walter de Gruyter, Berlin.

Nutrition and the Brain, Vol. 7, edited by
R. J. Wurtman and J. J. Wurtman. Raven Press,
New York © 1986.

Monoamine Precursors in the Treatment of Psychiatric Disorders

H. M. van Praag and C. Lemus

Department of Psychiatry, Albert Einstein College of Medicine/Montefiore Medical Center, Bronx, New York 10467

I. RATIONALE FOR THE MONOAMINE-PRECURSOR STRATEGY

Precursors of monoamines (MAs) have been applied in depression ever since the introduction of the classic antidepressants in 1958; yet the number of properly designed studies is surprisingly small. As far as the precursors of serotonin (5-hydroxytryptamine; 5-HT) are concerned, they are marginally sufficient for some cautious conclusions. The number of studies with catecholamine (CA) precursors is even smaller, barely enough for even tentative conclusions.

The therapeutic use of MA precursors in depression was prompted by two sets of observations/deliberations. First, there are findings indicative of disturbed metabolism of MA, in particular 5-HT and norepinephrine (NE) in depression (11,197). Most findings suggested decreased MA metabolism. These have been interpreted in two ways. First, they indicate a primary decreased MA metabolism leading to diminution of MA-ergic function. The second hypothesis postulates a primary hyperactive MA-ergic system (as a result of hypersensitive postsynaptic MA receptors) leading to compensatory diminution of MA metabolism. Assuming that the MA-ergic dysfunction is causally related to the depressive state, strategies designed to increase MA availability would make sense. According to the first theory, this would increase the functional activity of MA systems; according to the latter theory, it would downregulate the hypersensitive postsynaptic MA receptors.

The second set of observations pertained to the phenomenon of antidepressant-resistant depression. Abundant evidence accumulated that antidepressants are not equally effective in all types of depression. Most antidepressants are preferentially active in the syndrome of vital depression (102,194,218), a syndrome similar to the one described in the British literature under the heading of endogenous depression. The best-fitting DSM-III (46) diagnosis is Major Depressive Episode, Melancholic Type (161). Only drugs that are MA oxidase inhibitors (MAOIs) were, in general, active in the so-called atypical depressions, as described mostly in the British literature. The syndrome differs from the vital/endogenous syndrome, which is apparently considered as a more genuine type of depression; it is roughly similar to the syndrome otherwise termed personal (194) reactive and neurotic. The closest DSM-III diagnosis is Dysthymic Disorder.

Although most antidepressants acted preferentially in vital depression, approximately 30 to 40 % of patients with this depression type turned out to be unresponsive to them. The explanation could not be found in pharmacokinetic factors. Another possibility was that the biochemical characteristics of the antidepressant and the biochemical characteristics of the depression did not "fit." In its simplest form, a depression in which 5-HT metabolism is predominantly disturbed would require a 5-HT-potentiating compound and could not be expected to benefit substantially from a compound that acted mainly to increase the availability of CA. The reverse would be likely for more "NE-related depressions." Since synthetic drugs with selectivity toward one particular MA became available only recently, MA precursors were resorted to in order to increase the concentrations of 5-HT or CAs selectively.

In the next sections, the following issues are reviewed: (i) Is the oral administration of MA precursors an appropriate way to increase central MA synthesis? (ii) Do MA precursors have antidepressant potential? (iii) Is their antidepressant effect, if any, related to prior signs of disturbed metabolism of a particular MA? (iv) Is the effect of MA precursors on central MA really selective? (v) Is increased selectivity of antidepressants an appropriate goal, or would treatments that enhance both 5-HT- and CA-driven systems provide the best conditions for therapeutic efficacy? MA precursors have been used chiefly in mood disorders. Would it make sense to explore other indications? This question is also discussed below.

II. L-TRYPTOPHAN

A. Rationale

Tryptophan hydroxylase catalyzes the hydroxylation of L-tryptophan— the ultimate precursor of 5-HT—to 5-hydroxytryptophan (5-HTP). Since tryptophan passes the blood-brain barrier, and because tryptophan hydroxylase is unsaturated and restricted to serotonergic neurons, oral administration of L-tryptophan gives rise to selective increases in 5-HT's synthesis in and release from serotoninergic neurons (49,54,57,66,177,229).

In humans, oral administration of L-tryptophan leads to increased baseline concentrations of 5-hydroxyindoleacetic acid (5-HIAA), the main degradation product of 5-HT, in cerebrospinal fluid (CSF), and to increased 5-HIAA accumulation after probenecid loading (48,138,209) (Fig. 1). Probenecid blocks the efflux of acid MA metabolites, such as 5-HIAA, from the central nervous system (CNS), including CSF, to the bloodstream. The accumulation of the metabolites is a crude indicator of the degradation of the mother amine in the CNS as a whole. Increased postprobenecid 5-HIAA accumulation constitutes suggestive evidence for increased 5-HT metabolism (42,109,190).

Even though L-tryptophan is transformed to 5-HT only in serotoninergic neurons, exogenous L-tryptophan can influence central CA metabolism, particularly if it is administered in large quantities. L-Tryptophan competes with other large neutral amino acids (LNAAs) for transport from the blood into the CNS (55,230). To the group of LNAAs also belong inter alias leucine, isoleucine, valine, phenylalanine, and tyrosine, the latter being the circulating precursor for CAs. Surplus L-tryptophan will interfere with tyrosine transport into the CNS and thus diminish CA synthesis. This has been demonstrated to occur in animals (77,175,229), but there is no direct evidence that the same effect occurs in humans (199). The level of CSF tyrosine does not decrease after an oral L-tryptophan load (209). Moreover, both after a single L-tryptophan load of 5 g and after treatment with 5 g L-tryptophan per day for 1 week, the concentration of homovanillic acid (HVA) and 3-methoxy-4-hydroxyphenylglycol (MHPG) in CSF failed to change. In the CNS, HVA is the main degradation product of dopamine (DA) and MHPG of NE. The CSF concentrations were studied after probenecid administration. The postprobenecid accu-

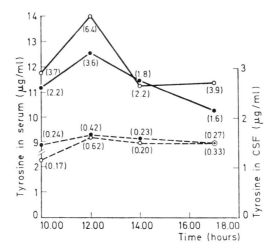

FIG. 1. Tyrosine concentration (mean ± SD) in serum and CSF before and after oral loading of 5 g L-tryptophan. Figures in parentheses indicate the standard deviation. ●——●, Serum concentration before tryptophan loading; ○——○, serum concentration after tryptophan loading; ●----●, CSF concentration before tryptophan loading; ○----○, CSF concentration after tryptophan loading. (From ref. 209, with permission.)

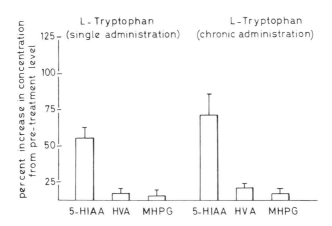

FIG. 2. Percentage increase in the concentrations of 5-HIAA, HVA, and MHPG in lumbar CSF after administration to test subjects of a single dose of L-tryptophan (5 g orally) and after administration of the same dose for 1 week. In all cases, the increase in 5-HIAA concentration in relation to the medication-free period was significant. Changes in postprobenecid HVA and baseline MHPG were insignificant. Lumbar CSF was withdrawn after probenecid loading (5 g/5 hr), 8 hr after starting the load. (From ref. 200, with permission.)

mulation of 5-HIAA in both cases increased substantially, indicating augmentation of 5-HT metabolism (Fig. 2).

L-Tryptophan administration affects other systems as well (236). No more than 3% of dietary L-tryptophan is converted to 5-HT. Most of it is metabolized by the liver enzyme tryptophan pyrrolase to the B-vitamin nicotinic acid via intermediate formation of kynurenine. Some tryptophan is used for protein synthesis, and a small fraction is probably converted to tryptamine. Tryptophan pyrrolase is induced by L-tryptophan administration (107) and also by cortisol (108), a hormone that is secreted in excess by a considerable percentage of patients with vital (endogenous) depression (167). The so-called kynurenine shunt can be assumed to be augmented in depressed patients during L-tryptophan treatment.

In summary, the evidence that oral administration of L-tryptophan to humans leads to increased 5-HT availability in the CNS is substantial. The effect, however, is probably not selective. Both CA-ergic and non-MA-ergic systems may be affected as well.

B. Outcome in Depression

The results with L-tryptophan in depression are conflicting. In eight studies, L-tryptophan was tested against placebo. In four, a parallel placebo group was used (38,131,182,202) and, in the others, placebo substitution of L-tryptophan (27,47,53,138). In no more than two of these studies did L-tryptophan prove to be superior to placebo. Murphy et al. (138) found L-tryptophan to be effective in bipolar but not unipolar depressives. Tryptophan doses ranged from 3 to 16 g/day and were generally high, i.e., >6 g/day. In the study by Thompson et al. (182), L-tryptophan was superior to placebo in patients suffering from a (mild) major depressive disorder.

Eleven studies compared L-tryptophan with a tricyclic antidepressant in a double-blind design. In nine, the two compounds were found to be equivalent (22,35,41,91,96,106,118,182); in two studies, L-tryptophan was inferior (120,228). Two studies report decreasing efficacy of L-tryptophan after 2 weeks of treatment (35,91). Quadbeck et al. (157), in a controlled study, compared moderate doses of L-tryptophan (3 g/day) with modest doses of the new antidepressant nomifensine; they concluded that both were equally effective.

In the largest and best designed L-tryptophan study to date, either L-tryptophan (3 g/day), amitriptyline (150 mg/day), the combination of the two compounds, or placebo was administered using a double-blind design for 12 weeks (182). A total of 115 mildly to moderately depressed outpatients were involved. The great majority were suffering from a major depressive disorder, according to the DSM-III criteria. All were treated by general practitioners. L-Tryptophan and amitriptyline were found to be equipotent and superior to placebo; the combination treatment was superior to either of the compounds alone (Fig. 3).

One double-blind study compared L-tryptophan and placebo with the combination of L-tryptophan and lithium in patients with "uni- and bipolar manic-depressive

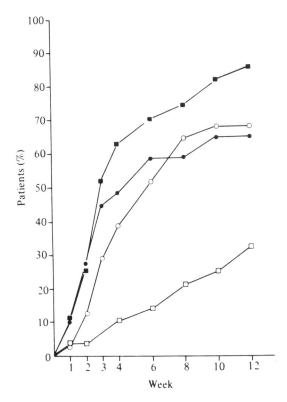

FIG. 3. Comparison of treatments showing the cumulative percentage of patients in each group in remission, defined as reaching a score of 0 (not depressed) on the global rating scale. ●, Tryptophan; ○, amitriptyline; ■, tryptophan–amitriptyline combination; □, placebo. (From ref. 182, with permission.)

psychosis" (228). As mentioned, L-tryptophan showed no antidepressant effect; the combination treatment did. It is impossible to deduce from this study whether the lithium/tryptophan combination was any better than lithium alone, in other words, whether L-tryptophan potentiated the therapeutic effects of lithium. The study of Brewerton and Reus (21) indicates that it does. These authors compared lithium and placebo with lithium and L-tryptophan in manic patients with a diagnosis of bipolar disorder ($n = 9$) or schizoaffective psychosis ($n = 7$). Therapeutic results were superior in the lithium/tryptophan group. The results may have been compounded by the greater doses of neuroleptics that had been administered to the group receiving L-tryptophan prior to the trial. Chouinard et al. (35) reported potentiation of the therapeutic effect of lithium by L-tryptophan, in particular among bipolar depressed patients. This study, however, was not controlled.

In four open studies, the efficacy of L-tryptophan was compared with that of electroconvulsive treatment (ECT). In two of them, L-tryptophan had no antidepressant effect, in contrast to ECT (31,90). One study considered both treatments as equipotent (40). MacSweeney's study (125) found L-tryptophan superior to ECT. L-Tryptophan appeared to have no practical value for potentiating the antidepressant efficacy of ECT (44,101).

The four controlled studies in which either L-tryptophan or placebo was combined with a MAOI all found L-tryptophan to be superior in potentiating the antidepressant response (10,39,71,151). The combination studies with tricyclic antidepressants, on the other hand, were inconclusive. In three, no potentiation was found (35,123,171), in four, L-tryptophan seemed to be better than placebo (163,223–225). The tricyclics used were amitriptyline, imipramine, desmethylimipramine, and clomipramine. Clomipramine, more so than the other three, is a strong and moderately selective inhibitor of 5-HT uptake. There was no indication that the combination of tryptophan with this drug was more efficacious than its combination with other tricyclics. The selective 5-HT reuptake inhibitor zimelidine was found not to be potentiated by L-tryptophan (222,223).

C. Strategies Used to Increase the Efficacy of L-Tryptophan

The kynurenine shunt shifts tryptophan away from 5-HT synthesis, and kynurenine may also interfere with the passage of tryptophan into the brain. (The evidence for such interference is, at best, marginal). In order to circumvent the degradation of tryptophan by the kynurenine pathway, the combined administration of L-tryptophan and a pyrrolase inhibitor, such as allopurinol or nicotinamide, has been suggested. Both compounds have been used in conjunction with L-tryptophan (35,125,172); however, since a tryptophan/placebo group was lacking in these studies, the usefulness of these compounds was not clarified.

Quadbeck et al. (157), in a controlled study, compared L-tryptophan (3 g/day) plus placebo, or the same dose of L-tryptophan combined with low doses of L-5-HTP (150 mg/day given without a peripheral decarboxylase inhibitor). The combination treatment was shown to be superior. This effect was attributed to an alleged pyrrolase-inhibiting effect of L-5-HTP, a claim, however, that was not substantiated.

To decrease the tryptophan-depleting effect of the kynurenine pathway, additional administration of vitamin B6 has been suggested (75). It was hypothesized that the large increase in kynurenine concentration, in both plasma and urine, caused by giving L-tryptophan reflected a relative saturation of the kynurenine pathway, possibly due to vitamin B6 depletion, since many of the degradative enzymes down the pathway are B6-dependent (76). (In that case, giving B6 might be expected to *accelerate* the degradation of tryptophan, which would be opposite to the desired effect.) In addition, B6 is also needed for the decarboxylation of L-5-HTP to 5-HT. Thus a relative B6 deficit could directly diminish the efficacy of L-tryptophan treatment. In support of this hypothesis, Green and Aronson (75) found that combining L-tryptophan with pyridoxine led to a substantial reduction of both plasma and urinary concentrations of kynurenine. [Wurtman *(unpublished observations)* found the opposite in rats: giving B6 with tryptophan increased the amino acid's catabolism in the periphery and diminished its ability to increase brain 5-HT.] Controlled studies on the antidepressive effects of giving L-tryptophan with and without vitamin B6 have not yet been conducted.

D. Discussion

From the placebo-controlled studies, L-tryptophan emerges as a placebo, but from the antidepressant-controlled studies, it has the properties of an active substance. The data derived from the first group of studies are weightier than those of the latter, first because most of the tricyclic-controlled studies used fewer than 20 patients. Since approximately 25% of potentially antidepressant-responsive patients are apt to respond to placebo as well as a truly effective treatment, and because the percentage of antidepressant responders in the group of vital (endogenous) depression is not greater than approximately 60 to 65%, a possible difference in the therapeutic potential of two test substances would easily be blurred in studies using small samples.

Moreover, one must take into account that in most studies, tricyclic antidepressants were administered in rather low doses (150 mg/day). Their apparent efficacy could have been a placebo effect, and a comparative study using two placebos would not be expected to yield striking differences.

For several reasons, it is premature to dismiss L-tryptophan as a mere placebo. Many of the studies suffer from methodological weaknesses. Some mentioned above include small sample size and use of inadequate doses of the comparative antidepressant. Most studies were performed before the DSM-III (46) and Research Diagnostic Criteria (161) were available. Consequently, the diagnostic nomenclature used in them is variable; diagnostic criteria remain frequently unstated; and inclusion criteria are often vague ("various forms of depression"). Tryptophan-responsive subcategories of patients could easily have been buried under averaged ratings in ill-defined groups. Another methodological flaw is the brief duration of several of the placebo-controlled trials (3 weeks or less), which may be too brief for a robust effect to develop. In addition, doses used in the studies varied widely, from 3 to 16 g/day. As discussed in Section II.A, tryptophan competes with tyrosine for entering into the brain. High doses of tryptophan could thus have interfered with tyrosine entrance to such a degree that CA synthesis diminished. Since a CA deficit is also considered to be a depressogenic factor, this effect could counteract the beneficial effects of increased 5-HT availability. Chouinard et al. (33) found evidence that a "therapeutic window" exists for L-tryptophan. The therapeutic potential of L-tryptophan would subside both with decreasing as well as with increasing (>6 g/day) doses. Hypothetically, the latter phenomenon could be related to an evolving CA deficit.

Dose may be related to tryptophan effects in yet another way. L-Tryptophan induces tryptophan pyrrolase in the liver (107). With increasing dose, more tryptophan is shunted into the kynurenine pathway, leaving proportionately if not absolutely less tryptophan for 5-HT synthesis. The surplus kynurenine might compete with tryptophan for entry in the brain. Similar mechanisms may explain the observations by Singleton and Marsden (173) that the rise in brain tryptophan in mice seen after 3 days on a high L-tryptophan diet had largely disappeared by the 18th day on such a diet. (Another explanation may be that they ate less.) It should be noted that it has never been shown that giving humans higher tryptophan doses causes smaller increases in plasma tryptophan.

A last reason why dismissal of L-tryptophan as a mere placebo would be premature is that all studies but one have failed to consider 5-HT-related variables, measured before treatment, in the analysis of treatment outcome. A number of observations suggest that 5-HT metabolism can be disturbed in depression: lowered baseline (6) and postprobenecid (201) CSF 5-HIAA levels; lowered ratio of tryptophan/LNAA in plasma (135); lowered imipramine binding (112) and decreased 5-HT uptake in blood platelets (164); subnormal 5-HT content of blood platelets (79); blunted response of prolactin to a L-tryptophan load (89); and therapeutic efficacy of drugs with a highly selective inhibiting effect on 5-HT uptake in nerve terminals, the so-called selective 5-HT reuptake inhibitors (45,88,97,146,147,152, 217). Finally, tryptophan depletion induced via ingestion of tryptophan-free amino acid mixtures led to rapid mood lowering in normal males (235).

Most findings suggest a decreased availability of synaptic 5-HT in some patients with depression. There is no consensus about these findings (11): Conflicting evidence exists, but we maintain that the statement is supported by a majority of studies (205).

It is logical to assume that depressed patients in whom 5-HT metabolism is measurably disturbed will respond preferentially to compounds such as L-tryptophan that increase 5-HT availability in the brain. Møller et al. (134) indeed found evidence that depressed patients with a low plasma tryptophan/LNAA ratio are most responsive to L-tryptophan treatment. They also found evidence that some depressed patients show elevated plasma levels of LNAAs, which might be attributed to disturbed tissue uptake or metabolism of these compounds. A decreased tryptophan/LNAA ratio could have led to diminished tryptophan entry into the CNS and reduced 5-HT synthesis. Unfortunately, no studies have been done regarding the relationship of the tryptophan/LNAA ratio and CSF 5-HIAA.

It is conceivable that the so-called 5-HT-disturbed subgroup of vital (endogenous) depression is preferentially responsive to L-tryptophan and that failure to classify patients accordingly has blurred the potentially therapeutic value of this compound (210).

E. Conclusions on L-Tryptophan in Depression

The status of L-tryptophan in depression treatment is still unsettled. Tricyclic-controlled studies qualify L-tryptophan as an active compound; placebo-controlled studies are overwhelmingly negative. The discrepancy can be explained by methodological flaws. In order to solve the issue, in future research the following conditions should be fulfilled: (i) large enough sample size, (ii) careful patient classification in terms of syndrome and severity, (iii) correlation of treatment outcome with 5-HT-related variables measured before treatment, such as CSF 5-HIAA and the ratio of tryptophan to LNAA, (iv) monitoring of the plasma ratio of tryptophan to LNAA, and of kynurenine, during treatment, and adjustment of the L-tryptophan dose to minimize competition with tyrosine for crossing the blood-brain barrier, and (v) potentiation of tryptophan uptake in the brain by high-carbohydrate meals. [Carbohydrates increase insulin secretion. Insulin has little influence on plasma tryptophan but greatly lowers plasma levels of other LNAAs by facilitating their uptake into skeletal muscle (87,126,229)].

Adding L-tryptophan to a MAOI seems to potentiate the therapeutic efficacy of both compounds. The results of combination treatment with tricyclic antidepressants tend to be inconclusive. Why MAOIs and tricyclics differ in this respect is unclear. Preliminary evidence suggests that L-tryptophan potentiates the therapeutic effects of lithium in both manic and depressed patients. Such combination studies are sufficiently encouraging to warrant large-scale replication.

Finally, it would make sense to study whether combining L-tryptophan with a pyrrolase inhibitor, vitamin B6, or tyrosine will increase its efficacy (see also Section VI.C).

F. Prophylactic Value of L-Tryptophan

Scattered data suggest L-tryptophan to be of prophylactic value in depression (16,35). No systematic study has been undertaken.

G. L-Tryptophan in Mania

There is suggestive evidence that L-tryptophan in high dosages (6 g/day or more) can cause improvement in (hypo)manic patients. Murphy et al. (138) treated 10 manic and hypomanic patients with L-tryptophan (9.6 ± 0.4 g/day for an average of 20 days) and placebo in a crossover design. Seven patients responded to tryptophan; three relapsed with placebo. Hypomanic patients did better than manic patients. One nonresponder became worse, more delusional, and disorganized on L-tryptophan. Chouinard et al. (34) found L-tryptophan, 12 g/day for 1 week, effective in controlling manic symptoms in 24 patients. In the second week, half the patients continued tryptophan while the others were switched to placebo under double-blind conditions. The tryptophan group remained well; the placebo group worsened, although not significantly so ($p<0.10$). Another double-blind placebo-controlled study failed to demonstrate tryptophan to be therapeutically active in mania (32). The dose used, however, was lower.

Prange et al. (155), using a similar design, compared L-tryptophan with chlorpromazine in 10 manic patients. The doses of both chlorpromazine and tryptophan were related to body weight; a 67.8 kg patient received 400 mg chlorpromazine daily or 6 g L-tryptophan. On most measures, tryptophan was superior to chlorpromazine, but the differences did not reach statistical significance. One must take into account the fact that the dose of chlorpromazine used was substantially less than that usually needed in manic states. Since in all three positive studies on mania, the dose of L-tryptophan used was high, one must consider the possibility that it acts not by increasing brain 5-HT synthesis but by decreasing the synthesis of CA by competition with tyrosine for uptake into the CNS.

Since the present evidence for an antimanic effect of tryptophan is at best tentative, larger scale replication studies are indicated.

H. L-Tryptophan in Schizophrenia

Studies on the use of tryptophan to treat schizophrenia are scarce. Bowers (20) treated six schizophrenic patients with 2 to 4 g L-tryptophan per day for 8 to 12 days. Tryptophan was combined with 100 mg/day pyridoxine. A tranquilizing effect was observed, but the therapeutic response was less than when phenothiazines were subsequently given. Gillin et al. (69), in a double-blind placebo-controlled study, found L-tryptophan, 9 to 20 g/day for 11 to 28 days, ineffective in eight chronic schizophrenics. (Tryptophan was also combined with B6, 100 mg/day, which may, as discussed above, have increased or even decreased its effect on brain 5-HT.) On the other hand, Chouinard et al. did observe a slight therapeutic effect of L-tryptophan, of gradual and slow onset, in 16 chronic schizophrenic patients. The authors compared L-tryptophan (2–6 g/day) combined with benserazide (to inhibit tryptophan pyrrolase in the liver but which also can inhibit 5-HT decarboxylase) with chlorpromazine (300–900 mg/day). The chlorpromazine effect was superior. Since the study lacked a placebo group, it is not possible to conclude that the tryptophan had been therapeutically active. The combination of tryptophan and the MAOI iproniazide reportedly elicits an increase in activity and in affect among chronic, withdrawn schizophrenics (154). In a similar study conducted by Lauer et al. (114), this combination resulted mainly in increased anxiety and agitation. There apparently are no studies indicating the usefulness of 5-HTP in schizophrenia (102). The few data available do not suggest a therapeutic role for 5-HT precursors in schizophrenia. There is hardly any theoretical basis for this use in schizophrenia.

III. L-5-HTP

A. Rationale

In the CNS of test animals, exogenous L-5-HTP—being an intermediate product in 5-HT synthesis—is readily transformed into 5-HT (59). The relevant enzyme, 5-HTP decarboxylase, is found not only in nerve cells that contain tryptophan hydroxylase but also in those containing tyrosine hydroxylase (124,237) and supposedly in nerve cells devoid of those enzymes as well (94). A substantial proportion of L-5-HTP administered orally to rats is, however, converted to 5-HT in serotoninergic neurons. Korf et al. (110) treated intact rats, and rats in which the raphe nuclei had been destroyed stereotactically, with small doses of L-5-HTP (12 mg/kg) combined with a peripheral decarboxylase inhibitor. Both groups showed increased 5-HT and 5-HIAA concentrations in the brain, but the increase was much more marked in the intact rats than in those with destroyed serotoninergic neurons (Fig. 4).

Orally administered L-5-HTP is transformed to 5-HT in CA-ergic neurons as well. Conceivably, extraneous 5-HT acts as a false transmitter, decreasing CA-ergic transmission (59). The increased synthesis of both DA and NE after L-5-HTP administration (8,51) can be viewed as compensatory, i.e., an attempt to overcome a functional block. Thus L-5-HTP may have a dual effect on CA-ergic systems: formation of false transmitter and a change in neuronal firing. The net effect of L-5-HTP brain CA-mediated neurotransmission is not known.

In humans, L-5-HTP combined with a peripheral decarboxylase inhibitor gives rise to a substantial rise in plasma L-5-HTP (227) (Fig. 5), baseline CSF 5-HIAA, and postprobenecid CSF 5-HIAA (199) (Fig. 6), indicating augmentation of CNS 5-HT synthesis and metabolism. If a peripheral decarboxylase inhibitor is omitted, the rise in plasma L-5-HTP is approximately 300% less (227) (Fig. 5). CSF data suggestive of an increase in central 5-HT metabolism under these circumstances are not available.

L-5-HTP increases not only the release of 5-HT but also that of DA and NE (Fig. 6). Both after single administration of L-5-HTP and when the substance was given for 1 week, significant increases occurred in CSF HVA and MHPG (203). CSF metabolites were studied after probenecid administration, and the L-5-HTP·

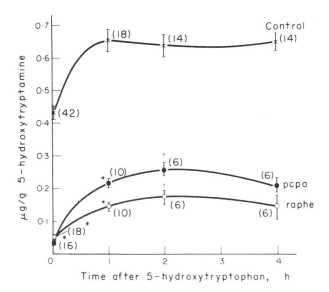

FIG. 4. Time course of 5-HT levels in the cerebral cortex after L-5-HTP (12 mg/kg i.v.). All rats were pretreated with a peripheral decarboxylase inhibitor (MK 486, 100 mg/kg). Three groups of rats were compared: controls; raphe, subjects with a chronic destruction of the raphe nucleus; pcpa, rats treated with PCPA. In the three groups of rats there was a significant increase of 5-HT after 5-HTP. The 5-HT increase is significantly less in the raphe rats compared with the nonlesioned rats. No. of animals in parentheses. (From ref. 110, with permission.)

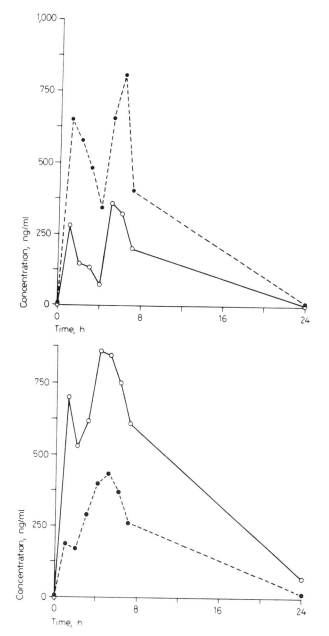

FIG. 5. Top: Plasma concentration–time of 5-HTP (○) and 5-HIAA (●) after oral administration of 200 mg L-5-HTP without pretreatment. **Bottom:** Plasma concentration–time curves of 5-HTP (○) and 5-HIAA (●) after oral administration of 200 mg L-5-HTP after pretreatment with carbidopa (150 mg/day) during 3 days. (From ref. 227, with permission.)

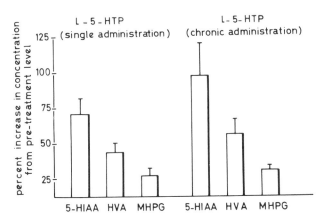

FIG. 6. Percentage increase in the concentration of 5-HIAA, HVA, and MHPG in lumbar CSF after administration to test subjects of a single dose of L-5-HTP (200 mg orally) and after administration of the same dose for 1 week. In the acute experiment, the patients were pretreated with carbidopa (150 mg/day) for 3 days. In the chronic experiment, L-5-HTP was combined with carbidopa in the same dose. In all cases, the increase in concentration in relation to the medication-free period was significant. Lumbar CSF was withdrawn after probenecid loading (5 g/5 hr), 8 hr after starting the load. (From ref. 199, with permission.) ·

was always combined with a peripheral decarboxylase inhibitor. Thus human findings are consistent with animal data.

B. Outcome in Depression

In 1963, Kline and Sacks (104) described antidepressant effects after a single intravenous dose of small amounts of DL-5-HTP in patients concurrently under treatment with a MAOI. However, the authors were subsequently unable to confirm this observation (105).

In the late 1960s, we started systematic studies on the use of L-5-HTP in depression. Before using the precursor therapeutically, we made the following preliminary observations (191): (i) Oral L-5-HTP increased the probenecid-induced accumulation of 5-HIAA in CSF, indicating augmented 5-HT metabolism in the CNS. (ii) Depressed patients with diminished CSF 5-HIAA accumulation after probenecid are able to transform L-5-HTP to 5-HT. This was concluded from the observation that an oral L-5-HTP load increased CSF 5-HIAA accumulation after probenecid to the same degree in patients with normal and subnormal 5-HIAA responses to probenecid. (iii) In rat brain, L-5-HTP is transformed into 5-HT at least in part within serotoninergic neurons (110) (Fig. 4). (iv) Combination of L-5-HTP with a peripheral decarboxylase inhibitor greatly enhances its efficiency (227) (Fig. 5).

In several double-blind studies controlled with placebo (195,214) and/or a tricyclic antidepressant (195,219), we demonstrated that L-5-HTP in combination with a peripheral decarboxylase inhibitor is superior to a placebo and equipotent with the tricyclic antidepressant clomipramine (Anafranil). The combination of L-5-HTP and a tricyclic was superior to either compound alone (Fig. 7). Patients who had had a subnormal CSF 5-HIAA response to probenecid before treatment responded preferentially to L-5-HTP (Fig. 8) (211). Several uncontrolled (Table 1) and controlled (Table 2) studies confirmed our therapeutic findings (196). The study relating pretreatment CSF 5-HIAA to treatment outcome has not yet been replicated.

Three studies (one open, two placebo-controlled) have so far yielded negative results. The open study (180) focused on brief therapy (7 days) with small doses of L-5-HTP. The study of Brodie et al. (24) was placebo-controlled but concerned only seven patients, who likewise were treated (too) briefly (1–15 days). Mendlewicz and Youdim (132) compared the antidepressant effects of three medications: a MAOI combined with L-5-HTP, L-5-HTP alone, and a placebo. The combined therapy was superior to that with the placebo. The effect of L-5-HTP alone did not significantly differ from that obtained with the combination. Nevertheless, the difference between L-5-HTP and the placebo was not significant. A possible explanation is that the groups studied were small, and the number of responders in the placebo group was unusually large.

Few antidepressants have been tested in combination with L-5-HTP. The therapeutic effect of the tricyclic antidepressant clomipramine is potentiated by L-5-

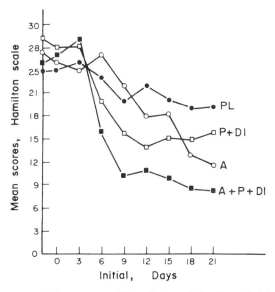

FIG. 7. Hamilton scores in four groups of 10 patients suffering from vital depression with uni- and bipolar course, before and during a 3-week treatment period with 5-HT-potentiating compounds. The groups consisted of 10 patients each, treated, respectively, with clomipramine alone (A; 225 mg/day), L-5-HTP alone (P; 200 mg/day, in combination with 150 mg MK 486, a peripheral decarboxylase inhibitor; DI), the combination of clomipramine with 5-HTP and placebo (PL). The design was double blind. (From ref. 194, with permission.)

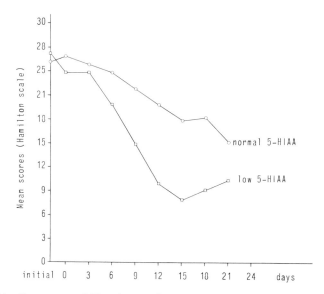

FIG. 8. Hamilton scores of 30 patients suffering from vital depression with uni- and bipolar course before and during a 3-week treatment period with 5-HT-potentiating compounds, i.e., clomipramine alone, L-5-HTP (together with a peripheral decarboxylase inhibitor) alone, and those drugs in combination. *Lower curve*, treatment results in patients with subnormal pretreatment 5-HIAA response to probenecid ($n = 13$); *upper curve*, results for patients with normal pretreatment 5-HIAA responses ($n = 17$). (From ref. 194, with permission.)

HTP in combination with carbidopa (206,219) and by L-5-HTP alone (142). Some striking results have been obtained with this combination in therapy-resistant vital (endogenous) depressions (219). No other tricyclic antidepressant has yet been tested in combination with L-5-HTP.

Two MAOIs, nialamide and deprenyl, have been tested in this context. The effect of the former is potentiated by L-5-HTP (122). Mendlewicz and Youdim (132) found that deprenyl in combination with L-5-HTP was more effective than L-5-HTP alone or placebo. A group of patients given deprenyl alone was not included in the design. Strictly speaking, therefore, the conclusion that L-5-HTP potentiated the MAOI is not warranted. Deprenyl is a selective inhibitor of MAO-B, while 5-HT is a selective substrate for MAO-A. Another preferred substrate for MAO-A is NE; DA and tryptamine are preferred substrates for MAO-B. Thus it is possible that the actions of L-5-HTP are mediated in part through release of the latter amines (12) (see also Section IV.B).

C. Dosage

Different dosages were used in the various 5-HTP studies; consequently, it is not yet possible to give firm guidelines on dosage. Only the following points were established with certainty: (i) A given dosage scheme leads to widely different blood 5-HTP levels in different subjects. Since nothing is known yet about a minimum (and possibly a

TABLE 1. *Survey of open studies into the efficacy of 5-HTP in depressions*[a]

Reference	Patients		5-HTP dosage (mg/day)	Duration of treatment (days)	Results
	n	Diagnosis[b]			
Sano (168)	107	Endogenous depression	50–300	7–35	74/107 markedly improved
Fujiwara and Otsuki (58)	20	Endogenous depression	50–200	7–28	10/20 improved
Matussek et al. (127)	23	Unipolar depression, 13; bipolar depression, 1; involutional depression, 8; schizoaffective depression, 1	100–300[c]	4–20	7/23 markedly improved
Takahashi et al. (179)	24	Unipolar depression, 20; involutional depression, 2; neurotic depression, 1; psychotic depression, 1	300	14	7/20 in the unipolar group markedly improved
Nakajima et al. (141)	59	Mixed group in which 8 different types of depression are distinguished	150–300	21 or more	13/59 markedly improved 27/59 moderately improved
van Hiele (187)	99	Vital depressions, 44; depressions with vital features, 24; personal depressions, 31	50–600[c]	14 or more	37/68 in the vital group and 6/31 in the personal group markedly improved
Kaneko et al. (99)	18	Endogenous depression	150–300	10–28	10/18 markedly improved
Total	350			191/350 improved	

[a]Listing only those studies that involved at least 14 days' 5-HTP medication at a daily dosage of at least 50 mg L-5-HTP was used in all studies.
[b]Terminology as used by the authors.
[c]5-HTP was given in combination with a peripheral decarboxylase inhibitor.

maximum) therapeutic dose, this makes it necessary to determine dosages individually on the basis of clinical findings. (ii) L-5-HTP should be given along with a peripheral decarboxylase inhibitor in order to reduce dosage and to minimize its side effects. (iii) The disappearance of 5-HTP from the blood is rapid; hence the compound should be administered at least three times per day (220).

We tentatively suggest that a daily dose of 200 mg L-5-HTP in combination with 150 mg carbidopa is acceptable as a gross average. However, many patients can do with less, and many require more (up to 500 mg/day) (187).

It is advisable to increase the 5-HTP dosage gradually in order to reduce the risk of gastrointestinal side effects. We usually start with 25 mg/day and, in the course of 10 to 14 days, increase this to an average of 200 mg/day. A therapeutic effect (if any) usually does not occur immediately but only after 5 to 20 days.

TABLE 2. *Survey of double-blind controlled studies into the efficacy of 5-HTP in depression[a]*

Reference	Patients		5-HTP dosage (mg/day)	Duration of treatment (days)	Design	Results
	n	Diagnosis[b]				
van Praag et al. (214)	5	Vital depression (unipolar and bipolar)	200–3,000	21	5-HTP/placebo	3/5 improved
Brodie et al. (24)	7	Psychotic depression, 6; schizoaffective psychosis, 1	250–3,250[c]	1–15	5-HTP/placebo	1/7 moderately improved
Bartlet and Pailard (15)	25	Melancholia, 4; involutional depression, 7; reactive depression, 8; neurotic depression, 6	200–800	10–240	5-HTP/placebo	19/25 improved
Lopez Ibor et al. (122)	14	Endogenous depression	50–300	15–20	5-HTP/ nialamide	12/15 markedly improved
Angst et al. (5)	36	Ill-defined; probably vital (endogenous) depressions	200–1,200[c]	At least 20 days	5-HTP/ imipramine	5-HTP and imipramine equally effective; number of improved patients not stated
van Praag (195)	20	Vital depression (unipolar and bipolar)	200[c]	21	5-HTP/ placebo/ clomipramine	11/20 markedly improved; 5-HTP and clomipramine equally effective
van Praag (201)	15	Vital depression (unipolar and bipolar)	200[c]	28	5-HTP/ tryptophan/ placebo	8/15 markedly improved; 5-HTP more effective than tryptophan and placebo
Mendlewicz and Youdim (132)	39	Bipolar 24 Unipolar 15	300[c]	32	5-HTP and deprenyl/5-HTP/placebo	13/21 responded to 5-HTP alone
Total (excluding study of Angst et al.)	125					67/125 improved

[a]DL-5-HTP was used in the study by van Praag et al. (214). L-5-HTP was used in all other studies.
[b]Terminology as used by the authors.
[c]5-HTP was given in combination with a peripheral decarboxylase inhibitor.

D. Conclusions

The number of controlled studies comparing L-5-HTP with a placebo or with a standard antidepressant is still small. A final evaluation, therefore, is not yet possible. The results obtained so far indicate that L-5-HTP may have antidepressant properties, and that the combination of L-5-HTP with clomipramine or with the MAOIs nialamide and deprenyl may be superior, therapeutically, to either of these substances separately. Whether this potentiating effect also applies to other tricyclic compounds and MAOIs remains to be established. In any case, this combined medication merits consideration in depressions of the vital (endogenous) type that show an insufficient response to traditional antidepressants.

Two other observations indicate an influence of L-5-HTP on mood: (i) L-5-HTP was found to have a euphoric effect on normal test subjects (156,185). (ii) When used as a therapeutic in myoclonus patients (181,221), L-5-HTP was found to cause (hypo)manic disinhibition as a frequent side effect.

Considering group averages, L-5-HTP can be described as roughly equal in therapeutic efficacy to traditional antidepressants. If the observation that the low 5-HIAA subgroup of vital depressions preferentially responds to L-5-HTP (194,195) can be confirmed, then the net yield of 5-HTP therapy could probably be increased by measuring the (postprobenecid) CSF 5-HIAA accumulation prior to starting treatment.

E. Prophylactic Use of L-5-HTP

So far, only one prophylactic study has been conducted in which L-5-HTP and placebo were compared in a double-blind crossover design (207). Three observations prompted this study. First, it was demonstrated that low postprobenecid CSF 5-HIAA is state independent in a majority of patients (184,191). Second, evidence showed that the subgroup of patients with vital (endogenous) depression exhibiting low 5-HIAA had an increased relapse risk (206) (Table 3). Finally, low CSF 5-HIAA was shown to correlate with increased depressive morbidity in the family (170) (Table 4). Those data suggested that low CSF 5-HIAA levels might be a depression-predisposing factor. If that were so, increasing 5-HT availability in the CNS could be expected to have a prophylactic effect.

The study of van Praag and de Haan (207) confirmed this prediction. In combination with a peripheral decarboxylase inhibitor, 5-HIAA was shown to be superior to placebo (Table 5) and equipotent to lithium in unipolar vital (endogenous) depression. In bipolar depression, L-5-HTP seemed inferior to lithium, probably because it did not prevent (hypo)manic episodes and, in fact, might have even provoked them (208).

This study has not yet been replicated. If confirmed, L-5-HTP prophylaxis would be the first form of aimed chemoprophylaxis in psychiatry [aimed at a suspected pathogenetic factor in certain types of vital (endogenous) depression].

TABLE 3. *Frequency of admissions for depression*

Patient groups	No. of admissions per patient					Total no. of admissions
	1	2	3	4	5	
Subnormal 5-HIAA group	5	9	12	5	2	89[a]
Normal 5-HIAA group	9	20	4	—	—	61

[a]The number of hospitalizations for depression in the subnormal 5-HIAA group significantly exceeds that in the normal 5-HIAA group ($p < 0.002$; Mann-Whitney U-test, two-tailed).
From ref. 206, with permission.

TABLE 4. *Relationship between 5-HIAA concentration in lumbar CSF and psychiatric family history*

5-HIAA concn. in CSF (pmole/ml)	No. of subjects		
	Psychiatric family history	No psychiatric family history	Total
Normal	16	31	47
High (>140)	8	0	8
Low (<70)	4	1	5
	28	32	60

In the subjects with a family history of psychiatric morbidity, there was a significantly greater variation in 5-HIAA than in the subjects lacking such a history. Subjects who had family members with schizophrenic psychosis had significantly higher 5-HIAA concentrations than subjects with depressive disorder in the family.

From ref. 170, with permission.

TABLE 5. *Patients who relapsed during 5-HTP periods: Comparison between patients with normal and those with subnormal postprobenecid CSF 5-HIAA concentrations*

Patient groups	No. of patients	Relapse during 5-HTP	No relapse during 5-HTP
Persistent normal postprobenecid CSF 5-HIAA	7	5	2
Persistent subnormal postprobenecid CSF 5-HIAA	13	1	12

The relapse rate in the 5-HT-deficient subgroup is significantly lower than that in the normoserotonergic subgroup ($p < 0.02$; Fisher's exact probability test; two-tailed). Persistent means during depressive episodes and in symptom-free intervals.

From ref. 207, with permission.

F. L-5-HTP in Mania

To the best of our knowledge, no studies on the effect of L-5-HTP in (hypo)mania have been published.

IV. COMPARISON OF L-5-HTP AND L-TRYPTOPHAN IN DEPRESSION

A. Therapeutic Comparison

The data on L-tryptophan in depression seem to be more ambiguous than those on L-5-HTP. Therefore, we conducted a comparative study (202).

Forty-five patients were involved, all suffering from the syndrome of vital (endogenous) depression and satisfying the DSM-III criteria for Major Depressive Disorder, Melancholic Type. None of them displayed psychotic features. After a drug-free period of at least 10 days, they were randomly distributed among one of the following three treatment groups: L-tryptophan (5 g/day), L-5-HTP (200 mg/day) in combination with the peripheral decarboxylase inhibitor carbidopa (150 mg/day), or placebo. The groups were comparable with respect to severity of the depression, number of precipitated and nonprecipitated depressions, ratio of first episode/unipolar/bipolar depressions, male/female ratio, and age (Table 6). The design was doubleblind, and the treatment period lasted for 4 weeks. Before treatment and weekly during treatment, the patients were rated according to the Hamilton Rating Scale for depression. Apart from a benzodiazepine hypnotic, if needed, no other medication was permitted.

L-Tryptophan was found to be slightly but not significantly superior to placebo. L-5-HTP, on the other hand, was found to be superior to both placebo and L-tryptophan (Fig. 9).

The study of Thomson et al. (182), cited by us in Section II.B as the best L-tryptophan study in depression, found L-tryptophan to be better than placebo and equal to amitriptyline. The authors studied mildly depressed outpatients, but we

TABLE 6. *Comparability of the patient groups treated with tryptophan, 5-HTP, or placebo*

Parameter	Tryptophan	5-HTP	Placebo
Severity (Hamilton scale)	26 ± 6	25 ± 5	23 ± 5
Precipitated/nonprecipitated	10/15	12/15	9/15
First episode/unipolar/bipolar	3/9/3	2/8/5	4/8/3
Male/female	4/11	6/9	4/11
Age (years)	21–64	19–62	24–63

There are no significant differences in a number of important variables. From ref. 202, with permission.

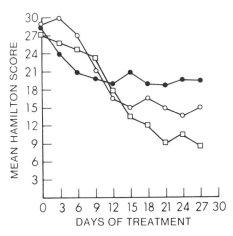

FIG. 9. Comparative controlled study of L-5-HTP (200 mg/day, □) in combination with carbidopa (150 mg/day), L-tryptophan (5 g/day, ○), and placebo (●) in patients suffering from the syndrome of vital (endogenous) depression. 5-HTP is significantly superior to tryptophan and placebo. Tryptophan treatment is not significantly different from placebo treatment. (From ref. 202, with permission.)

studied severely depressed inpatients. Their inclusion criteria were relatively broad (major depressive disorder), ours strict (major depressive disorder, melancholic type). Our data by no means exclude the possibility that L-tryptophan is a euphoriant in milder forms of depression.

B. Biochemical Comparisons

We were interested in the possible cause of the therapeutic discrepancy between the two 5-HT precursors in comparable types of depressive disorder. One possible explanation is that they influence CA metabolism differently. L-5-HTP increases the release of both 5-HT and CA, whereas L-tryptophan presumably augments 5-HT but not CA metabolism and may tend even to decrease the latter (see Sections II.A and III.A).

A second set of data support the notion that it could be the stimulating effect on both 5-HT and CA that gives L-5-HTP a therapeutic edge over L-tryptophan. In the 15 years that we have been studying L-5-HTP in depression, we observed that in approximately 20% of patients who respond initially, the therapeutic effect wears off after the first month of treatment (although seldom to the point of complete relapse). This effect could not be explained by pharmacokinetic factors, since plasma 5-HTP levels remained stable over time.

Next we studied whether the influence of L-5-HTP on central MA metabolism changes over time (199,202). In two independent studies, we demonstrated that while in the first month of 5-HTP treatment, CSF concentrations of 5-HT, DA, and NE metabolites are all increased, the situation in the second month of treatment is different. CSF 5-HIAA remains elevated: however, the concentration of the CA metabolites returns to pretreatment values.[1] This was the case in particular in patients who (partially) relapsed in the second month of L-5-HTP treatment (Fig. 10).

On the basis of these observations, we hypothesized that the antidepressant effect of L-5-HTP is based on its combined effect on 5-HT and CA metabolism; the diminution of the effect of L-5-HTP on CA after the first month is responsible for the partial relapse sometimes observed at this time; and the inferior therapeutic effects of L-tryptophan in comparison to L-5-HTP are related to the inability of the former amino acid to increase CA metabolism.

To verify these hypotheses, we examined the following questions: (i) Is the effect of L-5-HTP potentiated by L-tyrosine? (ii) In cases in which the therapeutic effect of L-5-HTP wears off, is L-tyrosine capable of restoring the original therapeutic yield? (iii) Is L-tyrosine able to augment the effect of L-tryptophan in depression?

---

[1] A possibly comparable phenomenon has been observed during treatment with neuroleptics. In the first few treatment weeks, the plasma prolactin concentration is increased, as is postprobenecid CSF HVA. The first phenomenon reflects blockade of postsynaptic DA receptors, the latter a (compensatory) increase in DA metabolism. The increase in prolactin persists over time. CSF HVA, on the other hand, returns to normal after the first treatment month (192). The "habituation" of DA metabolism to the state of receptor blockade could explain the delay between the start of neuroleptic medication and its full therapeutic impact. Only when the DA metabolism has returned to normal does the effect of the receptor blockade become maximal.

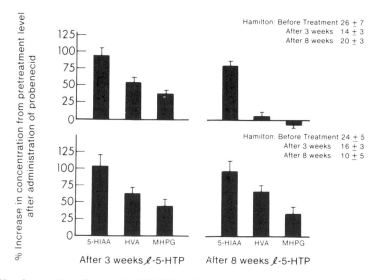

FIG. 10. Augmenting effect of L-5-HTP (200 mg/day in combination with carbidopa, 150 mg/day) on CA metabolism is transient in patients who relapsed in the first month of 5-HTP treatment **(top)**. In the first month of treatment, there is a substantial increase of HVA and MHPG in CSF after a probenecid load. In the second treatment month, the levels of those metabolites have returned to normal. The 5-HIAA response remains increased over time. In patients in whom the therapeutic response to 5-HTP continued, the effect on CA metabolites in CSF did not subside (199) **(bottom)**.

The admittedly preliminary findings justify affirmative answers to all three questions, indicating that simultaneous increases of 5-HT and CA provide the best conditions for antidepressant effect. (These findings raise doubts about the appropriateness of the tendency of pharmaceutical research to develop MA-specific compounds.) In Section VI, studies on these precursor combinations are discussed.

V. L-DOPA

A. Rationale

Exogenously administered L-DOPA increases DA levels and DA synthesis in DA-ergic neurons and supposedly enhances DA-ergic neurotransmission as well. Its effect on noradrenergic function is less clear. Brain NE levels do not change (52); release of NE increases somewhat (65), but it is unclear whether this is a direct consequence of increased precursor availability or a compensatory phenomenon: the consequence of surplus DA formation in noradrenergic neurons, DA acting there as a false transmitter. Probably the latter mechanism is the more important one, since the conversion of DA to NE through DA-β-hydroxylase is rate limiting (9,12,100). The net effect of L-DOPA on noradrenergic transmission remains unclear.

Since L-DOPA and L-5-HTP are decarboxylated by the same aromatic amino acid decarboxylase, L-DOPA entering serotoninergic neurons is transformed to DA, which probably functions as a false transmitter (143). While 5-HT release may initially increase as a result, brain 5-HT levels soon fall (52,100), probably because the L-DOPA decreases brain tryptophan uptake (162).

Findings in humans roughly parallel the animal data. L-DOPA combined with a peripheral decarboxylase inhibitor leads to increased postprobenecid accumulation of HVA in CSF (189,213). The effect on CSF MHPG is negligible, whereas the postprobenecid CSF 5-HIAA concentration decreases (193) (Fig. 11). Baseline CSF 5-HIAA does not change after L-DOPA (74).

B. Outcome in Depression

The overall effects of L-DOPA on depression have been described as unimpressive (27,30,47,74,103,131,139). The number of studies is small, and they suffer from the same imperfections as the tryptophan studies: small sample size, disparate dose regimens (varying from 100 mg–12 g/day), variable classification of depression, and variable and sometimes vague inclusion criteria.

Only one open study reports overall beneficial effects of L-DOPA in five depressed patients, all treated over several years with the conventional psychiatric methods with brief or negligible results. All recovered or improved markedly on treatment with L-DOPA. In four, however, the remission was temporary, and DOPA lost its effect after 3 to 4 months. The vanishing effect could not be influenced by increasing the dose of L-DOPA (153).

Several authors have reported a beneficial, albeit limited, effect of L-DOPA in retarded depression, i.e., motor activation and increased level of initiative (27, 73,74,153,189) without appreciable change in mood and vegetative symptoms.

We studied L-DOPA in 10 depressed patients. Five were selected because of their subnormal CSF HVA responses to probenecid; in the other five, this response

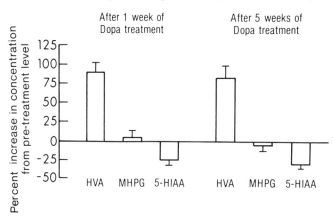

FIG. 11. L-DOPA (mean, 290 mg/day) in combination with the peripheral decarboxylase inhibitor MK 486 (150 mg/day) induced in five test persons a significant increase in postprobenecid CSF HVA. The concentration of MHPG did not change significantly, while postprobenecid 5-HIAA decreased slightly but consistently (in all test persons). CSF concentrations were measured before treatment and after 1 week and 5 weeks of DOPA treatment. The changes persisted over time.

was normal (189,212,213). This selection criterion was chosen because we had demonstrated that motor retardation in depression strongly correlates with low postprobenecid CSF HVA. CSF HVA can be lowered in retarded depression to the same degree as in Parkinson's disease. Hence we postulated that decreased DA metabolism is not specific for a particular disease, i.e., Parkinson's disease, but for a particular functional state, i.e., hypokinesia and anergia, irrespective of the nosological framework in which these symptoms occur (215). (In the study referred to above, it was also noted that motor retardation was most pronounced in the low HVA group.) The therapeutic (activating) effect of L-DOPA was evident only in the low HVA group. Under the influence of L-DOPA, postprobenecid CSF HVA rose to high-normal values (Table 7).

The relationship of DA-ergic function to psychomotor status is further supported by reports of increased agitation, switch into (hypo)mania, and agitated psychoses in some depressed patients given high doses of L-DOPA (27,74). Similarly, mood changes, agitation, and psychoses have been reported in parkinsonian patients treated with L-DOPA (133). Also in accordance with this hypothesis is the observation of Lindstrom (119) that low CSF HVA levels occur in schizophrenics, in particular among patients in whom vegetative symptoms, such as lassitude and slowness of movement, are prominent.

C. Conclusions

Although the data so far are limited, it seems fair to conclude that L-DOPA, although not being an antidepressant, may have therapeutic value in retarded depression as an activating agent. Its possible therapeutic usefulness has been underestimated and underanalyzed.

Investigators agree that L-DOPA lacks mood-elevating properties. This might be explained by the inability of L-DOPA to increase 5-HT and/or NE availability. As discussed, DA could conceivably act as a false transmitter in noradrenergic neurons, and has at best a modest influence on NE synthesis. The influence of DOPA on 5-HT systems is likewise depressing. DA formed in serotonergic cells could act as a false transmitter. 5-HT synthesis does not increase but, on the contrary, attenuates

TABLE 7. *DA metabolism before treatment and treatment response to L-DOPA in depression*

Patients	No.	HVA accumulation (ng/ml)[a]	Motor retardation[a]	
			Before treatment	After treatment
DA-deficient	5	74 (65–90)	6.8 (4–8)	2.7 (0.3)
Non-DA-deficient	5	121 (107–143)	2.1 (0–3)	2.4 (0.3)

[a]Group mean and range.
From ref. 213, with permission.

after DOPA administration, possibly because of diminished entry of tryptophan into the brain. Within the framework of the MA hypothesis of depression, one would thus expect L-DOPA to have a negative effect on mood. In future trials, it would seem appropriate to combine L-DOPA with a 5-HT precursor or a drug that increases 5-HT availability in the brain.

D. L-DOPA in Schizophrenia

According to several studies, L-DOPA can cause behavioral worsening in schizophrenia among patients treated (4,63) or not treated (28) with neuroleptics. In particular, the positive symptoms are adversely affected. According to Alpert et al. (3), the effect of DOPA in these cases is more a manifestation of toxicity than a genuine worsening of the schizophrenic syndrome. On the other hand, a few reports indicate that L-DOPA combined with neuroleptics can be advantageous in combating certain symptoms in schizophrenia, such as poor rapport and communication, emotional blunting, apathy, and tendency to isolation (93,148,234). An activating effect of L-DOPA has also been reported in retarded depression (see Section V.B). It is unclear how DOPA works when DA receptors are being blocked by neuroleptics.

VI. L-TYROSINE

A. Rationale

Tyrosine hydroxylase, the enzyme that converts tyrosine to DOPA, is restricted to CA-ergic neurons (140). Until recently, it was believed that this enzyme is fully saturated, and that tyrosine administration will not increase the production rate of DA and NE. Recent studies indicated that this enzyme is not fully saturated (29,232), and that administration of tyrosine, although not usually increasing CA levels, indeed does lead to increases in turnover and release of DA and NE (67,68,130,232). This effect is particularly marked in neurons that are activated, i.e., firing rapidly, such as after haloperidol blockade of postsynaptic CA receptors (169) or in spontaneously hypertensive rats (178). The ability of tyrosine to accelerate CA synthesis quantitatively depends on the firing rate of CA-ergic neurons (231). In disease states in which a deficiency of DA or NE occurs, CA neurons can be expected to be particularly sensitive to tyrosine. Large amounts of tyrosine can interfere with the synthesis of 5-HT (229) by competing with tryptophan for entry into the CNS.

Findings in humans corroborate the animal data. Oral doses of L-tyrosine increased plasma tyrosine, the plasma tyrosine/LNAA ratio (70), as well as plasma DA and NE concentrations in normal test persons (159). In patients with Parkinson's disease, L-tyrosine, in a dose of 100 mg/kg/day, significantly increased postprobenecid CSF HVA; CSF 5-HIAA levels did not change; and MHPG was not measured (78) (Fig. 12). We found that the same dose of L-tyrosine in depressed patients increased CSF concentrations of both HVA and MHPG after probenecid administration. CSF 5-HIAA dropped slightly but consistently (Fig. 13).

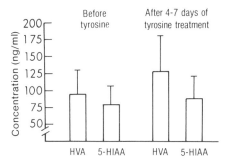

FIG. 12. Postprobenecid HVA and 5-HIAA levels in CSF before and during administration of L-tyrosine (100 mg/kg/day) for 4 to 7 days in nine patients with Parkinson's disease. MA metabolites were measured 2 hr after a dose of tyrosine. HVA concentration rose significantly; that of 5-HIAA did not change. (After ref. 78.)

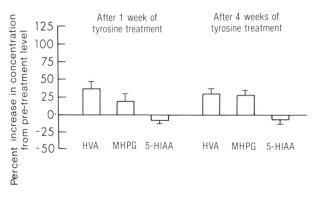

FIG. 13. Tyrosine (100 mg/kg/day) induced in five test persons a significant increase in CSF MHPG. CSF HVA increased significantly as well, but much less pronounced than after DOPA administration (see Fig. 11). CSF 5-HIAA did not change significantly. CSF concentrations were measured before treatment and after 1 and 4 weeks of tyrosine treatment. The changes persisted over time. CSF concentrations were measured after probenecid loading. Lumbar punctures were performed 2 hr after a dose of tyrosine.

These data indicate that tyrosine administration can lead to increased release of both DA and NE, and that, at least in certain individuals, 5-HT metabolism can be depressed. In animals, increased noradrenergic activity tends to facilitate 5-HT turnover and to increase 5-HT-mediated neurotransmission (43,95,160,166). That CSF 5-HIAA after oral L-tyrosine falls rather than rises could be considered as indirect evidence for diminished tryptophan supply to the CNS.

B. Outcome in Depression

The literature on tyrosine in depression is minimal and includes reports on three patients who had been successfully treated in an open fashion (62,72) and a few small controlled studies.

Gelenberg et al. (60,61) conducted a double-blind placebo-controlled study in 14 patients with major depressive disorder. L-Tyrosine was given for 4 weeks in a dose of 100 mg/kg/day. Five placebo nonresponders were likewise treated with L-tyrosine in an open trial. Although the numbers were too small for more definitive conclusions, the results were considered to be encouraging (Table 8). Urinary MHPG excretion increased an average of 24%. The increase of fasting plasma tyrosine averaged 27%. A trend toward a positive correlation between improvement and the rise in plasma tyrosine was noted.

van Praag (199) reported two studies in which L-5-HTP was combined with L-tyrosine. The rationale for the studies is described in Section IV.B. Briefly, the effect of 5-HTP on CA metabolism was observed to decline over time in some patients; this habituation was possibly related to diminishing the antidepressant efficacy of the 5-HTP. Accordingly, (re-)augmentation of CA metabolism could be expected to increase the efficacy of 5-HTP.

So far, two pilot experiments have been conducted. In one, four depressed patients were involved who had relapsed in the second month of treatment with L-5-HTP. From the end of the second month of 5-HTP treatment, L-tyrosine (100 mg/kg/day) or placebo was added in a cross-over design (Fig. 14). In all four patients, adding the L-tyrosine coincided with a remission. This was not the case with placebo. During tyrosine addition, both CSF HVA and MHPG rose significantly above baseline values (Fig. 15). The second was a two-group experiment involving six patients, all suffering from major depressive disorder, melancholic type. They were treated for 4 weeks with either L-5-HTP/carbidopa and L-tyrosine or L-5-HTP/carbidopa and placebo. The first combination was superior to the latter (Fig. 16).

C. L-Tyrosine and L-Tryptophan

Could the effect of tryptophan in depression be potentiated by tyrosine? What is the rationale? We had postulated that the inferior therapeutic effect of L-trypto-phan in comparison to L-5-HTP was related to the inability of the former to increase CA metabolism. This hypothesis would be supported by evidence that L-tyrosine potentiates the effect of L-tryptophan in depression (see also Section IV.B).

Ten patients were selected: six women and four men between the ages of 35 and 55 years. Two independent raters had diagnosed them as suffering from major

TABLE 8. *Double-blind 4-week controlled placebo/tyrosine study in 14 patients with major depressive disorders*

Study	No.	No. improved	No. not improved	Percent improved
Tyrosine (100 mg/kg/day, double-blind)	6	4	2	67
Tyrosine (100 mg/kg/day, open)	5	3	2	60
Placebo	8	3	5	38

From ref. 61, with permission.

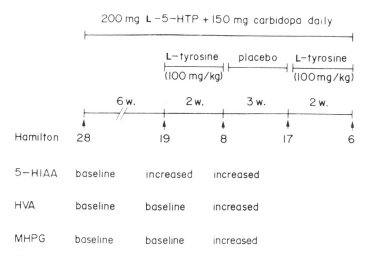

FIG. 14. Four patients who had been treated with L-5-HTP (200 mg/day) and carbidopa (150 mg/day) for 6 weeks and who had partially relapsed in the second month of treatment were given additionally L-tyrosine (100 mg/kg/day). Tyrosine was administered in a cross-over design. During the 5-HTP/tyrosine combination, all patients remitted, to relapse again in the 5-HTP/placebo period. During tyrosine administration, CSF HVA and MHPG rose significantly. (From ref. 199.)

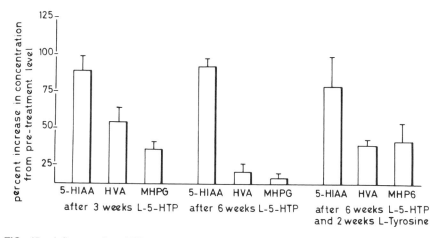

FIG. 15. Influence of L-5-HTP and the combination of L-5-HTP and L-tyrosine on postprobenecid CSF 5-HIAA and HVA and baseline MHPG in the patients depicted in Fig. 14. After 6 weeks of 5-HTP, CSF HVA and MHPG had "habituated." Both concentrations rose again after adding tyrosine. 5-HIAA remained high during the entire treatment period. (From ref. 199, with permission.)

depressive disorder, melancholic type. The average score on the Hamilton Rating Scale for depression the day prior to the initial treatment was 23 ± 4; thus the severity of the depressive syndrome was considerable. Psychotic features were absent. All had been admitted at least once for a similar syndrome. In three, (hypo)manic episodes had occurred in the past (bipolar depression). Seven patients

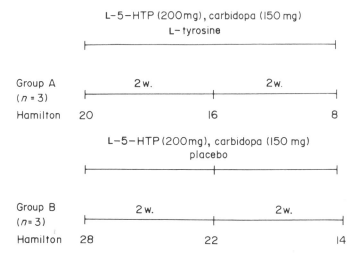

FIG. 16. Influence of L-tyrosine or placebo on the antidepressant effect of L-5-HTP in combination with the peripheral decarboxylase inhibitor carbidopa. (From ref. 199, with permission.)

had responded favorably to treatment with tricyclic antidepressants at previous admissions. Three patients had been treated with tricyclics on previous admissions, but also with ECT because of incomplete response to the antidepressants.

In the second week after admission, all patients were put on tryptophan in a dose of 3 g/day for 4 weeks. At the end of that period, the Hamilton score had declined systematically and significantly but modestly, so that all patients still had to be considered as considerably depressed. After having been treated for 4 weeks with tryptophan alone, tyrosine (100 mg/kg/day) was added in five patients, and placebo in the remaining five. The dichotomy was made at random. In the tryptophan/tyrosine group, the Hamilton scores declined gradually. At the end of the fourth week, three patients were symptom free, and in two, the depression had cleared substantially, although some residual symptoms remained, most notably decreased appetite and libido. In the placebo group, only one patient improved substantially (Fig. 17).

We concluded tentatively that tryptophan, in itself insufficiently effective in severe depression, is potentiated by tyrosine, supporting our hypothesis that increasing 5-HT and CA availability produces better conditions for improvement than raising 5-HT availability alone.

D. Conclusions

The only controlled study of tyrosine in depression suggests that the compound has antidepressant potential at least in outpatients with mild forms of major depressive disorder. In the few inpatients with more severe forms of major depression we have treated in an uncontrolled design, we did not observe any therapeutic effect. Three small but controlled studies indicate that the effect of 5-HT precursors

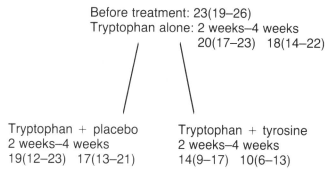

Before treatment: 23(19–26)
Tryptophan alone: 2 weeks–4 weeks
20(17–23) 18(14–22)

Tryptophan + placebo
2 weeks–4 weeks
19(12–23) 17(13–21)

Tryptophan + tyrosine
2 weeks–4 weeks
14(9–17) 10(6–13)

FIG. 17. Average Hamilton scores and range in 10 patients suffering from vital (endogenous) depression treated for 4 weeks with L-tryptophan. Subsequently 5 were treated for 4 weeks with L-tryptophan and placebo, the remaining with L-tryptophan and L-tyrosine *(unpublished results)*.

is potentiated by simultaneously administered tyrosine. This would support the hypothesis that increasing CA and 5-HT availability in the brain creates better conditions for therapeutic effects than increasing 5-HT alone. If confirmed, these data would raise questions about attempts of the pharmaceutical industry to develop compounds with specific effects on either 5-HT or CA, to heighten the drug's antidepressant potential and specificity (203).

One must keep in mind that data on tyrosine in depression are still so few, that conclusions about its therapeutic value remain premature.

VII. SIDE EFFECTS OF MONOAMINE PRECURSORS

Cole et al. (36) noted that side effects are rarely mentioned in the tryptophan/depression literature. They are probably rather few and usually mild. One cannot ignore the possibility, however, that the limited scope of many of the papers prevented the authors from discussing this issue thoroughly.

Mild gastrointestinal effects, in particular nausea, headache, and some sedation have been reported. High doses of L-tryptophan have been associated with tremor. The usual side effects of standard antidepressants, notably hypotension, impaired cardiac conduction, and parasympatholytic effects, are uncommon (12).

The literature includes rare cases of sexual excitation both in normals (149) and in depressed patients (50,92). Broadhurst and Rao (23), however, never saw that complication in 500 patients treated with L-tryptophan.

The combination of L-tryptophan with a MAOI can induce myoclonus (71). There have been reports of LSD-like psychotic reactions after this combination (188).

The only side effects of 5-HTP of practical importance are gastrointestinal in nature: nausea, vomiting, and diarrhea (174). These effects are dose dependent. Tolerance can be improved by coating the 5-HTP tablets (to prevent dissolution in the stomach), using a gradual build-up of the dosage, and simultaneous administration of a peripheral decarboxylase inhibitor (to reduce the 5-HTP dose).

The literature includes a patient with intention myoclonus who developed a scleroderma-like illness during treatment with L-5-HTP and carbidopa (176). He had received 1,400 mg L-5-HTP and 150 mg carbidopa per day over a period of 20 months. The 5-HTP dosage was significantly higher than that used in depression (50–500 mg daily). The patient had high plasma kynurenine levels, which remained high when the 5-HTP/carbidopa combination was discontinued. The levels rose further upon drug rechallenge, however, suggesting that the drug masked an abnormality in one of the enzymes that catabolizes kynurenine. Scleroderma-like syndromes have been associated with disorders of both the kynurenine and the 5-HT pathways of tryptophan metabolism.

In parkinsonian patients treated with L-DOPA, psychiatric side effects are common (113). Overall, they represent the third most common group of side effects after gastrointestinal and cardiovascular effects (74). Behavioral side effects are reported to occur in up to 36% of cases in some series (36). These effects include nightmares, depression, agitation, (hypo)mania, and psychotic episodes of a paranoid delusional type, sometimes with episodes of confusion.

Depression in DOPA-treated parkinsonian patients could conceivably be related to competitive inhibition of tryptophan or tyrosine influx into the CNS, resulting in decreased 5-HT or NE production. It is relevant in this context to note the following: Depression is frequent in parkinsonian patients. This complication is unlikely to be fully explained as a psychological reaction to a disabling disease (129). Postmortem studies have revealed not only a DA deficit but also a 5-HT deficit in the brains of parkinsonian patients (17). Accordingly, CSF 5-HIAA is decreased (111), while Mayeux et al. (128) demonstrated a correlation between lowered CSF 5-HIAA and signs of major depressive disorder in parkinsonian patients. Administering high doses of L-DOPA over long periods of time might critically lower an already marginal 5-HT supply.

In the few studies of DOPA treatment in depression, mention is made of a switch to hypomania, in particular among bipolar patients (27,139), and of the production of angry feelings and behavior (74). It should be noted that DOPA has been administered for depression only over short periods, in contrast to its use in the treatment of Parkinson's disease.

A transient elevation in blood pressure has been observed in patients treated with D,L-DOPA plus a MAOI. This occurred with doses as low as 50 mg oral DOPA. During these hypertensive episodes, sinus bradycardia also occurred (103). No side effects of significance have yet been reported after L-tyrosine administration.

VIII. OTHER POSSIBLE PSYCHIATRIC INDICATIONS FOR 5-HT PRECURSORS

A. L-Tryptophan in Aggression Disorders

Low CSF 5-HIAA concentrations, both baseline and after probenecid loading, have been reported in depression by several investigators (Fig. 18). These findings

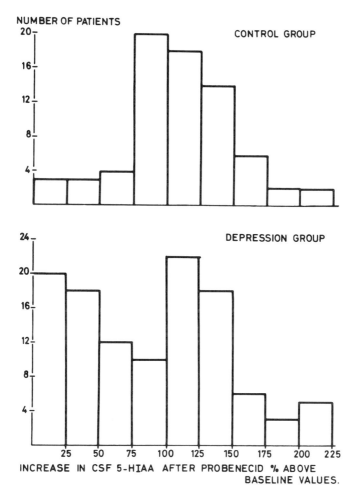

FIG. 18. Increase of CSF 5-HIAA concentration after probenecid in patients suffering from vital (endogenous) depression **(bottom)** and in a nonpsychiatric control group **(top).** The columns indicate the number of patients showing the increase in concentration given at the bottom of the column. The distribution in the depression group is bimodal. There is a significant increase in individuals with low CSF 5-HIAA. (From ref. 6, with permission.)

indicate decreased central 5-HT release or metabolism, either as a primary phe-nomenon or secondary to receptor disturbances (see Sections I and II.D). Lowered CSF 5-HIAA was found in particular in a subgroup of patients with major depressive disorders, melancholic type (197,198). Initially, no clear-cut psychopathological differences were found between patients that did or did not exhibit disturbances of central 5-HT metabolism, apart from a possible heightened anxiety level in the low 5-HIAA subgroup (14).

In 1976, Asberg et al. (7) reported that low levels of CSF 5-HIAA occurred in particular among depressed patients who had attempted suicide, often by violent means (Fig. 19). This observation has been confirmed by most (1,2,13,14,136,150,198) but not all (165) authors. Risk of violent suicide attempts has been shown to be distinctly greater in melancholic type patients with a major depressive disorder than in other depression categories (216) (Table 9). Therefore, it is impossible to decide whether the 5-HT abnormality relates to disordered regulation of aggression or of mood.

Other findings link CSF 5-HIAA and aggression. Low CSF 5-HIAA has also been reported to occur in nondepressed suicide attempters (183) and in nonde-pressed schizophrenics who had attempted suicide when ordered to do so ("voices")

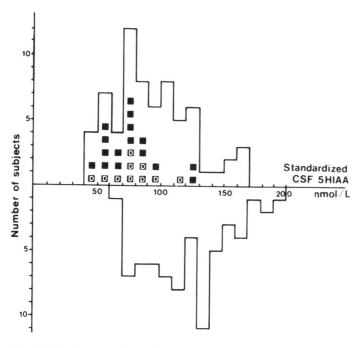

FIG. 19. Standardized concentrations of CSF 5-HIAA in patients who have attempted suicide *(upward)* and healthy volunteer control subjects *(downward)*. ■, Suicide attempts by a violent method (any method other than a drug overdose, taken by mouth, or a single wrist cut). D, a subject who subsequently died from suicide, in all cases but one within 1 year after the lumbar puncture. (From ref. 6, with permission.)

TABLE 9. *Syndromal depression diagnosis*

Suicide attempt	No.	Vital depression (n)	Other depression types (n)
Violent	31	26	5
Nonviolent	31	13	18

From ref. 216.

(145,200) (Fig. 20). Several studies found a negative correlation between CSF 5-HIAA and increased outward-directed aggression (19,25,26,116,121). The latter studies were conducted in convicted criminals (Fig. 21) and in severe borderline patients (Table 10). Finally, we compared two matched groups of patients with major depressive disorder, melancholic type, who did or did not have low postprobenecid CSF 5-HIAA levels, in terms of their ability to regulate aggression. We

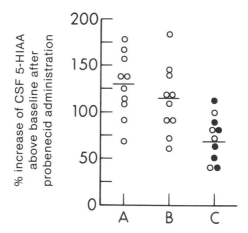

FIG. 20. Postprobenecid CSF 5-HIAA in nondepressed schizophrenic patients with (C) and without (B) suicidal histories and in nonpsychiatrically disturbed controls (A). The 5-HIAA levels in the suicidal group are significantly decreased. ○ Nonviolent suicide; ●, violent suicide. (From ref. 200, with permission.)

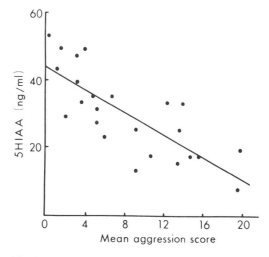

FIG. 21. Relationship of aggression scores in young military men to CSF 5-HIAA. The subjects had various personality disorders and difficulties adjusting to military life. Aggression scores showed a significant negative correlation with 5-HIAA ($r = -0.78$). (From ref. 26, with permission.)

TABLE 10. *Studies on CSF 5-HIAA and aggression[a]*

Reference	No.	Sex	Diagnosis	Measurement aggression	Assay CSF 5-HIAA	Postprobenecid or baseline 5-HIAA	Other MA metabolites in CSF
Brown et al. (26)	26	M	Personality disorder	Checklist lifetime history of aggressive acts	Flurometrically	Baseline	HVA unchanged MHPG increased
Brown et al. (25)	12	M	Borderline personality	Checklist lifetime history of aggressive acts Buss-Durkes Inventory MMPI	Mass fragmentography	Baseline	HVA unchanged MHPG unchanged
Bioulac et al. (19)	6	M	xyy Personality disorder	Lifetime history of aggressive behavior	Fluorometrically	Postprobenecid	HVA unchanged MHPG not measured
Linnoila et al. (121)[b]	36	M	Severe personality disorders	21 had killed; 15 had made attempts to kill; all were alcohol abusers	Liquid chromatography	Baseline	HVA unchanged MHPG unchanged
Lidberg et al. (116)	1 2	F M	Depression	Killed own child; subsequently attempted suicide	Not stated	Baseline	Not stated

[a]The two variables were negatively correlated in all studies.
[b]Low CSF 5-HIAA in impulsive violent offenders as opposed to those who had premeditated their acts.

found in the low 5-HIAA group not only increased suicidality but also signs of increased outward-directed aggression (204) (Table 11).

One should not overrate these findings. The biology of aggression is extremely difficult to study. This behavioral state is preeminently influenced by environmental factors, which are difficult to control in a laboratory situation. In addition, disturbances in aggression regulation are generally short lasting, in contrast to disturbances in mood regulation. Biologically, therefore, they are difficult to study.

With those restrictions in mind, we speculate that disturbed aggression regulation (and/or disturbed impulse control) is a behavioral correlate of low CSF 5-HIAA. These findings do not contradict a relationship between low CSF 5-HIAA and mood disorder. It is conceivable that disturbances in serotonin-mediated brain neurotransmission give rise to both mood and aggression dysregulation. Two observations favor this assumption. First, low CSF 5-HIAA has been found in depressed patients without suicidal histories (7,198). Second, CSF 5-HIAA values have been found to be lowest in depressed patients who had attempted suicide by violent means (183). A common factor in the brain mechanisms regulating mood and aggression would provide a biological explanation for the clinical observation that dysregulation of mood and dysregulation of aggression frequently go hand in hand (37,56,64,226).

In view of the above, it is sensible to study the antiaggressive effect of compounds, such as L-tryptophan, that increase the availability of 5-HT centrally. One preliminary study has suggested that L-tryptophan could indeed diminish the level of aggressivity in schizophrenics (137).

The second 5-HT precursor, L-5-HTP, seems to be a less suitable candidate for dealing with aggressive behaviors. It increases, as discussed below, 5-HT and CA release. The latter effects could, by increasing levels of arousal, motor activity, and initiative, overpower possibly beneficial effects of increased 5-HT availability (18).

TABLE 11. *Low 5-HIAA depressives compared to normal 5-HIAA depressives present*

Finding	*p*
More suicide attempts	<0.01
Greater number of contacts with police	<0.05
Increased arguments with	
relatives	<0.05
spouse	<0.01
colleagues	<0.05
friends	<0.05
More hostility at interview	<0.05
Impaired employment history (arguments)	<0.05

From ref. 204.

B. L-Tryptophan in Sleep Disorders and States of Hyperarousal

L--Tryptophan increases feelings of sleepiness, induces drowsiness, and reduces vigor and alertness (83,115). Since Hartmann's (80) original observation, approximately 40 relevant papers have appeared, recently reviewed by that author (81,82). The effect is dose dependent. Doses of 1 g or less may not be effective; 4 g L-tryptophan produces a definite effect. The range in between is insufficiently characterized (81). The effects of L-tryptophan are usually clearly present after 45 to 60 min and last for 2 hr (83).

L-Tryptophan, while inducing drowsiness, does not impair performance and had no effect on anxiety levels (117). These studies, however, were conducted in healthy controls in whom anxiety levels can be assumed to be low to minimal. The sedative qualities of L-tryptophan in patients suffering from anxiety disorder, or in non-psychiatric patients under severe stress, have not been studied. It would seem sensible to do so.

In addition, Hartmann et al. (84) demonstrated that L-tryptophan actually affects sleep. It reduces sleep latency and waking time while having little effect on the internal structure of sleep, i.e., on particular sleep states. Some negative reports have also appeared. In the study by Nicholson and Stone (144), test subjects had short sleep latencies (10–12 min) and almost no waking time during sleep, such that their initial values left little room for improvement (83). Despite the different methodologies used, there is overwhelming evidence that L-tryptophan can have a positive effect on sleep (Table 12).

The sleep effects are dose dependent. Doses lower than 1 g have negative or unclear effects. Higher doses usually cause positive effects. Figure 22, borrowed from Hartmann (83), depicts the effect of dose and severity of sleep disorder on the effect of L-tryptophan. It is clear that L-tryptophan is most effective in normal subjects with long sleep latencies and in mild insomnia. In more severe sleep disorders, its efficacy is less clear.

TABLE 12. *Numbers of controlled studies finding L-tryptophan versus placebo differences in five sleep-related variables*

Measure	Significant effect	Trend	No change	Opposite trend	Opposite significant effect
Reduced sleep latency	15	2	7	0	0
Reduced waking time or number of awakenings	9	3	6	0	0
Increased total sleep	8	4	7	0	0
Improvement in insomnia measures for the days after administration	3	0	0	0	0
Sleepiness scale (increased sleepiness)	2	1	1	0	0

From ref. 83.

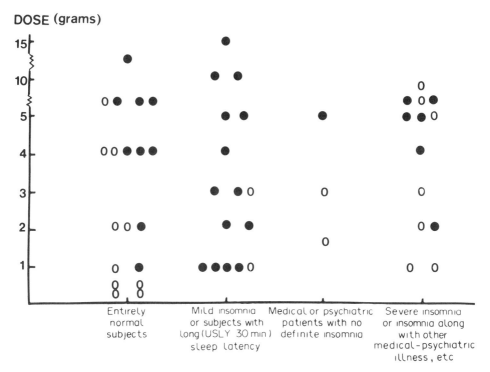

FIG. 22. Therapeutic effect of L-tryptophan *vis à vis* dose administered and severity of the insomnia. Each circle represents a study; ●,those with positive results; ○, those with negative or unclear results. (From ref. 83, with permission.)

More detailed studies of the usefulness of L-tryptophan in insomnia are indicated. How mild must a sleep disorder be in order to be responsive to L-tryptophan? Is there a subgroup of more severe insomniacs that is preferentially responsive to the amino acid? Is that subgroup characterized by disturbances in central 5-HT? This work seems all the more indicated, inasmuch as L-tryptophan may be free of hangover effects.

The mechanism by which tryptophan influences sleep has not been established. It is logical to assume that increased availability of brain 5-HT is responsible, since serotoninergic neurons participate in the regulation of sleep and since giving the tryptophan along with a dietary carbohydrate (which enhances its brain uptake) potentiates its antiinsomia effect (Wurtman, *unpublished observations*). In animals with lesioned midbrain raphe nuclei, time spent sleeping is greatly reduced. Systemic administration of parachlorophenylalanine (PCPA), an inhibitor of 5-HT synthesis, produces an even greater sleep deficit (98). Some data, however, question the view that the effects of tryptophan are mediated by 5-HT. The effects of tryptophan on sleep were not blocked by PCPA (233). Leucine, competing with tryptophan for transport into the brain, did not have an effect opposite to tryptophan

(85,86) but valine did in infants (234a). Other mechanisms could be relevant, such as decreased synthesis of DA and/or NE (via decreased access of tyrosine to the brain). In that case, tryptophan and leucine should have comparable effects on sleep variables.

The second 5-HT precursor, L-5-HTP, has hardly been studied in regard to its effects on sleep in humans. There are no indications that it increases sleepiness. The discrepancy between the two 5-HT precursors may be related to their differential effect on CA, 5-HTP increasing and tryptophan tending to decrease the release of these compounds within the CNS.

IX. SUMMARY AND CONCLUSIONS

5-HT precursors have therapeutic potential in depression, particularly in patients in whom the vital (endogenous) symptomatology is prominent. The data are most unequivocal for 5-HTP and more controversial for tryptophan.

In the only controlled comparative study of both 5-HT precursors, 5-HTP was superior to placebo; tryptophan was not. Two possible reasons for the discrepancy have been discussed: By decreasing the plasma tyrosine/LNAA ratio, tryptophan decreases tyrosine's entry in the CNS and, with that, CA synthesis. By increasing plasma kynurenine, tryptophan may also affect its own effects on brain 5-HT synthesis. Those effects could detract from the therapeutic efficacy of tryptophan. 5-HTP increases the release not only of brain 5-HT but also of CA. Tryptophan lacks the latter effect, which is likely to contribute to a lesser antidepressant potential.

If these considerations are valid, study of the combination of tryptophan and tyrosine is warranted. The first combination study of that kind indeed yielded positive results. In future studies, it will be important to monitor plasma tryptophan/LNAA and tyrosine/LNAA ratios and to titrate tryptophan and tyrosine doses in such a way that optimum entry of the MA precursor in the CNS is obtained.

In animals, brain serotonin release has been demonstrated to be involved in aggressive behaviors (186). Preliminary data indicate the same to be the case in humans, suggesting that studies on the clinical use of tryptophan in aggression disorders may be warranted. Furthermore, the therapeutic potential of L-tryptophan as a (mild) sedative and hypnotic should be explored systematically. The data available so far, although admittedly preliminary, are promising. The sedative effects of tryptophan could have been responsible for its therapeutic effects in depressed patients, as reported by some investigators. In favor of this hypothesis is the tendency for tryptophan to yield positive findings in studies involving mild depressive syndromes. (In the comparative tryptophan/5-HTP study mentioned above (202), the severity of the depression, as measured on the Hamilton scale, was considerably greater.)

The therapeutic effect of 5-HTP sometimes wears off in the second month of treatment. This effect may be related to a normalization of CA release. Combination of 5-HTP and a CA precursor, such as tyrosine, is warranted. Preliminary data tend to confirm this theoretical notion.

Another way to increase the yield of 5-HT precursor treatment is to differentiate patients with and without signs of disturbed central 5-HT metabolism, under the assumption that the former category will be more likely to be responsive. Few studies of that kind have been conducted, using postprobenecid CSF 5-HIAA accumulation and the plasma tryptophan/LNAA ratio as 5-HT indicators. The results are promising, in that these 5-HT-related variables seem to predict treatment outcome. These studies should be repeated and extended.

L-DOPA has been largely overlooked in depression studies, although the indications are strong that it merits consideration as an activating agent in retarded depression. Adding a 5-HT precursor might potentiate its mood-elevating efficacy. Further studies of L-DOPA alone and combined with a 5-HT precursor are needed.

The study of L-tyrosine in depression is in its infancy. Some preliminary data indicate that this amino acid can be of value in mild depression. The indications that it can potentiate the antidepressant effects of 5-HTP or tryptophan are somewhat stronger.

In summary, it is particularly the mixture of 5-HT and CA precursors that merits further study. All available evidence points in that direction. Thus far, MA precursors have been mainly studied in depressive disorders. Sufficient evidence exists to warrant systematic study of 5-HT precursors, in particular tryptophan, as possible antiaggression and tranquilizing/hypnotic agents.

Finally, the study of MA precursors in depression suggests increase of 5-HT and CA availability in the brain to provide the best conditions for antidepressant effects. It is argued that the tendency of pharmaceutical research to develop antidepressants with ever-increasing MA specificity is probably ill-advised. "Broad-spectrum antidepressants" are more desirable.

REFERENCES

1. Agren, H. (1980): Symptom patterns in unipolar and bipolar depression correlating with monoamine metabolism in the cerebrospinal fluid. *Psychiatr. Res.*, 3:225.
2. Agren, H. (1983): Life at risk: Markers of suicidality in depression. *Psychiatr. Dev.*, 1:87.
3. Alpert, M., Friedhoff, A. J., Marcos, L. R., and Diamond, F. (1978): Paradoxical reaction to L-dopa in schizophrenia patients. *Am. J. Psychiatry*, 135(11):1329–1332.
4. Angrist, B., Sathananthan, G., and Gershon, S. (1973): Behavioral effects of L-dopa in schizophrenia patients. *Psychopharmacologia*, 1:1–12.
5. Angst, J., Woggon, B., and Schoepf, J. (1977): The treatment of depression with L-5-hydroxytryptophan versus imipramine. *Arch. Psychiatr. Nervenkr.*, 224:175–186.
6. Asberg, M., Bertilsson, L., Martensson, B., Scalia-Tomba, G.-P., Thoren, P., and Traskman, L. (1984): CSF monoamine metabolites in melancholia. *Acta Psychiatr. Scand.*, 69:201–219.
7. Asberg, M., Traskman, L., and Thoren, P. (1976): Serotonin depression: A biochemical subgroup within the affective disorders? *Science*, 131:478–480.
8. Awazi, N., and Goldberg, H. C. (1978): On the interaction of 5-hydroxytryptophan and 5-hydroxytryptamine with dopamine metabolism in rat striatum. *Naunyn Schmeidebergs Arch. Pharmacol.*, 303:63–72.
9. Axelrod, J. (1972): Dopamine-beta-hydroxylase: Regulation of its synthesis and release from nerve terminals. *Pharmacol. Rev.*, 24:233–243.
10. Ayuso Gutierrez, J. L., and Lopez-Ibor, J. J. (1971): Tryptophan and an MAOI (Nialamide) in the treatment of depression. A double-blind study. *Int. Pharmacopsychiatry*, 6:92–97.
11. Baldessarini, R. J. (1983): *Biomedical Aspects of Depression*. American Academic Press, New York.

12. Baldessarini, R. J. (1984): Treatment of depression by altering monoamine metabolism: Precursors and metabolic inhibitors. *Psychopharmacol. Bull.*, 20:224–239.
13. Banki, C. M., and Arato, M. (1983): Amine metabolites and neuroendocrine responses related to depression and suicide. *J. Affective Disord.*, 5:223.
14. Banki, C. M., Molnar, G., and Vojnik, M. (1981): Cerebrospinal fluid amine metabolites, tryptophan and clinical parameters in depression: Psychopathological symptoms. *J. Affective Disord.*, 3:91.
15. Bartlet, P., and Pailard, P. (1973): Etude clinique du 5-hydroxytryptophane dans les etats depressifs du troisieme age. *Cah. Med. Lyon.*, 50:1985–1901.
16. Beitman, B. D., and Dunner, D. L. (1982): L-Tryptophan in the maintenance treatment of bipolar II manic-depressive illness. *Am. J. Psychiatry*, 139:1498–1499.
17. Bernheimer, H., Birkmayer, W., and Hornykiewicz, O. (1961): Verteilung des 5-hydroxytryptamine (serotonin) in Gehirn des Menschen und sem Verhalters bei Patients mit Parkinson-Syndrome. *Klin. Wirh.*, 39:1056–1059.
18. Bigelow, L. B., Walls, P., Gillin, J. C., and Wyatt, R. J. (1979): Clinical effects of L-5-hydroxytryptophan administration in chronic schizophrenic patients. *Biol. Psychiatry*, 14(1):53–67.
19. Bioulac, B., Benezich, M., Renaud, B., Noel, B., and Roche, D. (1980): Serotonergic functions in the 47, XYZ syndrome. *Biol. Psychiatry*, 15:917.
20. Bowers, M. B. (1970): Cerebrospinal fluid 5-hydroxyindoles and behavior after L-tryptophan and pyridoxine administration to psychiatric patients. *Neuropharmacology*, 9:599–604.
21. Brewerton, T. D., and Reus, V. I. (1983): Lithium carbonate and L-tryptophan in the treatment of bipolar and schizoaffective disorders. *Am. J. Psychiatry*, 140:757–760.
22. Broadhurst, A. D. (1970): L-tryptophan versus ECT. *Lancet*, I:1392–1393.
23. Broadhurst, A. D., and Rao, B. (1977): L-tryptophan and sexual behavior. *Br. Med. J.*, I:51–52.
24. Brodie, H. K. H., Sack, R., and Siever, L. (1973): Clinical studies of L-5-hydroxytryptophan in depression. In: *Serotonin and Behavior*, edited by J. Barchas and E. Usdin, pp. 549–559. Academic Press, New York.
25. Brown, G. L., Ebert, M. E., Goyer, P. F., Jimerson, D. C., Klein, W. J., Bunney, W. E., and Goodwin, F. K. (1982): Aggression, suicide, and serotonin: Relationships to CSF amine metabolites. *Am. J. Psychiatry*, 139:741.
26. Brown, G. L., Goodwin, F. K., Ballenger, J. C., Goyer, P. F., and Major, L. F. (1979): Aggression in humans correlates with cerebrospinal fluid metabolites. *Psychiatr. Res.*, 1:131.
27. Bunney, W. E., Brodie, H. K. H., Murphy, D. L., and Goodwin, F. K. (1971): Studies of alpha-methyl-para-tyrosine, L-dopa, and L-tryptophan in depression and mania. *Am. J. Psychiatry*, 127:872–881.
28. Calil, H. M., Yesavage, J. A., and Hollister, L. E. (1977): Low dose levodopa in schizophrenia. *Commun. Psychopharmacol.*, 1:593–596.
29. Carlsson, A., and Lindquist, M. (1978): Effects of antidepressant agents on the synthesis of brain monoamines. *J. Neural Transm.*, 42:73–91.
30. Carroll, B. J. (1972): Monoamine precursors in the treatment of depression. *Clin. Pharmacol. Ther.*, 12:743–761.
31. Carroll, B. J., Mowbray, R. M., and Davies, B. (1970): Sequential comparison of L-tryptophan with ECT in severe depression. *Lancet*, I:967–969.
32. Chambers, C. A., and Naylor, G. J. (1978): A controlled trial of L-tryptophan in mania. *Br. J. Psychiatry*, 132:555–559.
33. Chouinard, G., Jones, B. D., Young, S. N., and Annable, L. (1979): Potentiation of lithium by tryptophan in a patient with bipolar illness. *Am. J. Psychiatry*, 136:719–720.
34. Chouinard, G., Young, S. N., and Annable, L. (1985): A controlled clinical trial of L-tryptophan in acute mania. *Biol. Psychiatry (in press)*.
35. Chouinard, G., Young, S. N., Annable, L., and Sourkes, T. L. (1979): Tryptophan-nicotinamide, imipramine and their combination in depression. *Acta Psychiatr. Scand.*, 59:395–414.
36. Cole, J. O., Hartmann, E., and Brigham, P. (1980): L-tryptophan: Clinical studies. *McLean Hosp. J.*, 1:37–71.
37. Conte, H. R., and Plutchik, R. (1974): Personality and background characteristics of suicidal mental patients. *J. Psychiatr. Res.*, 10:181.
38. Cooper, A. J., and Datta, S. R. (1980): A placebo controlled evaluation of L-tryptophan in depression in the elderly. *Can. J. Psychiatry*, 25:386–390.

39. Coppen, A., Shaw, D. M., and Farrell, J. P. (1963): Potentiation of the antidepressive effect of a monoamine-oxidase inhibitor by tryptophan. *Lancet*, i:79–80.
40. Coppen, A., Shaw, D. M., Herzberg, B., and Maggs, R. (1967): Tryptophan in the treatment of depression. *Lancet*, ii:1178–1180.
41. Coppen, A., Whybrow, P. C., Noguera, R., Maggs, R., and Prange, A. J. (1972): The comparative antidepressant value of L-tryptophan and imipramine with and without attempted potentiation by liothyronine. *Arch. Gen. Psychiatry*, 26:234–241.
42. Cowdry, R. W., Ebert, M. H., van Kammen, D. P., Post, R. M., and Goodwin, F. K. (1983): Cerebrospinal fluid probenecid studies: A reinterpretation. *Biol. Psychiatry*, 18:1287–1299.
43. Cowen, P. J., Grahame-Smith, D. G., Green, A. R., and Heal, D. J. (1982): β-adrenoceptor agonists enhance 5-hydroxytryptamine-mediated behavioral responses. *Br. J. Pharmacol.*, 76:265–270.
44. D'Elia, G., Lehmann, J., and Raotma, H. (1977): Evaluation of the combination of tryptophan and ECT in the treatment of depression. 1.Clinical analysis. *Acta Psychiatr. Scand.*, 56:303–318.
45. De Wilde, J. E. M., and Doogan, D. P. (1982): Fluvoxamine and chlorimipramine in endogenous depression. *J. Affective Disord.*, 4:249–259.
46. *Diagnostic and Statistical Manual of Mental Disorders (DSM III)* (1980): 3rd edition, edited by J. B. W. Williams. American Psychiatric Association, Washington, D.C.
47. Dunner, D. L., and Fieve, R. R. (1975): Affective disorder: Studies with amine precursors. *Am. J. Psychiatry*, 132:180–183.
48. Dunner, D. L., and Goodwin, F. K. (1972): Effect of L-tryptophan on brain serotonin metabolism in depressed patients. *Arch. Gen. Psychiatry*, 26:364–366.
49. Ebert, M. H., Kartzinel, R., Cowdry, R. W., and Goodwin, F. K. (1980): Cerebrospinal fluid amine metabolites and the probenecid test. In: *Neurobiology of CSF*, edited by J. U. Wood. Plenum, New York.
50. Egan, G., and Hammand, G. (1976): Sexual disinhibition with L-tryptophan. *Br. Med. J.*, 2:701.
51. Everett, G. M. (1979): Effects of 5-hydroxytryptophan on brain levels of monoamines and the dopamine metabolite DOPAC. In: *Catecholamines: Basic and Clinical Frontiers*, edited by E. Usdin, I. J. Kopin, and J. Barchas. Pergamon, New York.
52. Everett, G. M., and Borcherding, J. W. (1970): L-Dopa: Effect on concentrations of dopamine, norepinephrine, and serotonin in brain of mice. *Science*, 168:849–850.
53. Farkas, T., Dunner, D. L., and Fieve, R. R. (1976): L-Tryptophan in depression. *Biol. Psychiatry*, 11:295–302.
54. Fernstrom, J. D., and Wurtman, R. J. (1971): Brain serotonin content: Physiological dependence of plasma tryptophan levels. *Science*, 173:149–152.
55. Fernstrom, J. D., and Wurtman, R. J. (1972): Brain serotonin content: Physiological regulation by plasma neutral amino acids. *Science*, 178:414–416.
56. Freud, S. (1956): Mourning and melancholia. In: *Collected Papers*, edited by J. E. London. Hogarth Press, pp. 237–259.
57. Friedman, P. A., Kappelman, A. H., and Kaufman, S. (1972): Partial purification and characterization of tryptophan hydroxylase from rabbit hindbrain. *J. Biol. Chem.*, 247:4165–4173.
58. Fujiwara, J., and Otsuki, S. (1974): Subtypes of affective psychoses classified by response in amine precursors and monoamine metabolism. *Folia Psychiatr. Neurol. Jpn.*, :93.
59. Fuxe, K., Butcher, L. L., and Engel, J. (1971): DL-5-hydroxytryptophan-induced changes in central monoamine neurons after peripheral decarboxylase inhibition. *J. Pharmacol.*, 23:420–424.
60. Gelenberg, A. J., Gibson, C. J., and Wojcik, J. D. (1982): Neurotransmitter precursors for the treatment of depression. *Psychopharmacol. Bull.*, 18:7–18.
61. Gelenberg, A. J., Wojcik, J. D., Gibson, C. J., and Wurtman, R. J. (1982): Tyrosine for the treatment of depression. In: *Research Strategies for Assessing the Behavioral Effects of Foods and Nutrients*, edited by H. R. Lieberman and R. J. Wurtman. Proceedings of a conference held at the Massachusetts Institute of Technology, Cambridge.
62. Gelenberg, A. J., Wojcik, J. D., Growdon, J. H., Sved, A. F., and Wurtman, R. J. (1980): Tyrosine for the treatment of depression. *Am. J. Psychiatry*, 137:622–623.
63. Gerlach, J., and Luhdorf, K. (1975): The effect of L-dopa on young patients with simple schizophrenia, treated with neuroleptic drugs. *Psychopharmacologia*, 44:105–110.
64. Gershon, E. S., Cromer, M., and Klerman, G. L. (1968): Hostility and depression. *Psychiatry*, 31:224.

65. Gershon, E. S., Goodwin, F. K., and Gold, P. (1970): Effects of L-tyrosine and L-dopa on norepinephrine (NE) turnover in rat brain in vivo. *Pharmacologist*, 12:268.
66. Gibson, C. J. (1983): Control of monoamine synthesis by amino acid precursors. In: *Management of Depression with Monomaine Precursors*, edited by H. M. van Praag and J. Mendlewicz. Karger, Basel.
67. Gibson, C. J., and Wurtman, R. J. (1977): Physiological control of brain catechol synthesis by brain tyrosine concentration. *Biochem. Pharmacol.*, 26:1137–1142.
68. Gibson, C. J., and Wurtman, R. J. (1978): Physiological control of brain norepinephrine synthesis by brain tyrosine concentration. *Life Sci.*, 22:1399–1406.
69. Gillin, J., Kaplan, J., and Wyatt, R. (1976): Clinical effects of tryptophan in chronic schizophrenic patients. *Biol. Psychiatry*, 11:635–639.
70. Glaeser, B. S., Melamed, E., Growdon, J. H., and Wurtman, R. J. (1979): Elevation of plasma tyrosine after a single oral dose of L-tyrosine, *Life Sci.*, 25:265–272.
71. Glassman, A. H., and Platman, S. (1969): Potentiation of a monoamine oxidase inhibitor by tryptophan. *J. Psychiatr. Res.*, 7:83–88.
72. Goldberg, I. K. (1980): L-Tyrosine in depression. *Lancet*, I:364.
73. Goodwin, F. K., and Bunney, W. E. (1973): A psychobiological approach to affective illness. *Psychiatric Annals*, 3:49–56.
74. Goodwin, F. K., Murphy, D. L., Brodie, H. K. H., and Bunney, W. E. (1971): Levo-Dopa: Alterations in behavior. *Clin. Pharmacol. Ther.*, 12:383–396.
75. Green, A. R., and Aronson, J. K. (1983): The pharmacokinetics of oral L-tryptophan: Effects of dose and of concomitant pyridozine, allopurinol or nicotinamide administration. *Adv. Biol. Psychiatry*, 10:67–81.
76. Green, A. R., Bloomfield, M. R., Woods, H. F., and Seed, M. (1978): Metabolism of an oral tryptophan load by women and evidence against the induction of tryptophan pyrrolase by oral contraceptives. *Br. J. Clin. Pharmacol.*, 5:233–241.
77. Green, H., Greenberg, S. M., and Erickson, R. W. (1962): Effect of dietary phenylalanine and tryptophan upon the rat brain amine levels. *J. Pharmacol. Exp. Ther.*, 136:174–178.
78. Growdon, J. H., Melamed, E., Logue, M., Hefti, F., and Wurtman, R. J. (1982): Effects of oral L-tyrosine administration on CSF tyrosine and homovanillic acid levels in patients with Parkinson's Disease. *Life Sci.*, 30:827–832.
79. Hanh Le Quan-Bui, K., Plaisant, O., Leboyer, M., Gay, C., Kamal, L., Devynck, M-A., and Meyer, P. (1984): Reduced platelet serotonin in depression. *Psychiatr. Res.*, 13:129–139.
80. Hartmann, E. (1967): The effect of L-tryptophan on the sleep-dream cycle in man. *Psychosom. Sci.*, 8:479–480.
81. Hartmann, E. (1979): L-Tryptophan as a hypnotic agent: A review. *Waking Sleep*, 1:155–161.
82. Hartmann, E. (1981): Tryptophan and sleep: Who responds to tryptophan? *Biol. Psychiatry*, 613–621.
83. Hartmann, E. (1982/1983): Effects of L-tryptophan on sleepiness and on sleep. *J. Psychiatr. Res.*, 17:107–113.
84. Hartmann, E., Chung, R., and Chien, C. (1971): L-tryptophan and sleep. *Psychopharmacologia*, 19:114–127.
85. Hartmann, E., and Cravens, J. (1976): Amino acids and human sleep: The effects of L-tryptophan, glycine, L-leucine and placebo. *Sleep Res.*, 5:54.
86. Hartmann, E., Spinweber, C. L., and Ware, C. (1976): L-tryptophan, L-leucine, and placebo: Effects on subjective alertness. *Sleep Res.*, 5:57.
87. Hedaya, R. J. (1984): Pharmacokinetic factors in the clinical use of tryptophan. *J. Clin. Psychopharmacol.*, 4:347–348.
88. Heel, R. C., Morley, P. A., Brogden, R. N., Carmine, A. A., Speight, T. M., and Avery, G. S. (1982): Zimelidine: A review of its pharmacological properties and therapeutic efficacy in depressive illness. *Drugs*, 24:169–206.
89. Heninger, G. R., Charney, D. S., and Sternberg, D. E. (1984): Serotonergic function in depression. *Arch. Gen. Psychiatry*, 41:398–402.
90. Herrington, R. N., Bruce, A., Johnstone, E. C., and Lader, M. H. (1974): Comparative trial of L-tryptophan and ECT in severe depressive illness. *Lancet*, ii:731–734.
91. Herrington, R. N., Bruce, A., Johnstone, E. C., and Lader, M. H. (1976): Comparative trial of L-tryptophan and amitriptyline in depression illnesses. *Psychol. Med.*, 6:673–678.
92. Hullin, R., and Jarram, T. (1976): Sexual disinhibition with L-tryptophan. *Br. Med. J.*, 2:1010.

93. Inanaga, K., and Tanaka, M. (1973): Effects of L-dopa on schizophrenia. In: *Sexual Disorders and Drug Abuse*, edited by T. A. Ban, et al., pp. 229–233. Amsterdam, North-Holland Publishing Co.

94. Jaeger, C. B., Teitelman, G., Joh, T. H., Albert, V. R., Park, D. H., and Reis, D. J. (1983): Some neurons of the rat central nervous system contain aromatic-L-amino acid decarboxylase but not monoamine. *Science*, 219:1233–1235.

95. Janowsky, A., Okada, F., Manier, D. H., Applegate, C. D., Sulser, F., and Steranka, L. R. (1982): Role of serotonergic input in the regulation of the β-adrenergic receptor-coupled adenylate cyclase system. *Science*, 218:900–901.

96. Jensen, K., Freunsgaard, K., Ahlfors, U. G., Pinkanen, T. A., Tuomikoski, S., Ose, E., Dencker, S. J., Lindberg, D., and Nagy, A. (1975): Tryptophan/imipramine in depression. *Lancet*, i:920.

97. Jouvent, R., Rodier, C., Baruch, P., Hardy, M. C., Lemperiere, T., and Widlocher, D. (1984): Indalpine, a specific 5-HT uptake inhibitor, in delusional depression. *Psychiatr. Res.*, 11:365–366.

98. Jouvet, M. (1977): Neuropharmacology of the sleep-waking cycle. In: *Handbook of Psychopharmacology*, edited by L. L. Iversen, S. D. Iversen, and S. U. Snyder. Plenum, New York, pp. 187–276.

99. Kaneko, M., Kumashiro, H., Takahashi, Y., and Hoshino, Y. (1979): L-5-HTP treatment and serum 5-HT level after L-5-HTP loading on depressed patients. *Neuropsychobiology*, 5:232.

100. Karobath, M., Diaz, J. L., and Huttunen, M. O. (1971): The effect of L-dopa on the concentrations of tryptophan, tyrosine, and serotonin in the rat brain. *Eur. J. Pharmacol.*, 14:393–396.

101. Kirkgaard, C., Møller, S. E., and Bjørum, N. (1978): Addition of L-tryptophan to electroconvulsive treatment in endogenous depression. A double-blind study. *Acta Psychiatr. Scand.*, 58:457–462.

102. Klein, D. F., Gittelman, R., Quitkin, F., and Rifkin, A. (1980): *Diagnosis and Drug Therapy of Psychiatric Disorders: Adults and Children*, 2nd edition. Williams & Wilkins, Baltimore.

103. Klerman, G. L., Schildkraut, J. J., Hasenbush, L. L., Greenblatt, M., and Friend, D. G. (1963): Clinical experience with dihydroxyphenylalanine (DOPA). *J. Psychiatr. Res.*, 1:289–297.

104. Kline, N. S., and Sacks, W. (1963): Relief of depression within one day using an MAO inhibitor and intravenous 5-HTP. *Am. J. Psychiatry*, 120:274–275.

105. Kline, N. S., Sacks, W., and Simpson, G. M. (1964): Further studies on one day treatment of depression with 5-HTP. *Am. J. Psychiatry*, 121:379–381.

106. Kline, N. S., and Shah, B. K. (1973): Comparable therapeutic efficacy of tryptophan and imipramine: Average therapeutic ratings versus "true" equivalence. An important difference. *Curr. Ther. Res.*, 15:484–487.

107. Knox, W. E. (1951): Two mechanisms which increase in vivo the liver tryptophan peroxidase activity: Specific enzyme adaption and stimulation of the pituitary adrenal system. *Br. J. Exp. Pathol.*, 32:462–469.

108. Knox, W. E., and Auerbach, V. H. (1955): The hormonal control of tryptophan peroxidase in the rat. *J. Biol. Chem.*, 214:307–313.

109. Korf, J., and van Praag, H. M. (1971): Amine metabolism in the human brain: Further evaluation of the probenecid test. *Brain Res.*, 35:221–230.

110. Korf, J., Venema, K., and Postema, F. (1974): Decarboxylation of exogenous L-5-hydroxytryptophan after destruction of the cerebral raphe system. *J. Neurochem.*, 23:249–252.

111. Lakke, J. P. W. F., Korf, J., van Praag, H. M., and Schut, T. (1972): Predictive value of the probenecid test for the effect of L-dopa therapy in Parkinson's Disease. *Nature [New Biol.]*, 236:208–209.

112. Langer, S. Z., and Briley, M. (1981): High-affinity ^{3}H-imipramine binding: A new biological tool for studies in depression. *Trends Neurosci.*, 4:28.

113. Langrall, H. M., and Joseph, C. (1972): State of the clinical evaluation of L-dopa in the treatment of Parkinson's disease and syndrome. *Clin. Pharmacol. Ther.*, 12:323–331.

114. Lauer, J. W., Inskip, W. M., Bernsohn, J., and Zeller, E. A. (1958): Observations on schizophrenic patients after iproniazid and tryptophan. *Arch Neurol. Psychiatry*, 80:122–130.

115. Leathwood, P. D., and Pollet, P. (1982/1983): Diet-induced mood changes in normal populations. *J. Psychiatr. Res.*, 17:147–154.

116. Lidberg, L., Asberg, M., and Sundqvist-Stensman, U. B. (1984): 5-Hydroxyindoleacetic acid levels in attempted suicides who have killed their children. *Lancet*, ii:928–929.

117. Lieberman, H. R., Corkin, S., Spring, B. J., Growdon, J. H., and Wurtman, R. J. (1982/1983):

Mood, performance, and pain sensitivity: Changes induced by food constituents. *J. Psychiatr. Res.*, 17:135–145.

118. Lindberg, D., Ahlfors, U. G., Dencker, S. J., Fruensgaard, K., Hansten, S., Jensen, K., Ose, E., and Pinkanes, T. A. (1979): Symptom reduction in depression after treatment with L-tryptophan or imipramine. *Acta Psychiatr. Scand.*, 60:287–294.

119. Lindstrom, L. H. (1985): Low HVA and normal 5-HIAA CSF levels in drug free schizophrenic patients compared to healthy volunteers: Correlations to symptomatology and heredity. *Psychiatry Res.*, 14:265–274

120. Linnoila, M., Seppala, T., Mattila, M. J., Vihko, R., Pakarinen, A., and Skinner, J. T. (1980): Clomipramine and dexepin in depressive neurosis. *Arch. Gen. Psychiatry*, 37:1295–1299.

121. Linnoila, M., Virkkunen, M., Scheinin, M., Nuutila, A., Rimon, R., and Goodwin, F. K. (1983): Low cerebrospinal fluid 5-hydroxyindoleacetic acid concentration differentiates impulsive violent behavior. *Life Sci.*, 33:2609–2614.

122. Lopez-Ibor Alino, J. J., Ayuso Guttierrez, J. L., and Iglesisa, M. L. M. M. (1976): 5-Hydroxy-tryptophan (5-HTP) and a MAO I (nialamide) in the treatment of depression. A double-blind controlled study. *Int. Pharmacopsychiatry*, II:8–15.

123. Lopez-Ibor Alino, J. J., Ayuso Guttierrez, J. L., and Montejo, M. L. (1973): Tryptophan and amitriptyline in the treatment of depression. A double-blind study. *Int. Pharmacopsychiatry*, 8:145–151.

124. Lovenberg, W., Weissbach, H., and Undenfriend, S. (1962): Aromatic L-amino acid decarboxylase. *J. Biol. Chem.*, 237:89–93.

125. MacSweeney, D. A. (1975): Treatment of unipolar depression. *Lancet*, ii:510–511.

126. Madras, B. K., Cohen, E. L., Fernstrom, J. D., Larin, F., Muncro, H. N., and Wurtman, R. J. (1973): Dietary carbohydrate increases brain tryptophan and decreases free plasma tryptophan. *Nature*, 244:34–35.

127. Matussek, N., Angst, J., Benkert, O., Gmur, N., Papousek, M., Ruther, E., and Woggon, B. (1974): The effect of L-5-hydroxytryptophan alone and in combination with a decarboxylase inhibitor (Ro 4-4602) in depressive patients. *Adv. Biochem. Psychopharmacol.*, 11:399.

128. Mayeux, R., Stern, Y., Cote., L., and Williams, J. B. W. (1984): Altered serotonin metabolism in depressed patients with Parkinson's disease. *Neurology*, 34:(5)642–646.

129. Mayeux, R., Stern, Y., Rosen, J., and Leventhal, J. (1981): Depression, intellectual impairment and Parkinson's disease. *Neurology*, 31:645–650.

130. Melamed, E., Hefti, F., and Wurtman, R. J. (1980): Tyrosine administration increases striatal dopamine release in rats with partial nigrostriatal lesions. *N.Y. Acad. Sci.*, 77:4305–4309.

131. Mendels, J., Stinnett, J. L., Burns, D., and Frazer, A. (1975): Amine precursors and depression. *Arch. Gen. Psychiatry*, 32:22–30.

132. Mendlewicz, J., and Youdim, M. B. H. (1980): Antidepressant potentiation of 5-hydroxytryptophan by L-deprenil in affective illness. *J. Affective Disord.*, 2:137–146.

133. Mindham, R. H. S., Marsden, C. D., and Parkes, J. D. (1976): Psychiatric symptoms during L-dopa therapy for Parkinson's disease and their relationship to physical disability. *Psychol. Med.*, 6:23–33.

134. Møller, S. E., Kirk, L., Brandup, E., Hollnagel, M., Kaldan, B., and Ødum, K. (1983): Tryptophan availability in endogenous depression—relation to efficacy of L-tryptophan treatment. *Adv. Biol. Psychiatry*, 10:30–46.

135. Møller, S. E., Kirk, L., and Fremming, K. H. (1976): Plasma amino acids as an index for subgroups in manic-depressive psychosis: Correlation to effect of tryptophan. *Psychopharmacologia*, 49:205–213.

136. Montgomery, S. A., and Montgomery, D. (1982): Pharmacological prevention of suicidal behavior. *J. Affective Disord.*, 4:291.

137. Morand, C., Young, S. N., and Ervin, F. R. (1983): Clinical response of aggressive schizophrenics to oral tryptophan. *Biol. Psychiatry*, 18:575–578.

138. Murphy, D. L., Baker, M., Goodwin, F. K., Miller, H., Kotkin, J., and Bunney, W. E. (1974): L-Tryptophan in affective disorders: Indoleamine changes and differential clinical effects. *Psychopharmacologia*, 34:11–20.

139. Murphy, D. L., Goodwin, F. K., Brodie, H. K. H., and Bunney, W. E. (1973): L-dopa, dopamine, and hypomania. *Am. J. Psychiatry*, 130:79–82.

140. Nagatsu, T., Levitt, M., and Underfriend, S. (1964): Tyrosine hydroxylase: The initial step in norepinephrine biosynthesis. *J. Biol. Chem.*, 239:2910–2917.

141. Nakajima, T., Kudo, Y., and Kaneko, A. (1978): Clinical evaluation of 5-hydroxy-L-tryptophan as an antidepressant drug. *Folia Psychiatr. Neurol. Jpn.*, 32:223.
142. Nardini, M., DeStafano, R., Iannuccelli, M., Borghesi, R., and Battistini, N. (1983): Treatment of depression with L-5-hydroxytryptophan combined with chlorimipramine, a double-blind study. *Int. J. Clin. Pharmacol. Res.*, III:239–250.
143. Ng, K. Y., Chase, T. N., Colburn, R. W., and Kopin, I. J. (1970): L-Dopa induced release of cerebral monoamines. *Science*, 170:76–77.
144. Nicholson, A. N., and Stone, B. M. (1979): L-Tryptophan and sleep in healthy man. *Electroencephalogr. Clin. Neurophysiol.*, 47:539–545.
145. Ninan, P. T., van Kammen, D. P., Scheinin, M., Linnoila, M., Bunney, W. E., and Goodwin, F. K. (1984): CSF 5-hydroxyindoleacetic acid levels in suicidal schizophrenic patients. *Am. J. Psychiatry*, 141:(4)566–569.
146. Norman, T. R., Burrows, G. D., Marriot, P. F., McIntyre, I. M., Davies, B. M., and Moore, R. G. (1983): Zimelidine: A placebo-controlled trial in depression. *Psychiatr. Res.*, 8:95–103.
147. Ogren, S-O., Holm, A-C., Hall, H., and Lindberg, U. H. (1984): Alaproclate, a new selective 5-HT uptake inhibitor with therapeutic potential in depression and senile dementia. *J. Neural Transm.*, 59:265–288.
148. Ogura, C., Kishimoto, A., and Nakao, T. (1976): Clinical effect of L-dopa on schizophrenia. *Curr. Ther. Res.*, 20:(3)308–318.
149. Oswald, I., Ashcroft, G., Berger, R., Eccleston, D., Evans, J. F., and Thacore, V. R. (1966): Some experiments in the chemistry of normal sleep. *Br. J. Psychiatry*, 112:391–399.
150. Palaniappan, V., Ramachandran, V., and Somasundaram, O. (1983): Suicidal ideation and biogenic amines in depression. *Indian J. Psychiatry*, 25:286–292.
151. Pare, C. M. B. (1963): Potentiation of monoamine-oxidase inhibitors by tryptophan. *Lancet*, ii:527–528.
152. Pederson, O. L., Kragh-Sørensen, P., Bjerre, M., Overø, K. F., and Gram, L. F. (1982): Citalopram, a selective serotonin reuptake inhibitor: Clinical antidepressive and long-term effect—a phase II study. *Psychopharmacology*, 77:199–204.
153. Persson, T., and Walinder, J. (1971): L-dopa in the treatment of depressive symptoms. *Br. J. Psychiatry*, 119:277–278.
154. Pollin, W., Cardon, P. V., and Kety, S. S. (1961): Effects of amino acid feedings in schizophrenic patients treated with iproniazid. *Science*, 133:104–105.
155. Prange, A. J., Wilson, I. C., Lynn, C. W., Alltop, L. B., and Stikeleather, R. A. (1974): L-Tryptophan in mania. *Arch. Gen. Psychiatry*, 30:56–62.
156. Puhringe, W., Wirx-Justice, A., Graw, P., Lacoste, V., and Gastpar, M. (1976): Intravenous L-5-hydroxytryptophan in normal subjects: An interdisciplinary precursor loading study. I. Implication of reproducible mood elevation. *Pharmakopsychiatrie*, 9:260–268.
157. Quadbeck, H., Lehmann, E., and Tegeler, J. (1984): Comparison of the antidepressant action of tryptophan, tryptophan/5-hydroxytryptophan combination and nomifensine. *Neuropsychobiology*, 11:111–115.
158. Rao, B., and Broadhurst, A. D. (1976): Tryptophan and depression. *Br. Med. J.*, I:460.
159. Rasmussin, D. D., Ishizuka, B., Quigley, M. E., and Yen, S. S. C. (1983): Effects of tyrosine and tryptophan ingestion on plasma catecholamine and 3,4-dihydroxyphenylacetic acid concentrations. *J. Clin. Endocrinol. Metab.*, 57:760–763.
160. Reinhard, J. F., Galloway, M. P., and Roth, R. H. (1983): Noradrenergic modulation of serotonin synthesis and metabolism. II. Stimulation by 3-isobutyl-1-methylxanthine. *J. Pharmacol. Exp. Ther.*, 226:764.
161. *Research Diagnostic Criteria for a Selected Group of Functional Disorders* (1978): Edited by R. L. Spitzer, J. Endicott, and E. Robins. New York Psychiatric Institute, New York.
162. Rieder, E. R. (1980): L-Dopa competes with tyrosine and tryptophan for human brain uptake. *Nutr. Metab.*, 24:417–423.
163. Roos, B. E. (1976): Tryptophan, 5-hydroxytryptophan and tricyclic antidepressants in the treatment of depression. *Monogr. Neural Sci.*, 3:23–25.
164. Rotman, A. (1983): Blood platelets in psychopharmacological research. *Prog. Neuropsychopharmacol. Biol. Psychiatry*, 7:135–151.
165. Roy-Byrne, P., Post, R. M., Rubinow, D. R., Linnoila, M., Savard, R., and Davis, D. (1983): CSF 5-HIAA and personal and family history of suicide in affectively ill patients: A negative study. *Psychiatr. Res.*, 10:263–274.

166. Rudorfer, M. V., Scheinin, M., Karoum, F., Ross, R. J., Potter, W. Z., and Linnoila, M. (1984): Reduction of norepinephrine turnover by serotonergic drugs in man. *Biol. Psychiat.*, 19:179–193.
167. Sachar, E. J., Hellman, L., Roffwarg, H. P., Halpern, F. S., Fukushima, D. K., and Gallagher, T. F. (1973): Disrupted 24-hour patterns of cortisol secretion in psychotic depression. *Arch. Gen. Psychiatry*, 28:19–24.
168. Sano, I. (1972): L-5-Hydroxytryptophan (L-5-HTP) therapy. *Folia Psychiatr. Neurol. Jpn.*, 26:7.
169. Scally, M. D., Ulus, I. H., and Wurtman, R. J. (1977): Brain tyrosine levels control striatal dopamine synthesis in haloperidol-treated rats. *J. Neural Transm.*, 41:1–6.
170. Sedvall, G., Fyro, B., Gullberg, B., Nyback, H., Wiesel, F. A., and Wode-Helgodt, B. (1980): Relationships in healthy volunteers between concentration of monoamine metabolites in cerebrospinal fluid and family history of psychiatric morbidity. *Br. J. Psychiatry*, 136:366–374.
171. Shaw, D. M., MacSweeney, D. A., Hewland, R., and Johnson, A. L. (1975): Tricyclic antidepressants and tryptophan in unipolar depression. *Psychol. Med.*, 5:276–278.
172. Shopsin, B. (1978): Enhancement of the antidepressant response to L-tryptophan by a liver pyrrolase inhibitor: A rational treatment approach. *Neuropsychobiology*, 4:188–192.
173. Singleton, L., and Marsden, C. A. (1979): Increased responsiveness to 5-methoxy, N.N.-dimethyl tryptamine in mice on a high tryptophan diet. *Neuropharmacology*, 18:569–572.
174. Sourkes, T. L. (1983): Toxicology of serotonin precursors. *Adv. Biol. Psychiatry*, 10:160–175.
175. Sourkes, T. L., Murphy, G. F., and Chavez, B. (1961): The action of some alpha-methyl and other acids on cerebral catecholamines. *J. Neurochem.*, 8:109–115.
176. Sternberg, E., van Woert, M. H., Young, S. N., Magnussen, J., Baker, H., Gauthier, S., and Osterland, C. K. (1980): Development of a sclerodermalike illness during therapy with L-5-hydroxytryptophan and carbidopa. *N. Engl. J. Med.*, 303:782–787.
177. Sved, A. F. (1983): Precursor control of the function of monoaminergic neurons. In: *Nutrition and the Brain*, edited by R. J. Wurtman and J. J. Wurtman, Vol. 6, pp. 223–275. Raven Press, New York.
178. Sved, A. F., Fernstrom, J. D., and Wurtman, R. J. (1979): Tyrosine administration reduces blood pressure and enhances brain norepinephrine release in spontaneously-hypertensive rats. *Proc. Natl. Acad. Sci. USA*, 76:3511–3514.
179. Takahashi, S., Kondo, H., and Kato, N. (1975): Effect of L-5-hydroxytryptophan on brain monoamine metabolism and evaluation of its clinical effect in depressed patients. *J. Psychiatr. Res.*, 12:177.
180. Takahashi, S., Takahashi, R., Masamura, I., and Miike, A. (1976): Measurement of 5-hydroxyindole compounds during 5-HTP treatment in depressed patients. *Folia Psychiatr. Neurol. Jpn.*, 30:463–473.
181. Thal, L. J., Sharpless, N. S., Wolfsen, L., and Katzman, R. (1980): Treatment of myoclonus with L-5-hydroxytryptophan and carbidopa. Clinical, electrophysiological and biochemical observation. *Ann. Neurol.*, 7:570–576.
182. Thomson, J., Rankin, H., Ashcroft, G. W., Yates, C. M., McQueen, J. K., and Cummings, S. W. (1982): The treatment of depression in general practice: A comparison of L-tryptophan, amitriptyline, and a combination of L-tryptophan and amitriptyline with placebo. *Psychol. Med.*, 12:741–751.
183. Traskman, L., Asberg, M., Bertilsson, L., and Sjostrand, L. (1981): Monoamine metabolites in CSF and suicidal behavior. *Arch. Gen. Psychiatry*, 38:631–636.
184. Traskman, L., Asberg, M., Bertilsson, L., and Thoren, P. (1984): CSF monoamine metabolites of depressed patients during illness and after recovery. *Acta Psychiatr. Scand.*, 69:333–342.
185. Trimble, M., Chadwick, D., Reynolds, E., and Marsden, C. D. (1975): L-5-Hydroxytryptophan and mood. *Lancet*, I:583.
186. Valzelli, L. (1981): *Psychobiology of Aggression and Violence.* Raven Press, New York.
187. van Hiele, L. J. (1980): L-5-Hydroxytryptophan in depression. The first substitution therapy in psychiatry? *Neuropsychobiology*, 6:230–241.
188. van Praag, H. M. (1962): Monoamine oxidase inhibition as a therapeutic principle in the treatment of depression. Doctoral dissertation, Utrect.
189. van Praag, H. M. (1974): Towards a biochemical typology of depression. *Pharmakopsychiatrie*, 7:281–292.
190. van Praag, H. M. (1977): *Depression and Schizophrenia. A Contribution on Their Chemical Pathologies.* Spectrum, New York.

191. van Praag, H. M. (1977): Significance of biochemical parameters in the diagnosis, treatment and prevention of depressive disorders. *Biol. Psychiatry*, 12:101–131.

192. van Praag, H. M. (1977): The significance of dopamine from the mode of action of neuroleptics and the pathogenesis of schizophrenia. *Br. J. Psychiatry*, 130:463–474.

193. van Praag, H. M. (1978): Amine hypothesis of affective disorders. In: *Handbook of Psychopharmacology, Vol. 13. Biology of Mood and Anti-Anxiety Drugs*, edited by L. L. Iversen, S. D. Iversen, and S. H. Snyder. Plenum, New York, pp. 189–276.

194. van Praag, H. M. (1978): *Psychotropic Drugs. A Guide for the Practitioner*. Bruner/Mazel, New York.

195. van Praag, H. M. (1979): Central serotonin: Its relation to depression vulnerability and depression prophylaxis. In: *Biological Psychiatry Today*, edited by J. Obiols, C. Ballus, E. Gonzalez Monclus, and J. Pujol. Elsevier/North-Holland, Amsterdam, pp. 485–498.

196. van Praag, H. M. (1981): Management of depression with serotonin precursors. *Biol. Psychiatry*, 16:291–310.

197. van Praag, H. M. (1982): Neurotransmitters and CNS disease: Depression. *Lancet*, II:1259–1264.

198. van Praag, H. M. (1982): Depression, suicide and the metabolism of serotonin in the brain. *J. Affective Disord.*, 4:275–290.

199. van Praag, H. M. (1983): In search of the action mechanism of antidepressants, 5-HTP/tyrosine mixtures in depression. *Neuropharmacology*, 22:433–440.

200. van Praag, H. M. (1983): CSF 5-HIAA and suicide in non-depressed schizophrenics. *Lancet*, II:977–978.

201. van Praag, H. M. (1984): Precursors of serotonin, dopamine and norepinephrine in the treatment of depression. In: *Proceedings of the Second World Conference on Clinical Pharmacology and Therapeutics*, edited by L. Lemberger and M. M. Reidenberg, p. 541. American Society for Pharmacology and Experimental Therapeutics, Maryland.

202. van Praag, H. M. (1984): Studies in the mechanism of action of serotonin precursors in depression. *Psychopharmacol. Bull.*, 20:599–602.

203. van Praag, H. M. (1984): Antidepressants today: Critical evaluation of some "established concepts." In: *Clinical Neuropharmacology, Vol. 7*, edited by G. Racagni, R. Paoletti, and P. Kielholz, pp. 322–323. Raven Press, New York.

204. van Praag, H. M. (1985): Brain serotonin and human (auto) aggression. In: Perspectives on Psychopharmacology, edited by W. E. Bunney and J. D. Barchas, Alan R. Liss, New York. *(in press)*.

205. van Praag, H. M. (1985): Monoamines and depression: The present state of the art. In: *Biological Foundation of Emotion*, edited by R. Plutchik and H. Kellerman. Academic Press, New York. *(in press)*

206. van Praag, H. M., and de Haan, S. (1979): Central serotonin metabolism and frequency of depression. *Psychiatr. Res.*, I:219–224.

207. van Praag, H. M., and de Haan, S. (1980): Depression vulnerability and 5-hydroxytryptophan prophylaxis. *Psychiatr. Res.*, 3:75–83.

208. van Praag, H. M., and de Haan, S. (1981): Chemoprophylaxis of depression. An attempt to compare lithium with 5-hydroxytryptophan. *Acta Psychiatr. Scand. [Suppl.]*, 290:191–205.

209. van Praag, H. M., Flentge, F., Korf, J., Dols, L. C. W., and Schut, T. (1973): The influence of probenecid on the metabolism of serotonin, dopamine, and their precursors in man. *Psychopharmacologia*, 33:141–151.

210. van Praag, H. M., and Korf, J. (1970): L-Tryptophan in depression. *Lancet*, II:612.

211. van Praag, H. M., and Korf, J. (1971): Endogenous depressions with and without disturbances in the 5-hydroxytryptamine metabolism: A biochemical classification? *Psychopharmacologia*, 19:148–152.

212. van Praag, H. M., and Korf, J. (1971): Retarded depression and the dopamine metabolism. *Psychopharmacologia*, 19:199–203.

213. van Praag, H. M., and Korf, J. (1975): Central monoamine deficiency in depression: Causative or secondary phenomenon. *Pharmakopsychiatrie*, 8:321–326.

214. van Praag, H. M., Korf, J., Dols, L. C. W., and Schut, T. (1972): A pilot study of the predictive value of the probenecid test in the application of 5-hydroxytryptophan as an antidepressant. *Psychopharmacologia*, 25:14–21.

215. van Praag, H. M., Korf, J., Lakke, J. P. W. F., and Schut, T. (1975): Dopamine metabolism in depressions, psychosis, and Parkinson's disease: The problem of the specificity of biological variables in behavior disorders. *Psychol. Med.*, 5:138–146.

216. van Praag, H. M., and Plutchik, R. (1984): Depression-type and depression-severity in relation to risk of violent suicide attempt. *Psychiatr. Res.*, 12:333–338.
217. van Praag, H. M., Schut, T., Bosma, E., and van den Bergh, R. (1971): A comparative study of the therapeutic effects of some 4-chlorinated amphetamine derivatives in depressive patients. *Psychopharmacologia*, 20:66–76.
218. van Praag, H. M., Uleman, A. M., and Spitz, J. C. (1965): The vital syndrome interview. A structured standard interview for the recognition and registration of the vital depressive symptom complex. *Psychiatr. Neurol. Neurochir.*, 68:329–346.
219. van Praag, H. M., van den Burg, W., Bos, E. R. H., and Dols, L. C. W. (1974): 5-Hydroxytryptophan in combination with clomipramine in "therapy-resistant" depression. *Psychopharmacologia*, 38:267–269.
220. van Praag, H. M., and Westenberg, H. G. M. (1983): Treatment of depression with L-hydroxytryptophan. In: *The Treatment of Depression with Monoamine Precursors*, edited by H. M. van Praag and J. Mendlewicz. Karger, Basel, pp. 94–128.
221. van Woert, M. H., Rosenbaum, D., Howieson, J., and Bowers, M. B. (1977): Long-term therapy of myoclonus and other neurological disorders with L-5-hydroxytryptophan and carbidopa. *N. Engl. J. Med.*, 296:70–75.
222. Walinder, J. (1983): Combination of tryptophan with MAO inhibitors, tricyclic antidepressants, and selective 5-HT reuptake inhibitors. *Adv. Biol. Psychiatry*, 10:82–93.
223. Walinder, J., Carlsson, A., and Persson, R. (1981): 5-HT reuptake inhibitors plus tryptophan in endogenous depression. *Acta Psychiatr. Scand.*, 63:179–190.
224. Walinder, J., Skott, A., and Carlsson, A. (1963): Potentiation of the antidepressant action of clomipramine by tryptophan. *Lancet*, I:79–81.
225. Walinder, J., Skott, A., Carlsson, A., Nagy, A., and Roos, B. E. (1976): Potentiation of the antidepressant action of clomipramine by tryptophan. *Arch. Gen. Psychiatry*, 33:1384–1389.
226. Weissman, M., Fox, K., and Klerman, J. L. (1973): Hostility and depression associated with suicide attempts. *Am. J. Psychiatry*, 130:450.
227. Westenberg, H. G. M., Gerritsen, T. W., Meijer, B. A., and van Praag, H. M. (1982): Kinetics of L-5-hydroxytryptophan in healthy subjects. *Psychiatr. Res.*, 7:373–385.
228. Worrall, E. P., Moody, J. P., Peet, M., Dick, P., Smith, A., Chambers, C., Adams, M., and Naylor, G. J. (1979): Controlled studies of the acute antidepressant affects of lithium. *Br. J. Psychiatry*, 135:255–262.
229. Wurtman, R. J. (1982): Nutrients that modify brain function. *Sci. Am.*, 246:42–51.
230. Wurtman, R. J. (1982/1983): Introduction. *J. Psychiatr. Res.*, 17:103–105.
231. Wurtman, R. J., Hefti, F., and Melamed, E. (1981): Precursor control of neurotransmitter synthesis. *Pharmacol. Rev.*, 32:315–335.
232. Wurtman, R. J., Larin, F., Mostafapour, S., and Fernstrom, J. D. (1974): Brain catechol synthesis: Control by brain tyrosine concentration. *Science*, 185:183–184.
233. Wyatt, R. J., Engelman, K., Kupper, D. J., Fram, D. H., Sjoerdsma, A., and Snyder, F. (1970): Effects of L-tryptophan (a natural sedative) on human sleep. *Lancet*, II:842–846.
234. Yaryura-Tobias, J. A., Wolpert, A., and Dana, L. (1970): Action of L-dopa in drug-induced extrapyramidalism. *Dis. Nerv. Syst.*, 31:60–63.
234a. Yogman, M. W., and Zeisel, S. H. (1983): Diet and sleep patterns in newborn infants. *N. Engl. J. Med.*, 309:1147–1149.
235. Young, S. N., Smith, S., Pihl, R. O., and Ervin, F. R. (1985): Tryptophan depletion causes a rapid lowering of mood in normal males. *Psychopharmacology (in press)*.
236. Young, S. N., and Sourkes, T. L. (1977): Tryptophan in the central nervous system: Regulation and significance. *Adv. Neurochem.*, 2:133–191.
237. Yuwiler, A., Geller, E., and Eiduson, S. (1959): Studies on 5-hydroxytryptophan decarboxylase. I. In vitro inhibition and substrate interaction. *Arch. Biochem.*, 80:162–173.

Nutrition and the Brain, Vol. 7, edited by
R. J. Wurtman and J. J. Wurtman. Raven Press,
New York © 1986.

Bulimia, Carbohydrate Craving, and Depression: A Central Connection?

Norman E. Rosenthal and Margaret M. Heffernan

Department of Health and Human Services, Public Health Service, National Institutes of Health, Bethesda, Maryland 20205

I. INTRODUCTION

> Stay me with flagons, comfort me with apples:
> for I am sick of love.
> *Song of Solomon*, 2:4–5

Since ancient times popular belief has held that what we eat affects the way we feel. Conversely, our mood may determine what (and how much) we choose to eat. In this chapter, we explore the relationship between regulation of eating behavior and mood, using for the most part information derived from patients in whom these functions are disturbed.

Disturbances of mood regulation are generally referred to as the affective disorders. As the plural form of the term implies, these disorders consist of more than one entity. The classification of the affective disorders has been a subject of long-standing debate, the most recent distillation of which has found expression in the third edition of the Diagnostic and Statistical Manual (DSM-III) of psychiatric disorders (3). In this chapter, we discuss the classification of depressive subgroups according to differences in patterns of eating behavior. Such an emphasis, while unorthodox, focuses on the importance of eating patterns as a clue to underlying disturbances of brain physiology.

The major eating disorders are anorexia nervosa and bulimia. Anorexia nervosa is discussed in a separate chapter in this volume. Bulimia, a condition characterized by binge eating, is more prevalent than was previously recognized and is reported to occur in 19% of college women (33). The binges may occur in patients of average weight, a condition we refer to as normal-weight bulimia, as distinct from binges that occur in patients who are suffering from anorexia nervosa. The latter group maintain their weight at abnormally low levels by inducing vomiting or abusing laxatives or diuretics as opposed to those anorectics who restrict their food intake. We refer to these two groups as bulimic and nonbulimic anorectics, respectively. Although we shall not be dealing with obesity in depth, we discuss a group of obese patients who experience marked cravings for carbohydrates, a symptom also found in certain depressives.

An issue that has been raised by eating disorder researchers is whether these disorders may actually be variants of affective disorders (11). Psychiatric researchers have long been preoccupied with how to classify a variety of conditions of unknown etiology. Guidelines for classification of patients into discrete syndromes were outlined in the frequently cited paper by Feighner and colleagues (24). They suggested that clinical presentation, both similarities and differences, family history, clinical course (which includes response to pharmacological interventions), and laboratory studies should be taken into account in order to distinguish meaningful patient subgroups. In this chapter we review the evidence for considering the eating disorders mentioned above as variants of the affective disorders.

Research into the eating disorders is relatively new compared to affective disorder research. The strategies that have profitably been employed by those researching the eating disorders have in many instances been borrowed from research in the affective disorders. However, students of the affective disorders frequently fail to take the pattern of their patients' eating behavior seriously enough and may thereby be missing important clues to the understanding of the pathophysiology of their patients' symptoms. These researchers would benefit by taking into account strategies that have been developed by researchers in the eating disorders (discussed below).

We briefly review and discuss possible neurophysiological associations between the regulation of eating and of mood and speculate about how derangements of these shared systems may produce both affective and eating behavior disturbances.

II. CLINICAL PICTURE: AFFECTIVE DISTURBANCES
IN THE EATING DISORDERS

In order to compare reports on the clinical profiles of patients seen by different groups of researchers, standardized criteria are required to ensure that the same types of patients are being considered. Consensus about such standardized criteria has only recently been available for bulimia and does not yet exist for carbohydrate-craving obesity. Solid data on depressive symptomatology in the former condition have been available only since 1980 with the advent of DSM-III (3); data about depression in the latter condition have not yet been published. In evaluating depression in patients with eating disorders, it is important to distinguish between depression as a symptom and depression as a syndrome as defined by standardized criteria. The latter is a more meaningful concept, carrying with it implications with respect to treatment, family history, pharmacological response, and prognosis.

A. Bulimia

The DSM-III defines bulimia as a condition characterized by the following: (i) the rapid consumption of food in a discrete period of time, usually less than 2 hr; (ii) awareness that the bingeing pattern is abnormal and fear of not being able to stop voluntarily; (iii) depressive and self-deprecating thoughts after bingeing episodes; (iv) repeated attempts to lose weight through dieting, self-induced vomiting, or use of laxatives or diuretics; and (v) frequent weight fluctuations.

As one might expect from the above criteria, depressive symptoms are present in a high percentage of patients with bulimia (1,23,32,35,36,42,44–46,54,55, 69,78,95). Bulimic patients have also frequently been found to have concurrent or prior episodes of depressive disorder. Thus Herzog (36) reported that six of eight adolescents with bulimia met DSM-III criteria for major depressive episode.

Hudson et al. (42) interviewed 49 patients with a lifetime history of normal-weight bulimia and 25 patients with a lifetime history of both bulimia and anorexia nervosa and found that 73% of the former group and 92% of the latter group had lifetime histories of major affective disorder. Walsh et al. (92) studied 50 bulimic patients and found that 30% met DSM-III criteria for concurrent major depression, and 70% met criteria for a lifetime history of major depression. Walsh et al. included patients with both diagnoses in their sample and found no difference in the frequency of major depression in patients with bulimia alone and those with coexisting bulimia and anorexia nervosa.

Whenever there is a statistical association between two disorders, the question arises as to what causal and temporal relationships exist between the disorders. If we are dealing with two associated disorders, A and B, it is of interest to know whether A causes B, whether B causes A, or whether both A and B are due to some process, C, and are not causally related to each other. If there is a causal connection, it is useful to search for the intervening variables between A and B. Since in clinical research it is extremely difficult to establish causal connections, one must often be content with establishing temporal relationships. If A precedes B, A may have causal significance; if A follows B, however, A is unlikely to have caused B. This *ABC* paradigm will recur several times in this chapter as it does in clinical research.

The specific instance to be considered at this point is whether bulimia causes depression, whether depression causes bulimia, or whether they both reflect an underlying pathophysiological process and are not causally related to each other. Hudson et al. (42) addressed this question by looking at the temporal relationship between the eating disorder and the affective disorder in those patients afflicted by both illnesses (79). Of the 69 patients with a lifetime history of major affective disorder, the onset of the affective disorder preceded the onset of the eating disorder by at least 1 year in 34 (49%), occurred within the same year in 21 (30%), and followed the onset of the eating disorder by at least 1 year in 14 (20%). Walsh et al. (92) examined this same relationship in their population and found that in 26 of 35 patients (74%), the first episode of major depression had occurred simultaneously with or had followed the onset of the eating disorder, and that nine patients (26%) had had an episode of major depression prior to the beginning of their eating disorder. The mean interval between the episode of major depression and the onset of eating disorder in these nine patients was 3 years.

Although it is clearly important that this type of temporal information should be collected, it is apparent that even if figures were available on larger numbers of cases, we would be far from disentangling the causal connections between bulimia and the affective disorders.

The same cause-and-effect questions have been asked about the relationship between the dysphoric or unpleasant subjective experiences reported by bulimics and their episodes of bingeing and purging. These patients report not only depressed feelings but wide fluctuations of mood (27,45), irritability, and anxiety. Are these patients experiencing unpleasant feelings as a result of their uncontrollable eating patterns *(A)*, are they eating uncontrollably in an attempt to alleviate these feelings *(B)*, or are both the unpleasant feelings and the binges different manifestations of a central pathophysiological disturbance *(C)*?

We will ignore for the moment the possibility that the two sets of phenomena have nothing to do with each other. Possibility *A* could be explained on either psychological grounds (e.g., guilt at being out of control, worries about getting fat) or physiological grounds (e.g., biochemical disturbances resulting from the ingestion of large quantities of food in a short period of time, or from vomiting). Possibility *B* raises the interesting notion of a homeostatic feedback mechanism existing to restore to normality a biochemical abnormality in the brain by inducing the biochemical changes that follow bingeing and vomiting. This mechanism is compatible with viewing bulimia as a type of drug abuse, with food as the drug. It is an appealing model for those clinicians who work with bulimics and have noted in them the cravings, uncontrollable behavior, and secretiveness associated with other types of drug abuse. An extension of this hypothesis is that specific types of foods may normalize certain neurobiological abnormalities, and that these abnormalities may be experienced by the patient in a variety of ways, one of which may be a craving for the nutrient in question. We expand on this idea later in the chapter.

Three studies have examined the temporal relationships between the subjective feelings of bulimic patients and their bingeing behavior (1,45,49). Johnson and Larson (45) studied patterns of mood and bingeing in 15 normal-weight bulimics. They used electronic pagers and paged their subjects at random intervals to inquire about their feelings and eating behavior at that moment. In analyzing their data, the authors found that before a binge, patients reported feeling more irritable, weak, hungry, inadequate, and out of control than usual. During the binge, their mood states worsened, and guilt, shame, and anger were significantly greater than normal. The mood state during their purges seemed somewhat different. Although subjects remained sad and weak, they reported feeling more alert and less angry. During the immediate postbinge period, patients reported feeling significantly sadder, drowsier, weaker, and more bored than usual. Their self-reported levels of control and adequacy remained significantly below average, although they were less extreme than during the binge and purge. Reported guilt and shame also remained high. It should be emphasized that the data on bingeing and purging were derived from only 29 of a total of 673 reports (4.3%).

Johnson and Larson (45) postulate the drug addiction model as an explanation for the binges and purges, suggesting that bulimics go through certain stages in the course of their condition: (i) a stage of food addiction (bingeing) with undesirable consequences (obesity); (ii) food addiction without obesity, which is controlled by purging; and (iii) escalating bingeing and purging, which results in feelings of inadequacy and loss of self-control and for which patients seek treatment. Clearly this theory could not reasonably be derived solely from the above-mentioned paper. It presupposes that the patients in that study have gone beyond the stage where the binge provides them with feelings of relief and have reached the point where the bingeing results only in feelings of inadequacy and loss of control. It could be argued that the purging, by restoring the sense of control, makes patients feel better. However, there are alternative explanations. The ingestion of huge quantities of nutrients may create biochemical changes which produce the reported feelings. The purge itself may produce pleasurable chemical changes and thus may be an addictive behavior in certain cases rather than merely a mechanism for weight control. Finally, it is unclear to what extent some of the feelings reported may have been the result of being paged and disturbed in the middle of a binge or a purge.

Abraham and Beaumont (1) administered a questionnaire to 32 normal-weight bulimics, inquiring about their patterns of bingeing and purging. Feelings or events most likely to precipitate a binge were (in order of frequency) tension, eating something, being alone, thinking of food, craving specific foods, going home, and feeling bored and lonely. Feeling hungry ranked lower than all the above factors. All patients said they usually felt anxious and tense before a binge, and 80% described physical concomitants of anxiety. Feelings of depersonalization and de-realization were reported by 75%. Approximately one-third described relief from anxiety during the binge, and two-thirds described relief after the binge was over. Almost three-quarters reported an absence of "negative" mood states during a binge, and 44% reported that "negative" mood states occurred frequently after the binge was over. Thoughts of suicide were common (70%), and seven patients actually made suicide attempts shortly after a binge. Five of the 32 patients reported relief of anxiety only after inducing vomiting and not following the binge itself. The data of Abraham and Beaumont (1) substantiate the drug addiction model of bingeing suggested by Larson and Johnson (45) and concur with the observations of these latter authors that for some bulimics it is vomiting rather than bingeing that has a stress-relieving effect.

Most recently, Kaye and Gwirtsman (49) studied 12 normal-weight bulimics by observing them during bingeing and vomiting episodes and measuring their mood by the objective Brief Psychiatric Rating Scale (BPRS) and subjective visual analog scales before and after bingeing and purging. Before bingeing, most patients rated themselves as being more anxious than calm and more depressed than happy. A similar pattern was seen on the BPRS. Patients reported feeling significantly more satiated for 1 hr and significantly less anxious for 2 hr after bingeing and vomiting. There were no significant changes on any of the other subscales. Analysis of the BPRS revealed a significant decrease in three of the subscales: anxiety and tension ($p<0.01$) and guilt ($p<0.05$). The authors noted that the baseline scores for tension and anxiety were relatively low, and that these patients were not clinically particularly anxious. In only five of the 12 subjects did improved mood coincide with terminating cycles of bingeing and vomiting. An additional five subjects had a mood improvement during their bingeing and vomiting yet continued to do so. The remaining two subjects did not show a mood improvement either during or after their episodes.

In summary, it is clear that before bingeing and vomiting episodes, many bulimics experience dysphoric feelings, such as tension and anxiety, which are relieved by either bingeing or vomiting, or both. The drug addiction model of bulimia seems to fit this group quite well. However, other patients do not experience improvements in mood or may actually feel worse during or after episodes of bingeing and purging. For these people, the drug addiction model seems less applicable unless one speculates that they are being observed at a time when bingeing and purging no longer yield the improvement in anxiety and tension that may have occurred earlier in the course of the illness.

Although some bulimics claim that they binge predominantly on carbohydrates, the three studies that have evaluated the composition of foods chosen for binges have all shown that large quantities of protein and fat are also present in the selected food (1,49,62).

B. Obesity with Carbohydrate Craving

Wurtman and colleagues (99) have had a long-standing interest in the existence of and neurochemical substrates for specific types of appetitive behavior. They recently described a group of obese (at least 18% above normal body weight) patients who report cravings specifically for high-carbohydrate foods, which they eat in large quantities for snacks (99). These patients differ from bulimics in that their eating habits are more moderate. They do not generally binge to the same degree as bulimics, are not as secretive about their eating habits, and do not induce vomiting. Spring and colleagues (88) have shown that meals that are high in carbohydrates tend to make people feel sleepy. Recently, Lieberman and Wurtman *(personal communication)* fed high-carbohydrate meals to their population of carbohydrate cravers and found that, in contrast to its effects on normal subjects, the high-carbohydrate meal tends to make their patients feel more alert. They also had their own control population, a group of obese patients who craved and snacked on combinations of protein and carbohydrate foods, and found that these controls resembled the normals described by Spring et. al (88) in that they became drowsy after high-carbohydrate meals. This is an exciting preliminary finding as it provides a measurable correlate of the history of food preference, which may reflect a specific disturbance in brain biochemistry. The abnormal behavior may represent an attempt on the part of the individual to correct this disturbance. This concept is discussed in greater detail later in the chapter.

In selecting their population of carbohydrate cravers, Wurtman and colleagues screened out patients with obvious psychopathology at the time of the screening interview. Once patients were admitted to their program, they administered to them the Schedule for Affective Disorders and Schizophrenia (SADS) (22a) and made Research Diagnostic Criteria (RDC) (87) diagnoses on the basis of these interviews. The investigators again used as a control population patients who were equally obese but reported craving and snacking on foods that were not high in carbohydrates.

Wurtman, Mark, and Rosenthal and colleagues *(unpublished observation)* found that 44 of 63 carbohydrate cravers (70%) met criteria for major depression at some time in their lives. A similarly high frequency of major depression (13 of 22; 59%) was found in the noncarbohydrate-craving control population. Both these figures are higher than one would expect to find in the population as a whole but are not as high as the figures for major depression reported in bulimic populations. This finding suggests that obese patients with cravings (either for carbohydrates or other types of food) may have a vulnerability to depression between that found in the normal population and that which occurs in bulimics. In fact, the vulnerability may actually be higher in the obese cravers than Wurtman's findings suggest, as the more obviously depressed individuals were eliminated by the screening procedure.

In summary, there appears to be a history of major depression in a far higher percentage of bulimics and obese patients who crave carbohydrate or mixtures of carbohydrate and protein snacks than in normals. There is also an abnormally high incidence of depression in patients with anorexia nervosa (3,11,42). These findings suggest that the higher than normal incidence of depression observed in the eating disorders is not specific to any particular type of disorder. This observation must be taken into account in considering any theory that attempts to explain the widely reported association between the eating and affective disorders.

III. DISTURBANCES OF EATING BEHAVIOR AND WEIGHT IN THE AFFECTIVE DISORDERS

Just as disturbances of mood are common in the eating disorders, so are disturbances of appetite and weight regulation cardinal features of the affective disorders. Leckman and colleagues (56), in a recent large study, reported eating and weight disturbances in 70% of their depressed patients. Two main patterns of abnormal eating behavior and weight control occur in depressed patients: (i) anorexia and weight loss, and (ii) overeating and weight gain.

Weight loss during depression and weight gain on recovery were noted originally by Kraepelin (52) and later by Kraines (53). Anorexia and weight loss are generally found in conjuction with several other clinical features (see Table 1) in a syndrome called endogenous depression or melancholia. We use these descriptive terms interchangeably, although minor distinctions have been made between them. Although the term *endogenous* implies the absence of an environmental precipitant, this is by no means always the case. The term is currently used to refer to a type of depression associated with insomnia, particularly in the early morning hours, anhedonia, and lack of environmental reactivity. In its more severe form, it may require hospitalization and electroconvulsive treatment (ECT), although it will generally respond well to antidepressant medications. Diurnal variation is frequently present, and symptoms are generally worst in the morning hours. There is a seasonal variation in the incidence of this condition, with the peak occurring in the spring (77). Patients with this condition frequently fail to show normal suppression of cortisol secretion in response to the administration of a standardized oral dose of the powerful synthetic steroid dexamethasone (12), and some patients with endogenous depression have shown a blunted pituitary response to administration of thyrotrophin-releasing hormone (TRH) (51).

In contrast to endogenous depressives, some depressed patients have increased appetite, weight gain, and carbohydrate craving. These patients have been said to

TABLE 1. *Comparison between endogenous and atypical depression:*
Clustering of symptoms

Parameter	Endogenous	Atypical
Synonyms/subgroups	Melancholia, endogenomorphic, "psychotic"	Neurotic, reactive, SAD, hysteroid dysphoria
Sex ratio	Females less preponderant	Females more preponderant
Appetite	Decreased	Usually increased
Weight	Decreased	Increased
Carbohydrate craving	Absent	Present
Sleep	Decreased sleep length; middle and terminal insomnia	Increased sleep length; initial insomnia
Diurnal variation	Worse in morning	Worse later in the day
Severity	Severe; may be psychotic	Milder
Reactivity to environment	Absent	Present
Treatment setting	Hospital or outpatient	Outpatient
Treatment modalities	Antidepressants, lithium, ECT	Antidepressants (MAOIs may be superior); light (SAD)
Premenstrual mood problems	?	Often present
Seasonal occurrence	Spring peak	Fall and winter peak
Neuroendocrine studies	DST nonsuppression; TRH test, blunted response	Normal DST and TRH test results

suffer from "neurotic" or nonendogenous depression (37) or "atypical" depression (19). These patients have been regarded as neurotic perhaps because of their reactivity to psychological stresses, the relative mildness of their symptoms, which allows them to continue to function (albeit inadequately) at work and in their families, or perhaps because their symptoms tend to occur in less discrete episodes and appear instead as part of the daily fabric of their lives. In this category of depressives, women predominate over men to a greater degree than in melancholic patients. Sleep length may be increased (18,28), and insomnia, when present, may be more severe at sleep onset than in the early morning hours (2). Diurnal variation may occur; when it does, symptoms may be more severe in the later part of the day. Premenstrual mood problems are frequently present in menstruating patients (84). Seasonal fluctuations in incidence or severity, when present, seem to show a peak in the fall and winter (22). The dexamethasone suppression test (DST) and TRH stimulation test are frequently normal (75). Despite the use of the term *neurotic* to characterize these patients, there is no reason to believe that their symptoms are predominantly psychological in origin and lack a neurobiological substrate. However, the many clinical features that differentiate endogenous from atypical depressives suggest that the neurobiological disturbances responsible for these two conditions are probably quite different.

The condition of seasonal affective disorder (SAD) is a special type of atypical depression. It is characterized by annually occurring episodes of depression in the fall and winter alternating with periods of remission or hypomania in the spring and summer (74,75). Of 125 patients with SAD, 71% report a history of increased appetite during depression, whereas only 17% report an appetite decrease. Carbohydrate craving is reported by 67% of this population (76) and is one of the earliest symptoms of winter depression. The condition of SAD differs from some other types of atypical depression, in particular those studied by Liebowitz et al. (57), in that SAD patients are unusually sensitive not so much to psychological stimuli, such as attention or rejection, but to climatic stimuli, in particular the amount or duration of bright environmental light (76).

In patients with an eating disorder who also have a history of depression, it would be interesting to know what kind of depression had occurred, endogenous or atypical. As of the time of writing this chapter, only one study has examined this question systematically. Walsh et al. (92) questioned their patients carefully; in 31 of their bulimic subjects, they were able to obtain a sufficiently good history to categorize their depressions. In approximately one-third of their patients, the depression was endogenous and in one-third atypical, according to the criteria of Liebowitz et al. (57).

Research in the field of eating disorders is relatively recent compared to studies of the affective disorders, and students of the eating disorders have used many of the strategies developed in the earlier research. However, affective disorder researchers have not given sufficient attention to disturbed eating behavior as a possible clue to depressive subtypes and to the nature of the underlying neurobiological disturbances. Standard rating scales, such as the Hamilton Rating Scale

(HRS) (34) and Beck Depression Inventory (5), do not inquire specifically about overeating and weight gain. In fact, the HRS, geared as it is to endogenous depression, rates only decreased appetite and weight loss as depressive items, which would be unsuitable for atypical depressives, in whom such symptoms signal improvement rather than exacerbation. In our work on SAD, we have used a supplement to the HRS, which we have found to be quite useful (see Appendix 1). In addition to inquiring about the amount of food eaten, it is also important to inquire about food type, as this too may give a clue to the nature of the underlying neurobiological disturbance. In certain situations, actually measuring food intake may also be helpful.

In summary, depressive symptoms are common in the eating disorders, especially bulimia, and a history of affective episodes is present in a high percentage of cases. The temporal relationship of the depressive episode to the eating disorder is variable; it may occur before, during, or after the eating disorder. The nature of the depressive episode is not specific to the eating disorder, and both endogenous and atypical depressions have been reported to occur in bulimia. Disturbances of eating behavior and weight regulation are similarly common in the affective disorders. Patients may eat less and lose weight, or crave carbohydrates, eat more, and gain weight.

Despite the clear symptomatic overlap between the eating and affective disorders, the clinician will usually confidently make the diagnosis of one or the other. The melancholic depressive generally does not have the type of distorted body image characteristic of the anorectic and will accept that he or she has lost a great deal of weight and looks too thin. In the atypical depressive, the eating disturbances will generally be only part of the total clinical picture and not overwhelm it, as in the case of the bulimic. Yet there are some cases in which the syndromes may coexist, follow one another, or even be difficult to differentiate. The best explanation for the symptomatic overlap is that eating behavior and mood regulation probably share neurobiological substrates that, when disturbed, produce both types of symptoms. The underlying disturbances in these two groups of disorders are probably similar but not identical. We can probably learn as much from studying how these syndromes differ as we can from understanding their similarities. In studying symptoms, we recognize that we have only a dim reflection of the underlying neurochemical processes. At present, we know little about how mood and eating behavior are regulated in humans. We have some knowledge about the underlying neurobiology of eating behavior in animals, and this is briefly summarized in the following section.

IV. NEUROREGULATION OF EATING BEHAVIOR AND MOOD

The regulation of eating behavior in animals has been well reviewed by Morley and Levine (64). Early researchers believed that the ventral hypothalamus had two centers that regulated eating, one to stimulate appetite and one to signal satiety. More recent research has shown this to be a gross oversimplification, and Rolls

(73) has reviewed the reasons that this model is no longer tenable. However, the hypothalamus continues to be regarded as an important modulator of appetite and eating behavior. The ventromedial hypothalamus, formerly regarded as the satiety center, has a serotonergic tract and a noradrenergic tract coursing through it. The ventrolateral hypothalamus, formerly regarded as the hunger center, is associated with the dopaminergic nigrostriatal tract.

Although most studies of neural control of feeding have been performed on rats, some studies have involved nonhuman primates. These studies in particular should be regarded as having some relevance for explaining the control of feeding and body weight in humans (73). The small amount of direct evidence available in humans is consistent with the more ample evidence from animal studies. For example, Reeves and Plum (71) described a patient with a ventromedial hypothalamic tumor who had severe hyperphagia and weight gain. Quaade et al. (70) electrically stimulated the lateral hypothalamus in five obese patients and reported "convincing hunger responses" in three. In two obese patients, unilateral lateral hypothalamic lesions produced a transient suppression of feeding but no significant weight reduction.

Many studies in animals have explored what chemicals or neurotransmitters are involved in mediating feeding behavior and weight regulation. The role of nutrients as cues to hunger and feeding behavior was first advanced by Carlson (cited in ref. 64), who suggested that when blood glucose levels fell below a certain threshold, hunger might be produced (64). Subsequent researchers have proposed that other nutrients, such as fatty acids and amino acids, have a role in modulating feeding behavior. Theories involving nutrients as controlling eating behavior have an appeal, especially as they are compatible with the observations that animals select a proper balance of macronutrients and micronutrients when feeding. Given that these nutrients may serve as peripheral cues influencing feeding behavior, what neurotransmitters within the central nervous system (CNS) may be involved in this process? Several candidates have been proposed, including monoamines, opioid peptides and other neuropeptides, and γ-aminobutyric acid (64). It is beyond the scope of this chapter to review in detail the evidence for evaluating the importance of all the nutrients and neurotransmitters that may be involved in regulating feeding behavior (for review, see ref. 9).

We deal with two areas related to the neurophysiological control of mood and feeding in view of their particular relevance to the subject of this discussion: first, the role of the amino acid tryptophan in regulating CNS serotonin metabolism, a mechanism that has been postulated to underlie carbohydrate craving; and second, the possible role of the monoamines in the affective and eating disorders in general, since these are known to be affected by drugs that modify both mood and eating behavior in humans, and since disturbances of monoamine metabolism have been extensively explored as being of possible significance in both affective and eating disorders.

A. Carbohydrate Intake, Tryptophan, and CNS Serotonin Metabolism

The consumption of carbohydrate in the diet and the desire to eat carbohydrate have been associated with brain serotonin metabolism by Wurtman and colleagues (98,100) in a series of studies, initially in rats but more recently in humans. Studies in rats showed that consumption of a high-carbohydrate, low-protein diet for 1 to 2 hr accelerates serotonin synthesis and release from brain neurons of fasting rats (25). The mechanism for this effect appears to be as follows: The carbohydrate elicits insulin secretion, which markedly reduces plasma levels of most large neutral amino acids (LNAAs) but not of tryptophan (100). This alters the ratio of tryptophan to other LNAAs in plasma, which facilitates the uptake of tryptophan into the brain (100). Tryptophan hydroxylase, the enzyme that converts tryptophan to 5-hydroxytryptophan, the initial step in the synthesis of serotonin, is normally unsaturated. Thus the increase in brain tryptophan that results from a change in the tryptophan/LNAA ratio accelerates serotonin synthesis. A high-protein meal has the opposite effect, because dietary proteins contribute much larger quantities of the other LNAAs than of tryptophan to the plasma.

Wurtman and Wurtman (98) have hypothesized that a specific appetite for carbohydrates may be regulated by serotonin metabolism in the brain by a complex nutrient–neurotransmitter feedback loop. An individual who is deficient in serotonin may experience this deficiency as a desire or craving for carbohydrates, which, when ingested, would accelerate serotonin synthesis. The authors have shown that carbohydrate intake by animals allowed to choose among foods that differ in nutrient content is preferentially suppressed by drugs that enhance serotonergic neurotransmission (98). Extending their studies in humans, they have shown that orally administered fenfluramine, a serotonin agonist, specifically decreased snacking on carbohydrate-rich foods in a group of obese patients with a history of carbohydrate craving (99). A separate group of carbohydrate cravers was given oral tryptophan (2.4 g/day). Although this did not produce a significant reduction in the consumption of carbohydrate snacks by the group as a whole, it did have a significant effect in three of eight subjects (99).

It is clear how an understanding of neurochemical mechanisms that regulate the appetite for a particular type of nutrient may provide insight into conditions that are characterized by a craving for that nutrient. Thus depressives with marked carbohydrate craving presumably differ in some fundamental way from those who do not show that symptom.

The condition of SAD is an example of a type of depression in which carbohydrate craving is a marked and early symptom (75). Patients with SAD are highly sensitive to changes in their physical environment. In a series of studies, Rosenthal and colleagues (74–76) have shown that patients with SAD respond favorably to being exposed to bright artificial light, which reverses depressive symptoms, including carbohydrate craving. It is conceivable that both the craving and the other

SAD symptoms correspond to a central serotonin deficiency, and that light treatment, by reversing this deficiency, might exert its therapeutic effect.

A similar type of reasoning inspired the formulation of the biogenic amine theories of depression, which have been the focus of extensive research over the past three decades. When tricyclic antidepressants (TCAs) and monoamine oxidase inhibitors (MAOIs) were shown to have antidepressant properties, their known effect on monoamine metabolism (namely, to increase the availability of monoamines at the synaptic level) were hypothesized to be responsible for their antidepressant effects. Conversely, amine-depleting drugs, such as reserpine, were observed to produce sedation and "depression" in animals. The monoamine theories of depression stated that a deficiency in the monoamines, most notably norepinephrine (NE) and serotonin, might exist in depression and might be responsible for the disorder (65).

B. Monoamine Theories of Depression: Their Association with Eating Regulation

In the 30 years that have elapsed since the monoamine theories were first proposed, there is still no clear consensus as to what role disturbances of monoamine metabolism may play in the pathogenesis of the affective disorders. Jimerson (43) has recently reviewed the area and has pointed out the many sources of variance involved in studying the monoamines and their metabolites in the affective disorders. These include heterogeneity of the condition being studied, differences in methods of diagnosis, phase of the illness, concomitant psychological or physical symptoms, age, sex, height, and body weight, medication status (it has recently become apparent that the standard 2-week withdrawal period from antidepressants may not be enough) (13), diet, motor activity, diurnal and seasonal rhythms, methods of sample collection, storage, and assay methodology. It is important that the normal control population be as similar as possible to the patient group, a matter that is difficult to achieve in practice.

Perhaps because of these many variables, the findings from various groups have been contradictory. We briefly summarize the findings related to NE and serotonin. In many cases, it is the metabolites of these neurotransmitters rather than the transmitters themselves that have been studied. The level of metabolites in plasma, urine, and cerebrospinal fluid (CSF) is believed to reflect the turnover of the neurotransmitters. More recent studies have focused on the receptors for these neurotransmitters. An abnormality of receptor functioning might account for alterations in neurotransmission in the absence of any abnormality of neurotransmitter turnover or metabolite levels. These receptor studies have been performed either *in vitro* (e.g., in postmortem brain specimens or in peripheral tissues, such as platelets) or *in vivo* in various challenge paradigms.

1. NE

A considerable amount of work in investigating disturbances of NE metabolism has involved 3-methoxy-4-hydroxyphenylglycol (MHPG), the major NE metabolite in the human brain (80), which can be measured in urine, plasma, or CSF. Recent work has shown that up to 80% of urinary MHPG is derived from NE released by the peripheral sympathetic nerves, and MHPG itself is substantially converted to another metabolite, vanillylmandelic acid (8). Despite these limitations, several investigators have found reduced urinary MHPG in bipolar depressed patients (depressives with a history of mania or hypomania), whereas only one group found a reduced level in unipolar depressives (80). To our knowledge, when studying metabolite levels, no one has specifically subdivided depressives into those who overeat and those who undereat.

Measurement of CSF levels of MHPG provides the best available index of central NE turnover (43). In the 12 or more CSF studies performed in depressed patients, there is little consistent evidence for reduced MHPG levels in the patients in comparison with control groups (80).

Several groups have studied adrenergic receptor functioning *in vivo* by administering a drug known to act on these receptors and measuring variables known to change as a result of the drug–receptor interaction. Thus in depressives, the responses in growth hormone secretion, pulse, and plasma MHPG are blunted in response to an infusion of the α_2-adrenoceptor agonist clonidine (15,59,83). In contrast, peripheral postsynaptic α-adrenergic responses to tyramine, NE, and phenylephrine are increased in depressed patients in comparison with normal controls (16). Both α_2- and β_2-adrenoceptors are thought to respond primarily to circulating epinephrine released from the adrenal medulla (4). It is possible that blunted responses to these receptors in depressed patients may simply reflect a reaction to increased levels of epinephrine released as a result due to the stress of being depressed, rather than a primary abnormality.

Clinical and animal studies do suggest that altered NE function plays a role in the response to antidepressant treatment, perhaps by increasing NE activity at the synapse (43). That three decades of work in this area have resulted in such tentative conclusions indicates the many difficulties involved in establishing cause-and-effect relationships between brain neurotransmitter systems and specific disease entities.

Kaye et al. (50) have studied CSF NE in anorectics and found a marked reduction in NE in recovered anorectics. They found no difference between bulimic and nonbulimic anorectic subtypes. To date, no studies of NE or its metabolites have been reported in bulimics.

2. Serotonin

The serotonin hypothesis of the affective disorders rests on three main elements (65): (i) Functional levels of brain serotonin may be reduced in patients with depression and may directly contribute or predispose to their symptoms. (ii) Increasing brain serotoninergic function by administering the serotonin precursors tryptophan or 5-hydroxytryptophan alone or in combination with other drugs that potentiate serotoninergic function is thought to have an antidepressant effect. (iii) Other drugs, such as lithium carbonate, the TCAs, and the MAOIs, which are therapeutic for the affective disorders, are thought to act (at least in part) via brain serotoninergic mechanisms.

The strongest support for the hypothesis comes from the repeated demonstration from different laboratories that levels of 5-hydroxyindoleacetic acid (5-HIAA), the major serotonin metabolite, are reduced approximately 30% in depressed patients compared to controls (65). Although there is evidence of reduced brain serotonin levels in postmortem specimens from suicide victims in three of six studies and reduced brain 5-HIAA levels in postmortem specimens in all four brain studies where this was measured, methodological issues make this evidence less powerful but at least consistent with the hypothesis. Assuming a deficiency in 5-HIAA exists in depression, it could arise via different mechanisms, including a deficiency in tryptophan hydroxylase or decreased tryptophan availability. This question requires further study.

There is evidence of tryptophan potentiation of TCA and MAOI efficacy (65) and, more persuasively, of reversal of the therapeutic effects of the tricyclic imipramine and the MAOI tranylcypromine by the serotonin synthesis inhibitor parachlorophenylalanine (81,82).

As with the NE system, recent studies have investigated receptor function by *in vivo* challenge tests. Thus cortisol responses to the serotonin precursor 5-hydroxytryptophan appear to be potentiated in depressed patients compared to controls (60). Such results could reflect compensatory increases in postsynaptic receptor sensitivity resulting from a prolonged deficiency in synaptic serotonin.

The way in which antidepressant drugs exert their clinical effects is still not completely understood. This may have something to do with the known effect of TCAs to inhibit serotonin reuptake from the synapse and the effects on inhibiting serotonin breakdown by the MAOIs. We know that animal studies have shown a decrease in the density of neuronal serotonin receptors in response to antidepressant treatment, although these effects are less consistent than the observed decreases in β-adrenoceptor responses. There is also evidence of increased functional responsiveness of postsynaptic serotonin neurons following antidepressant treatment (14). The well-documented lithium-induced potentiation of TCA treatment may reflect potentiation of serotonin responses (20).

Although no CSF neurotransmitter studies have been performed thus far on normal-weight bulimics, Kaye et al. (48) have reported differences in concentrations of CSF 5-HIAA in bingeing and nonbingeing patients with anorexia nervosa. After probenecid administration (which produces an accumulation of 5-HIAA in CSF), weight-recovered bulimic anorectics had lower concentrations of 5-HIAA than those weight-recovered nonbulimic anorectics. A decrease in brain serotonin in bulimic anorectics might result both in their need to binge, which would be compatible with what is known about the role of serotonin in satiety in animals (9), and in their tendency to become depressed.

V. THE USE OF ANTIDEPRESSANTS IN BULIMIA

The symptomatic overlap between bulimia and depression has encouraged researchers to study the effects of known antidepressants on the disturbed eating behavior of bulimics. The controlled studies in this area (see Table 2) indicate that these attempts have been highly successful. Pope et al. (68) treated 22 bulimics either with the TCA imipramine, in dosages of up to 200 mg/day, or with placebo. They found a 70% overall reduction in bingeing after 6 weeks of imipramine treatment, compared with virtually no change on placebo. Binges were less intense on imipramine, and patients reported less preoccupation with food. Follow-up on an open basis, using imipramine and other antidepressants, continued to show a moderate to marked reduction in bingeing in 18 of the 20 treated subjects (90%). Besides showing a decrease in the number of binges, Pope and colleagues (68) found a mean reduction of almost 50% in the HRS in patients on imipramine, compared to 1% in those on placebo. There was a significant correlation between improvement on the HRS and reduction in binge frequency. These authors concluded that the beneficial effects of imipramine in bulimia were probably attributable to its antidepressant actions.

Mitchell and Groat (61) also conducted a double-blind, placebo-controlled study on 32 normal-weight bulimics using amitriptyline in doses of 150 mg/day in 16

TABLE 2. *Treatment of bulimia with antidepressants in controlled trials[a]*

Reference	No. of patients	Drug and dosage (mg/day)	Duration (week)	Effects of drug on		Follow-up
				Eating behavior	Mood	
Pope et al. (68)	22 (9 on drug)	Imipramine, 200	6	70% reduction in binge frequency	50% reduction in HRS	1–8 months after study
Mitchell and Groat (61)	32 (16 on drug)	Amitriptyline, 150		No significant drug–placebo difference but trend favored active drug	Decrease in HRS by 63% on drug and 30% on placebo	—
Sabine et al. (79)	50	Mianserin, 60	8	Overall sample; no change	No drug–placebo difference in change on HRS	—
Walsh et al. (93)	20 (9 on drug)	Phenelzine, 60–90	6	Binge free 5; 50% decreased (4)	Significant drug–placebo difference in change on HRS	Of 8 drug-treated: 5 stopped drug and 3 of these relapsed; 1 of 3 who continued drug relapsed

[a]All studies were placebo-controlled, double-blind, parallel design.

subjects for 7 weeks following 1 week of medication adjustment. Both drug and placebo groups showed impressive responses. The drug group reported a 72% reduction in the number of binges and a 79% reduction in the number of vomiting episodes per week. The placebo group reported a 52% reduction in the number of binges and a 53% reduction in vomiting episodes per week. These differences did not reach statistical significance. However, there was a significant reduction in depression levels in those patients on amitriptyline. When these researchers compared depressed and nondepressed bulimics, they found that the latter group showed a greater improvement in eating behavior than the former. However, there was a significant correlation between improvement in eating behavior and certain of the Hamilton subscales (those measuring retardation and cognitive disturbance). The authors concluded that the most parsimonious explanation for these findings is that initial depression is a negative prognostic indicator in bulimia, but that improvement in eating dysfunction is the result of improvement in depression.

Several problems with this study may have contributed to the failure to demonstrate drug–placebo differences in eating behavior: (i) the choice of the drug, (ii) the dosage used, and (iii) the concurrent administration of a "minimal" behavioral treatment program. Amitriptyline has been reported to cause increased appetite and carbohydrate craving when used to treat depressives (66) in other studies, although the authors report that carbohydrate craving and weight gain did not occur in their population. A dosage of 150 mg/day would be considered inadequate in many depressed patients and may have been suboptimal for the control of bingeing and vomiting in this population. Amitriptyline blood levels were measured in only half the patients and were rather low in half these cases. The authors concede that the behavioral treatment regimen that they had originally regarded as minimal turned out to be unexpectedly effective and may have been responsible for the surprisingly good outcome in patients on placebo.

Sabine et al. (79) undertook a study of mianserin, the tetracyclic antidepressant, and placebo in 50 normal-weight bulimics. They found a general trend toward improvement over the 8 weeks of the trial but found no difference between drug and placebo. Possible reasons include the following: (i) the dose of drug used was relatively low; (ii) their patients appear to have been less severely affected and certainly less depressed than those in the studies discussed above; (iii) they did not measure binge frequency; and (iv) their choice of drug, mianserin, which may be less effective in treating bulimics than other antidepressants.

Walsh et al. (93) studied the effects of the MAOI phenelzine in the treatment of 20 normal-weight bulimic women. Five of the nine phenelzine-treated patients stopped bingeing entirely, and the other four reduced their binge frequency by 50% or more. The difference between the drug- and placebo-treated groups became significant 4 weeks after randomization and remained so for the rest of the study. Follow-up information on most of their patients showed that phenelzine remained effective in most of those who continued to take it, whereas three of five patients who discontinued it experienced complete relapses. Walsh and colleagues (93) noted that only one patient admitted to the study received a diagnosis of current major depression and that two of the five patients who were given phenelzine at randomization and had complete remissions had low HRS scores, indicating that they were not depressed. Walsh and colleagues suggested that MAOIs may be more effective than TCAs in the treatment of bulimia, but clearly it is too soon to provide a definitive answer to this question.

Several open trials of antidepressants have been performed (10,47,67). The results generally support the observations of their efficacy based on the controlled trials. It is less clear whether these medications work primarily by treating an underlying depression, which thereby enables patients to decrease their bingeing and vomiting, or whether the effect may be more direct. Some of the patients who benefit from antidepressants are not clinically depressed. Walsh and colleagues (93) have suggested that even in these patients, the tension, anxiety, and dysphoria that have been well described in bulimia may exist, and that perhaps the antibingeing effect is mediated by relief of these tensions. Before bulimic patients binge, they experience certain thoughts and feelings. They are aware of a desire to binge. Plans must be made, albeit often simple ones, such as getting to the food and securing privacy. Patients frequently feel anxious or dysphoric at the time, perhaps because of an underlying chemical disturbance (which may be related to the type of disturbance that occurs in affective disorder patients) or perhaps because of an awareness of what they are planning to do (feelings of being out of control, disgust with themselves). When it occurs, the binge or vomit may relieve some of the dysphoric feelings, especially those due to an underlying chemical disturbance. This would be compatible with the drug addiction model of bulimia. On the other hand, the binge may aggravate certain of these feelings, either by the chemical effects it causes or by its psychological impact.

The study by Pope et al. (68) noted that patients on imipramine were less preoccupied with food. It is reasonable to suggest that such a decrease in preoccupation allows patients to exert more self-control, binge less, and suffer less from the negative emotional and perhaps biochemical effects of bingeing. At the same time, those patients who are depressed at baseline experience a mood improvement as a result of the medication. The most parsimonious explanation for these observations is that depression and the wish to binge, and its associated dysphoric feelings, are different manifestations of related but not identical biochemical disturbances involving related but not identical neural pathways. That would explain why not all depressives are bulimic and not all bulimics are depressed, why there is a far greater coexistence of depressed and bulimic symptoms than would be predicted by chance alone, and why antidepressants are effective in the treatment of both disorders.

Just as the discovery of the antidepressant medications, which were known to have a powerful effect on biogenic amines, gave birth to the biogenic amine theories of depression, is it possible that we could determine the biochemical abnormalities involved in bulimia from the observation that antidepressants relieve symptoms in these patients? Over the past three decades, we have become more aware of the limitations of such an approach. Antidepressants do not act selectively at a single site but generally have several effects other than those involving biogenic amine metabolism, for example, anticholinergic and antihistaminic effects. Furthermore, we know that neurotransmitter systems are related to one another, and that effects on one system may affect other systems. We have become aware of a growing list of neurotransmitters and neuromodulators and do not know how these may be disturbed in depression or the complex ways in which they may be affected by antidepressants. We still do not know how the antidepressants exert their therapeutic effects in depression, and it is likely that the mechanism of their antibingeing effect will be similarly elusive.

VI. NEUROENDOCRINE STUDIES IN BULIMIA

In order to understand the neurobiological disturbances in depression, researchers have sought various biological markers of the condition. These could include physiological or biomedical abnormalities that occur in patients with the condition but not in normal controls, or in patients when they are in an acute affective episode but not when they are healthy. One heuristic approach has been to challenge the hypothalamus and pituitary by administering a drug and measuring the response in the periphery. This type of challenge paradigm resembles the *in vivo* receptor studies discussed previously. We deal here with two neuroendocrine tests that have been widely studied in depression and investigated to a lesser extent in patients with bulimia: the DST and the TRH stimulation test.

The DST involves the administration of a small dose of the powerful synthetic steroid dexamethasone in the evening and measurement of plasma cortisol the following afternoon. Under normal circumstances, the steroid, acting via the hypothalamus and pituitary, suppresses the endogenous production of cortisol from the adrenal, resulting in a low cortisol level the following afternoon. In endogenous depression, there is overactivity of the hypothalamic–adrenal–pituitary (HPA) axis and suppression does not occur, resulting in higher than normal cortisol levels the following afternoon, a condition known as DST nonsuppression. Carroll and colleagues (12) have reviewed this test extensively and have concluded that when it is carried out within certain constraints, nonsuppression is highly specific for endogenous depression and occurs in only 4% of normal subjects and psychiatric controls. Patients with atypical (nonendogenous) depression appear to respond normally to dexamethasone (75).

If bulimics were to show failure to suppress their cortisol secretion in response to dexamethasone, it could be argued that this would suggest a further biological overlap with major depression. Several investigators have administered the DST to normal-weight bulimics and have found a 47 to 67% incidence of DST nonsuppression (32,39,40,63). This would seem to be one further powerful indicator of the biological link between bulimia and depression were it not for several factors. First, since depression frequently coexists with bulimia, it is not clear to what extent the high incidence of abnormal DST results in bulimia reflects the presence of depression rather than of the eating disorder. Second, minor weight fluctuations have been reported to be associated with abnormal responses to the DST (6,7), and the likelihood of DST nonsuppression in bulimics may be inversely correlated with weight (32). Third, it has recently become apparent that DST nonsuppression is not in fact specific to major affective disorder but may occur in a variety of psychiatric and medical illnesses (21,85).

The TRH stimulation test involves the injection of a standard dose of TRH, which stimulates the pituitary to release thyroid-stimulating hormone (TSH), which is then measured in the plasma. Patients with major depression, especially the endogenous type, have been reported to have blunted TSH responses (51). Gwirtsman and colleagues (32) studied 10 normal-weight bulimics and found that eight of these patients had blunted responses similar to those found in depression. However, abnormal responses to the TRH stimulation test are also not specific for depression and have been reported to occur, for example, in alcoholic and manic patients (31,51).

There are other examples of neuroendocrine challenge tests which have been administered to depressed patients and which, no doubt, will be administered in time to patients with the eating disorders. Even if such tests are abnormal in both types of disorder, issues of specificity and confounding variables will presumably arise just as in the case of the DST and TRH test. Even if these issues can be resolved, the relationship between the observed neuroendocrine abnormality and the specific etiology of the condition may still be unclear, thus limiting the value of this approach.

VII. FAMILY STUDIES OF DEPRESSION AND BULIMIA

If the affective and eating disorders are related, as seems to be the case, perhaps by the involvement of common underlying neurochemical disturbances, it is reasonable to wonder whether these disturbances are heritable and whether the vulnerability to both types of disorder will be found in the same families. An analogous clustering of different types of psychiatric disorders has been described by Winokur (96), who coined the term *depressive spectrum disorder* to refer to a type of unipolar depression usually occurring in women, having an early onset, and characterized by a family history of alcoholism and sociopathy. Winokur suggested that in this condition, the same genetic vulnerability might find different forms of expression in different family members. In the case of depressive spectrum disorder, the alcoholism and sociopathy would be regarded as "depressive equivalents." It is possible that bulimia or carbohydrate craving might similarly be regarded genetically as depressive equivalents.

In an ideal study, relatives of probands (patients affected by the disease in question) and relatives of a control population are personally interviewed (family study method), and standardized diagnostic criteria are applied to ill relatives. The ratio of ill to well relatives is calculated and adjusted to take into account the age of relatives at the time of the interview; that adjusted ratio is called the morbid risk. Such rigorous methodology is not always possible; in some studies, researchers simply question affected probands (family history method) and may not have a control population but may rely instead on epidemiological data obtained from other sources. The morbid risk for affective disorder in relatives of patients with anorexia nervosa has been thoroughly studied and has been found to be considerably increased over the morbid risk for relatives of normal control populations (11,17,29,30,72,90,91,94,97). There is some controversy over whether the morbid risk for relatives of bingeing (bulimic) anorectics is higher than that for restricting anorectics (26,30,41,90), but the consensus at this time is that the morbid risk for affective disorder is equal in these two subtypes of anorexia, which are thus not thought to be genetically distinct subtypes (26,30,41). Probably because normal-weight bulimia is a more recently recognized entity, the nature and incidence of psychopathology among family members has been less well characterized.

To date, two good studies have been done on normal-weight bulimics, but their findings are unfortunately in disagreement with each other. Hudson and colleagues (41) questioned patients with normal-weight bulimia about their family histories and also questioned the relatives directly where possible. They used DSM-III diagnostic criteria in diagnosing psychopathology in relatives and had as control groups patients with anorexia nervosa, anorexia plus bulimia, bipolar affective disorder, schizophrenia, and borderline personality disorder. They evaluated 251 relatives of 55 patients with normal-weight bulimia and found the morbid risk for major affective disorder to be 26%. This did not differ significantly from the morbid risks for major affective disorder in relatives of patients with anorexia nervosa (31%), anorexia plus bulimia (28%), or bipolar affective disorder (12%) but did differ significantly from the morbid risks in relatives of patients with schizophrenia (1%) and borderline personality disorder (3%). There are two major limitations of this study: (i) The relatives were not interviewed directly; and (ii) the interviewers were not blind to the diagnoses of the patients being questioned.

In the second study, Stern and colleagues (89) interviewed at least one first-degree relative (usually the mother) of each of 27 normal-weight bulimics as well as the mothers of 27 normal controls about the family history of psychiatric illness. The interviewer was blind as to whether the relative was the parent of a proband or of a normal control. The probands were interviewed about their own psychiatric histories by a different interviewer. Contrary to their expectations, Stern and colleagues found no significant difference between the relatives of bulimic and control probands with respect to the lifetime prevalence of affective disorder. The morbid risk for major affective disorder was similar for the two groups: 14% for relatives of bulimic probands and 16% for relatives of control subjects. A personal lifetime history of affective disorder was present in 56% of the bulimics as opposed to 30% of the normal controls. In an earlier study by Hudson et al. (42), in which they inquired about a previous history of affective disorder in 49 bulimics (presumably a population overlapping the one used in the family history study), the authors found a lifetime history of major affective disorder in 73% of cases.

Pyle et al. (69), in the one other large family study on normal-weight bulimics, found a positive family history of affective disorder in about 50% of 33 bulimic probands. This corresponds more closely to the findings of Hudson et al. (41) than to those of Stern et al. (89). However, in the study by Pyle and colleagues, standardized criteria were not used. At this time, it would seem as though there is probably a higher than normal incidence of affective disorder in the families of bulimic patients, but more well-conducted studies are indicated.

VIII. CONCLUSION

In reviewing the symptoms, pharmacological responses, and neuroendocrine and family studies in the affective disorders and bulimia, we have attempted to show the many areas of overlap between these conditions. They are currently classified under separate diagnostic categories in the DSM-III and should probably remain so for the present. Indeed, in their pure form, they may appear clinically distinct from one another. However, there are many patients in whom the symptoms are mixed to the extent that a clear diagnosis of one or the other condition cannot be made. The condition may occur at different times in the life of a single patient; in such cases, the sequence in which the conditions appear seems variable. For unknown reasons, the affective disorders are more prevalent than the eating disorders in the population as a whole. The most parsimonious explanation of the similarities and differences between the two set of conditions is that the regulation of mood and eating behavior probably share neurochemical and neuroanatomical substrates which, when dysfunctional, may give rise to affective disorders and, less commonly, eating disorders. The affective disorders frequently manifest with disturbances of eating and the eating disorders with disturbances of mood regulation. The process of eating has feedback effects on the regulation of appetite and perhaps in certain people on the regulation of mood and may relieve feelings of anxiety, tension, or sadness. In these latter individuals, the choice of food may in some cases be specific, such as in the carbohydrate cravers, and in other cases nonspecific, such as in many bulimics. Presumably, different feedback mechanisms would be involved in cases that differ with respect to the type of food selected. In cases in which food is used to regulate mood rather than to fulfill nutritional needs, food may be conceptualized as a drug and the condition as a type of drug addiction. However, it is not always possible to explain the overeating and bingeing in terms of their regulatory effects on mood, since some bulimics seem to feel no better or even worse after they have binged. In these cases, the eating disturbance may be seen as primary and the mood changes as secondary to the resulting disturbances in brain chemistry or the psychological effects of the act of bingeing and vomiting. It may be difficult to separate what is primary from what is secondary in such cases. Indeed, both disturbances may be a function of a common underlying brain dysfunction.

The exact anatomical sites of the neurochemical disturbances in the affective and eating disorders are unknown, and we can do no more than speculate about these on the basis of the animal literature, largely in the area of eating behavior. Nevertheless, interesting theories involving biogenic amines and peptides have been proposed, and these can be tested clinically. One such approach has been taken by Wurtman and Wurtman (99) in the specific group of obese carbohydrate cravers where the serotonin system has been studied. Much may be gained by such an approach where a homogeneous population is used and a specific hypothesis tested.

Neuroendocrine studies offer an important approach to *in vivo* studies of brain function, but they are limited by problems of specificity and relevance to the core neurobiological disturbance of the disorder being studied.

Family studies are useful in determining whether the postulated neurochemical deficits involved in the two sets of disorders are cotransmitted or whether the disorders are different manifestations of the same genetic vulnerability, as has been proposed in the depressive spectrum disorders. It is too early to state whether there is in fact an increased genetic vulnerability to affective disorder in the families of bulimic subjects.

Researchers in the area of the eating disorders have benefited greatly from methodology established in earlier studies of the affective disorders and other psychiatric conditions. Over the years, the need for standardized criteria, discrimination between symptoms and syndrome, control populations, and many other methodological issues have become apparent, and this knowledge is being used to good effect in studies of the eating disorders. Researchers in the field of affective disorders should pay much more heed to disturbances of eating and inquire more carefully about, and even measure, the amount and type of food eaten. Division of depressives into overeating and undereating subgroups may lead to novel ways of examining biological data.

Appendix. Addendum to HRS

24. *Fatigability*

0. Does not get more tired than usual
1. Gets tired more easily than before but not for more than a few hours a day
2. Gets tired more easily than before for more than a few hours a day
3. Is tired most of the day
4. Too tired to do any tasks except for basic daily functions

25. *Social withdrawal*

0. Interacts with other people as usual
1. Less interested in socializing with others but continues to do so
2. Interacting less with other people in social (optional) situations
3. Interacting less with other people in work or family situations (i.e., where this is necessary)
4. Marked withdrawal from others in family or work situations

26. *Appetite increase*

0. No increase in appetite
1. Wants to eat a little more than usual
2. Wants to eat somewhat more than normal
3. Wants to eat much more than usual

27. *Increased eating*

0. Is not eating more than usual
1. Is eating a little more than usual

2. Is eating somewhat more than usual
3. Is eating much more than normal

28. *Carbohydrate craving* (in relation to total amount of food desired or eaten)

0. No change in food preference
1. Eating more carbohydrates (starches or sugars) than before
2. Eating much more carbohydrates than before
3. Irresistible craving for sweets or starches

29. *Weight gain*

0. No weight gain
1. Probable weight gain associated with present illness
2. Definite weight gain (according to patient)

30. *Hypersomnia* (compare sleep length to euthymic and not to hypomanic sleep
    length; if this cannot be established, use 8 hr)

0. No increase in sleep length
1. At least 1 hr increase in sleep length
2. 2 + hr increase
3. 3 + hr increase
4. 4 + hr increase in sleep length

Was euthymic sleep length used?   Yes _____ No _____
Was 8-hr sleep length used?   Yes _____ No _____

REFERENCES

 1. Abraham, S. F., and Beaumont, P. J. V. (1982): How patients describe bulimia or binge eating. *Psychol. Med.*, 12:625–635.
 2. Akiskal, H. S. (1983): Diagnosis and classification of affective disorders: New insights from clinical and laboratory approaches. *Psychiatr. Dev.*, 2:123–160.
 3. American Psychiatric Association: Task Force on Nomenclature and Statistics. (1980): *Diagnostic and Statistical Manual of Mental Disorders, Ed. 3.* Washington, D.C.
 4. Ariens, E. J., and Simonis, A. M. (1983): Physiological and pharmacological aspects of adrenergic receptor classification. *Biochem. Pharmacol.*, 32:1539–1545.
 5. Beck, A. T., Ward, C. H., Mendelson, M., Mock, J., and Erbaugh, J. (1961): An inventory for measuring depression. *Arch. Gen. Psychiatry*, 4:561–571.
 6. Berger, M., Doerr, P., Lund, R., Bronisch, T., and von Zerssen, D. (1982): Neuroendocrinological and neurophysiological studies in major depressive disorders. Are there biological markers for the endogenous subtype? *Biol. Psychiatry*, 17:1217–1239.
 7. Berger, M., Krieg, C., and Pirke, K. M. (1982): Is the positive dexamethasone test in depressed patients a consequence of weight loss? *Neuroendocrinol. Lett.*, 4:177.
 8. Blombery, P. A., Kopin, I. J., Gordon, E. K., Markey, S. P., and Ebert, M. H. (1980): Conversion of MHPG to vanillylmandelic acid. *Arch. Gen. Psychiatry*, 37:1095–1098.
 9. Blundell, J. E. (1983): Problems and processes underlying the control of food selection and nutrient intake. In: *Nutrition and the Brain, Vol. 6*, edited by R. Wurtman and J. Wurtman, pp. 163–222. Raven Press, New York.
10. Brotman, A. W., Herzog, D. B., and Woods, S. W. (1984): Antidepressant treatment of bulimia: the relationship between bingeing and depressive symptomatology. *J. Clin. Psychiatry*, 45:7–9.
11. Cantwell, D. P., Sturzenberger, S., Burroughs, J., Salkin, B., and Green, J. K. (1977): Anorexia nervosa: An affective disorder? *Arch. Gen. Psychiatry*, 34:1087–1093.
12. Carroll, B. J., Feinberg, M., Greden, J. F., Tarika, J., Albala, A. A., Haskett, R. F., James,

N. M., Dronfol, Z., Lohr, N., Steiner, M., de Vigne, J. P., and Young, E. (1981): A specific laboratory test for the diagnosis of melancholia. *Arch. Gen. Psychiatry*, 38:15–22.

13. Charney, D. S., Heninger, G. R., Sternberg, D. E., and Landis, H. (1982): Abrupt discontinuation of tricyclic antidepressant drugs: Evidence for noradrenergic hyperactivity. *Br. J. Psychiatry*, 141:377–386.

14. Charney, D. S., Menkes, D. B., and Heninger, G. R. (1981): Receptor sensitivity and the mechanism of action of antidepressant treatment: Implications for the etiology and therapy of depression. *Arch. Gen. Psychiatry*, 38:1160–1180.

15. Checkley, S. A., Slade, A. P., and Shur, E. (1981): Growth hormone and other responses to clonidine in patients with endogenous depression. *Br. J. Psychiatry*, 138:51–55.

16. Coppen, A., and Ghose, K. (1978): Peripheral alpha-adrenoreceptor and central dopamine receptor activity in depressive patients. *Psychopharmacology*, 59:171–177.

17. Crisp, A. H., Hsu, L. K., Harding, B., and Hartshorn, J. (1980): Clinical features of anorexia nervosa. *J. Psychosom. Res.*, 24:179–191.

18. Crisp, A. H., and Stonehill, E. (1973): Aspects of the relationships between sleep and nutrition: a study of 375 psychiatric outpatients. *Brit. J. Psychiatry*, 12:379–394.

19. Davidson, J. R. T., Miller, R. C., Turnbull, C. D., and Sullivan, J. (1982): Atypical depression. *Arch. Gen. Psychiatry*, 39:527–534.

20. de Montigny, C., Cournoyer, G., Morissette, R., Langlois, R., and Caille, G. (1983): Lithium carbonate addition in tricyclic antidepressant-resistant unipolar depression: Correlations with the neurobiologic actions of tricyclic antidepressant drugs and lithium ion on the serotonin system. *Arch. Gen. Psychiatry*, 40:1327–1334.

21. Dewan, M. J., Pandurangi, A. K., Boucher, M. L., Levy, B. F., and Major, L. F. (1982): Abnormal dexamethasone suppression test results in chronic schizophrenic patients. *Am. J. Psychiatry*, 139:1501–1503.

22. Eastwood, M. R., and Stiasny, S. (1978): Psychiatric disorder, hospital admission, and season. *Arch. Gen. Psychiatry*, 35:769–771.

22a. Endicott, J., and Spitzer, R. L. (1978): A diagnostic interview: The schedule for affective disorders and schizophrenia. *Arch. Gen. Psychiatry*, 35:837–844.

23. Fairburn, C. G., and Cooper, P. J. (1984): The clinical features of bulimia nervosa. *Br. J. Psychiatry*, 144:238–246.

24. Feighner, J. P., Robins, E., Guze, S. B., Woodruff, R. A., Winokur, G., and Munoz, R. (1972): Diagnostic criteria for use in psychiatric research. *Arch. Gen. Psychiatry*, 26:57–63.

25. Fernstrom, J. D., and Wurtman, R. J. (1972): Brain serotonin content: Physiological regulation by plasma neutral amino acids. *Science*, 178:414–416.

26. Garfinkel, P. E., Moldofsky, H., and Garner, D. M. (1980): The heterogeneity of anorexia nervosa: Bulimia as a distinct subgroup. *Arch. Gen. Psychiatry*, 37:1036–1040.

27. Garner, D. M., Garfinkel, P. E., and O'Shaughnessy, M. (1983): Clinical and psychometric comparison between bulimia in anorexia nervosa and bulimia in normal-weight women. *Report on the 4th Ross Conference on Medical Research*, pp. 6–11. Ross Laboratories, Columbus, Ohio.

28. Garvey, M. J., Mungas, D., and Tollefson, G. D. (1984): Hypersomnia in major depressive disorders. *J. Affective Disord.*, 6:283–286.

29. Gershon, E. S., Hamovit, J. R., Schrieber, J. L., Dibble, E. D., Kaye, W., Nurnberger, J. I., Andersen, A., and Ebert, M. (1983): Anorexia nervosa and major affective disorders associated in families: A preliminary report. In: *Childhood Psychopathology and Development*, edited by S. B. Guze, F. J. Earls, and J. E. Barrett, pp. 279–284. Raven Press, New York.

30. Gershon, E. S., Schreiber, J. L., Hamovit, J. R., Dibble, E. D., Kaye, W., Nurnberger, J. I., Andersen, A. E., and Ebert, M. (1984): Clinical findings in patients with anorexia nervosa and affective illness in their relatives, *Am. J. Psychiatry*, 141(11):1419–1422.

31. Gold, M. S., Pottash, A. L. C., Extein, I., Martin, D. M., Howard, E., Mueller, E. A., and Sweeney, D. R. (1981): The TRH test in the diagnosis of major and minor depression. *Psychoneuroendocrinology*, 6:159–169.

32. Gwirtsman, H. E., Roy-Byrne, P., Yager, J., and Gerner, R. H. (1983): Neuroendocrine abnormalities in bulimia. *Am. J. Psychiatry*, 140(5):559–563.

33. Halmi, K. A., Falk, J. R., and Schwartz, E. (1981): Binge-eating and vomiting: A survey of a college population. *Psychol. Med.*, 11:697–796.

34. Hamilton, M. (1967): Development of a rating scale for primary depressive illness. *Br. J. Soc. Clin. Psychol.*, 6:278–296.

35. Hatsukami, D. K., Mitchell, J. E., and Eckert, E. D. (1984): Eating disorders: A variant of mood disorders? *Psychiatr. Clin. North. Am.*, 7(2):349–365.

36. Herzog, D. B. (1982): Bulimia in the adolescent. *Am. J. Dis. Child.*, 136:985–989.

37. Hopkinson, G. (1981): A neurochemical theory of appetite and weight changes in depressive states. *Acta. Psychiatr. Scand.*, 64:217–225.

38. Deleted in proof.

39. Hudson, J. I., Laffer, P. S., and Pope, H. G. (1982): Bulimia related to affective disorder by family history and response to the dexamethasone suppression test. *Am. J. Psychiatry*, 139(5):685–687.

40. Hudson, J. I., Pope, H. G., Jonas, J. M., Laffer, P. S., Hudson, M. S., and Melby, J. C. (1983): Hypothalamic-pituitary-adrenal-axis hyperactivity in bulimia. *Psychiatr. Res.*, 8:111–117.

41. Hudson, J. I., Pope, H. G., Jonas, J. M., and Yurgelun-Todd, D. (1983): Family history study of anorexia nervosa and bulimia. *Br. J. Psychiatry*, 142:133–138.

42. Hudson, J. I., Pope, H. G., Jonas, J. M., and Yurgelun-Todd, D. (1983): Phenomenologic relationship of eating disorders to major affective disorder, *Psychiatr. Res.*, 9:345–354.

43. Jimerson, D. C. (1984): Neurotransmitter hypotheses of depression. *Psychiatr. Clin. North Am.*, 7(3):563–573.

44. Johnson, C., and Berndt, D. J. (1983): Preliminary investigation of bulimia and life adjustment. *Am. J. Psychiatry*, 140:774–777.

45. Johnson, C., and Larson, R. (1982): Bulimia: An analysis of moods and behavior. *Psychosom. Med.*, 44(4):341–351.

46. Johnson, C. L., Stuckey, M. K., Lewis, L. D., and Schwartz, D. M. (1982): Bulimia: A descriptive survey of 316 cases. *Int. J. Eating Disord.*, 2(1):3–16.

47. Jonas, J. M., Hudson, J. I., and Pope, H. G. (1985): Treatment of bulimia with MAO inhibitors. *J. Clin. Psychopharmacol. (in press).*

48. Kaye, W. H., Ebert, M. H., Gwirtsman, H. E., and Weiss, S. (1984): Differences in brain serotonergic metabolism between nonbulimic and bulimic patients with anorexia nervosa. *Am. J. Psychiatry*, 141(12):1598–1601.

49. Kaye, W. H., and Gwirtsman, H. E. (1985): Mood changes and patterns of food consumption during bingeing and purging: Are there underlying neurobiologic relationships? In: *Bulimia in Normal Weight Women: Physiology and Treatment*, edited by W. H. Kaye and H. E. Gwirtsman. American Psychiatric Press, Washington, D. C. (in press).

50. Kaye, W. H., Jimerson, D. C., Lake, C. R., and Ebert, M. H. (1985): Altered norepinephrine metabolism following long-term weight recovery in patients with anorexia nervosa. *Psychiatr. Res.*, 14(4):333–342.

51. Kirkegaard, C. (1981): The thyrotropin response to thyrotropin-releasing hormone in endogenous depression. *Psychoneuroendocrinology*, 6:182–212.

52. Kraepelin, E. (1921): *Manic Depressive Illness and Paranoia.* S. Livingstone, Edinburgh.

53. Kraines, S. H. (1972): Weight gain and other symptoms of the ascending depressive curve. *Psychosomatics*, 13:23–33.

54. Kumetz, N. F. (1983): Bulimia, a descriptive and treatment survey. *Dis. Ab. Int.*, 44(5).

55. Lacey, J. H. (1983): Bulimia nervosa, binge eating, and psychogenic vomiting: A controlled treatment study and long-term outcome. *Br. Med. J.*, 286:1609–1613.

56. Leckman, J. F., Caruso, K. A., Prusoff, B. A., Weissman, M. M., Merikangas, K. R., and Pauls, D. L. (1984): Appetite disturbance and excessive guilt in major depression: Use of family study data to define depressive subtypes. *Arch. Gen. Psychiatry*, 41:839–844.

57. Liebowitz, M. R., Quitkin, F. M., Stewart, J. W., McGrath, P. J., Harrison, W., Rabkin, J., Tricamo, E., Markowitz, J. S., and Klein, D. F. (1984): Phenelzine versus imipramine in atypical depression: a preliminary report. *Arch. Gen. Psychiatry*, 41:669–677.

58. Deleted in proof.

59. Matussek, N., Ackenheil, M., Hippius, H., Muller, F., Schroder, H.-Th., Schultes, H., and Wasilewski, B. (1980): Effect of clonidine on growth hormone release in psychiatric patients and controls. *Psychiatry Res.*, 2:25–36.

60. Meltzer, H. Y., Umberkoman-Wiita, B., Robertson, A., Tricou, B. J., Lowy, M., and Perline, R. (1984): Effect of 5-hydroxytryptophan on serum cortisol levels in major affective disorders. I. Enhanced response in depression and mania. *Arch. Gen. Psychiatry*, 41:366–374.

61. Mitchell, J. E., and Groat, R. (1984): A placebo-controlled, double-blind trial of amitriptyline in bulimia. *J. Clin. Psychopharmacol.*, 4:186–193.

62. Mitchell, J. E., Pyle, R. L., and Eckert, E. D. (1981): Frequency and duration of binge-eating episodes in patients with bulimia. *Am. J. Psychiatry*, 138:835–836.
63. Mitchell, J. E., Pyle, R. L., Hatsukami, D., and Bontacoff, L. I. (1984): The dexamethasone suppression test in patients with bulimia. *J. Clin. Psychiatry*, 45(12):508–511.
64. Morley, J. E., and Levine, A. S. (1983): The central control of appetite. *Lancet*, I, Feb. 19:398–401.
65. Murphy, D. L., Campbell, I., and Costa, J. L. (1978): Current status of the indolamine hypothesis of affective disorders. In: *Psychopharmacology: A Generation of Progress*, edited by M. A. DiMasco and A. Killam, pp. 1223–1234. Raven Press, New York.
66. Paykel, E. S., Mueller, P. S., and De la Vergne, P. M. (1973): Amitriptyline, weight gain, and carbohydrate craving: A side effect. *Br. J. Psychiatry*, 123:501–507.
67. Pope, H. G., and Hudson, J. I. (1982): Treatment of bulimia with antidepressants. *Psychopharmacology*, 78:176–179.
68. Pope, H. G., Hudson, J. I., Jonas, J. M., and Yurgelun-Todd, D. (1983): Bulimia treated with imipramine: A placebo-controlled, double-blind study. *Am. J. Psychiatry*, 140(5):554–558.
69. Pyle, R. L., Mitchell, J. E., and Eckert, E. D. (1981): Bulimia: A report of 34 cases. *J. Clin. Psychiatry*, 42(2):60–64.
70. Quaade, F., Vaernet, K., and Larsson, S. (1974): Stereotaxic stimulation and electrocoagulation of the lateral hypothalamus in obese humans. *Acta Neurochir. (Wien)*, 30:111–117.
71. Reeves, A. G., and Plum, F. (1969): Hyperphagia, rage, and dementia accompanying a ventromedial hypothalamic neoplasm. *Arch. Neurol.*, 20:616–624.
72. Rivinius, T. M., Biederman, J., Herzog, D. B., Kemper, K., Harper, G. P., Harmatz, J. S., and Houseworth, S. (1984): Anorexia nervosa and affective disorders: A controlled family history study. *Am. J. Psychiatry*, 141:1414–1418.
73. Rolls, E. T. (1981): Central nervous mechanisms related to feeding and appetite. *Br. Med. Bull.*, 37(2):131–134.
74. Rosenthal, N. E., Sack, D. A., Carpenter, C. J., Parry, B. L., Mendelson, W. B., and Wehr, T. A. (1985): Antidepressant effects of light in seasonal affective disorder. *Am. J. Psychiatry*, 142(2):163–170.
75. Rosenthal, N. E., Sack, D. A., Gillin, J. C., Lewy, A. J., Goodwin, F. K., Davenport, Y., Mueller, P. S., Newsome, D. A., and Wehr, T. A. (1984): Seasonal affective disorder: A description of the syndrome and preliminary findings with light therapy. *Arch. Gen Psychiatry*, 41:72–80.
76. Rosenthal, N. E., Sack, D. A., James, S. P., Parry, B. L., Mendelson, W. B., Tamarkin, L., and Wehr, T. A. (1984): Seasonal affective disorder and phototherapy. Presented at the New York Academy of Sciences, November, 1984.
77. Rosenthal, N. E., Sack, D. A., and Wehr, T. A. (1983): Seasonal variation in affective disorders. In: *Circadian Rhythms in Psychiatry*, edited by T. A. Wehr and F. K. Goodwin, pp. 185–201. Boxwood Press, Pacific Grove, California.
78. Russell, G. (1979): Bulimia nervosa: An ominous variant of anorexia nervosa. *Psychol. Med.*, 9:429–448.
79. Sabine, E. J., Yonace, A., Farrington, A. J., Barratt, K. H., and Wakeling, A. (1983): Bulimia nervosa: A placebo controlled double-blind therapeutic trial of mianserin. *Br. J. Clin. Pharmacol.*, 15:195S–202S.
80. Schildkraut, J. J. (1965): The catecholamine hypothesis of affective disorders: A review of supporting evidence. *Am. J. Psychiatry*, 122:509–522.
81. Shopsin, B., Friedman, E., and Gershon, S. (1976): Parachlorophenylalanine reversal of tranylcypromine effects in depressed patients. *Arch. Gen. Psychiatry*, 33:811–819.
82. Shopsin, B., Gershon, S., Goldstein, M., Friedman, E., and Wilk, S. (1975): Use of synthesis inhibitors in defining a role for biogenic amines during imipramine treatment in depressed patients. *Psychopharmacol. Commun.*, 1:239–249.
83. Siever, L. J., Uhde, T. W., Jimerson, D. C., Lake, C. R., Silberman, E. R., Post, R. M., and Murphy, D. L. (1984): Differential inhibitory noradrenergic responses to clonidine in 25 depressed patients and 25 normal control subjects. *Am. J. Psychiatry*, 141:733–741.
84. Smith, S. L., and Sauder, C. (1969): Food cravings, depression, and premenstrual problems. *Psychosom. Med.*, 31(4):281–287.
85. Spar, J. E., and Gerner, R. (1982): Does the dexamethasone suppression test distinguish dementia from depression? *Am. J. Psychaitry*, 139:238–249.
86. Deleted in proof.

87. Spitzer, R. L., Endicott, J., and Robins, E. (1978): Research and diagnostic criteria: rationale and reliability. *Arch. Gen. Psychiatry*, 35:773–782.

88. Spring, B., Maller, O., Wurtman, J., Digman, L., and Cozolino, L. (1983): Effects of protein carbohydrate meals on mood and performance: Interactions with sex and age. *J. Psychiatr. Res.*, 17:155–167.

89. Stern, S. L., Dixon, K. N., Nemzer, M. D., Lake, M. D., Sansone, R. A., Smeltzer, D. J., Lantz, S., and Schrier, S. S. (1985): Affective disorder in families of women with normal weight bulimia. *Am. J. Psychiatry*, 141(10):1224–1227.

90. Strober, M., Salkin, B., Burroughs, J., and Morrell, W. (1982): Validity of the bulimia restrictor distinction in anorexia nervosa: Parental personality characteristics and family psychiatric morbidity. *J. Ment. Nerv. Dis.*, 170(6):345–351.

91. Theander, S. (1970): Anorexia nervosa: A psychiatric investigation of 94 female patients. *Acta. Psychiatr. Scand. [Suppl. 214].*

92. Walsh, B. T., Roose, S. P., Glassman, A. H., Gladis, M., and Sadik, C. (1985): Bulimia and depression. *Psychosom. Med.*, 47(2):123–131.

93. Walsh, B. T., Stewart, J. W., Roose, S. P., Gladis, M., and Glassman, A. H. (1984): Treatment of bulimia with phenelyine. *Arch. Gen. Psychiatry*, 41(11):1105–1109.

94. Warren, W. (1968): A study of anorexia nervosa in young girls. *J. Child Psychol. Psychiatry*, 9:27–40.

95. Weiss, S. R., and Ebert, M. E. (1983): Psychological and behavioral characteristics of normal weight bulimics and normal weight controls. *Psychosom. Med.*, 45(2):293–303.

96. Winokur, G. (1974): The division of depressive illness into depression spectrum disease and pure depressive disease. *Int. Pharmacopsychiatry*, 9:5–13.

97. Winokur, G., March, V., and Mendels, J. (1980): Primary affective disorder in relatives of patients with anorexia nervosa. *Am. J. Psychiatry*, 137(6):695–698.

98. Wurtman, J. J., and Wurtman, R. J. (1984): Impaired control of appetite for carbohydrates in some patients with eating disorders: Treatment with pharmacologic agents. In: *The Psychobiology of Anorexia Nervosa*, edited by K. M. Pirke and D. Ploog, pp. 12–21. Springer-Verlag, Berlin.

99. Wurtman, J. J., Wurtman, R. J., Growdon, J. H., Henry, P., Lipscomb, A., and Zeisel, S. H. (1981): Carbohydrate craving in obese people: Suppression by treatments affecting serotoninergic transmission. *Int. J. Eating. Disord.*, 1:2–15.

100. Wurtman, R. J., and Wurtman, J. J. (1984): Nutritional control of central neurotransmitters. In: *The Psychobiology of Anorexia Nervosa*, edited by K. M. Pirke and D. Ploog, pp. 4–11. Springer-Verlag, Berlin.

Nutrition and the Brain, Vol. 7, edited by
R. J. Wurtman and J. J. Wurtman. Raven Press,
New York © 1986.

Psychobiology of Anorexia Nervosa

Karl M. Pirke and Detlev Ploog

Max-Planck-Institute für Psychiatrie, 8000 Munich 40, Federal Republic of Germany

I. THE SYNDROME OF ANOREXIA NERVOSA

A. Clinical Description

Anorexia nervosa is a psychosomatic syndrome that occurs mainly in adolescent girls from middle- and upper-class families. Five percent of all patients are male. Anorexia nervosa may occur, although less frequently, at ages other than adolescence (5). The disease was first described in England in the seventeenth century but incidence has increased during the last decades. For example, Crisp et al. (38) found the syndrome in one of 200 girls aged 12 to 18 years.

Various diagnostic criteria were applied in the past. Those of the American Psychiatric Association (DSM-III) (44) are probably the most frequently used criteria today:

1. "Intense fear of becoming obese, which does not diminish as weight loss progresses."

Disturbances in eating behavior and episodes of dieting inspired by the fear of becoming fat are reported by almost all girls (3) at some point during adolescence. While this remains a short episode in healthy individuals, anorectic girls continue to lose weight. This is achieved by different means. Approximately half the patients solely restrict their food intake and may take additional measures, such as severe exercise to burn energy. This subgroup has been classified as "restricters" (26). The other subgroup encompasses "vomiters." This group reports more or less frequent bouts of overeating (bingeing) that are followed by vomiting. Additional measures taken to lose weight include the use of diuretics, laxatives, and appetite-suppressing pills. On the average, the group of restricters is younger and is said to have a better prognosis (26). However, it is frequently observed that restricters become vomiters during the course of the disease.

2. "Disturbance of body image, e.g., claiming to 'feel fat', even when ema-ciated."

The fact that patients do not recognize their state of emaciation may be considered a part of their denial of illness (27,66). Numerous experimental studies have been conducted to measure the distorted body perception (58). Using such techniques, body image disturbance can be demonstrated in approximately half the patients with anorexia nervosa (59). Results vary greatly, depending on the techniques utilized (150). The tendency to overestimate body size correlates with a disturbance of interoception as measured by a satiety–aversion-to-sucrose test (61,62).

3. "Weight loss of at least 25% of original body weight, or if under 18 years of age, weight loss from original body weight plus projected weight gain ex-pected from growth charts may be combined to make the 25%."

This strict weight limit is currently under discussion and may soon be changed in favor of a more adequate definition of "underweight."

4. "Refusal to maintain body weight over a minimal normal weight for age and height."

5. "No known physical illness that would account for the weight loss."

Consuming diseases, such as carcinoma and gastrointestinal diseases, must be excluded. Pinealoma and other tumors in or in the vicinity of the hypothalamus may occasionally mimic anorexia nervosa (6,146,162). Other psychiatric diseases may also lead to emaciation; for example, a paranoid schizophrenic patient may stop eating for fear of being poisoned.

B. Eating Preferences

What do patients with anorexia nervosa eat? This question is of utmost impor-tance in view of the consequences of starvation. De Haven et al. (41) compared the effects of low-calorie, high-protein, and mixed diets. In contrast to the mixed diet, the high-protein diet caused greater sodium loss and a decrease of sympathetic nervous system activity with low plasma norepinephrine (NE) and orthostatic hypotension.

Crisp (33), Hurst et al. (83), and Russell (130) claimed that patients avoided carbohydrates and consumed relatively adequate amounts of protein and fat. In contrast to these reports, Beumont et al. (8) observed that the proportion of energy derived from protein was significantly higher, that from fat was lower, and that from carbohydrates was no different from that of controls. In a recent study by Huse and Lucas (84), it became apparent that food selection varies greatly in patients with anorexia nervosa. Only about one-third of the patients ate meals of satisfactory quality, that is, containing adequate amounts from the basic food groups (proteins, fats, and carbohydrates). Of 96 patients, 40 reported idiosyncratic food choices, such as vegetarianism, avoidance of red meat, and avoidance of sweets.

The great variety in metabolic and endocrine symptoms observed in anorexia nervosa and bulimia (120) may be the result of different food choices. Future studies on anorexia nervosa should take into account eating behavior and nutrient selection and avoidance. Such information can lead to studies on the relationship between patterns of calorie and nutrient intake and somatic and behavioral symptoms.

C. Etiology and Pathogenesis

The etiology of anorexia nervosa is unknown. The state of the art is best illustrated by a recent survey conducted by Slade *(personal communication)*. He asked qualified researchers in the field of eating disorders for their opinion on the etiology of anorexia nervosa. In this questionnaire, the following theories were offered:

1. Social cultural theory
2. Family pathology theory
3. Individual psychodynamic theory
4. Developmental psychobiological theory
5. Primary hypothalamic dysfunction theory
6. Cognitive dysfunction theory
7. Multifactorial model

Various attempts have been made to incorporate some of these theories into a multifactorial model (104,123). Figure 1 presents a multifactorial model proposed by Lucas (104) and slightly modified by Ploog (123). A genetic predisposition has been postulated based on two kinds of evidence. First, studies of twins (80) showed the concordance to be much higher in monozygotic than in heterozygotic twins. This fact cannot be considered as definite proof for a genetic predisposition. The authors (80) themselves indicate that the equal environment assumption made in twin research may be wrong in anorexia nervosa and that monozygotic twins are treated in a more similar manner than dizygote pairs. This report strongly suggests but does not prove genetic influences. Second, recent observations by Cantwell et

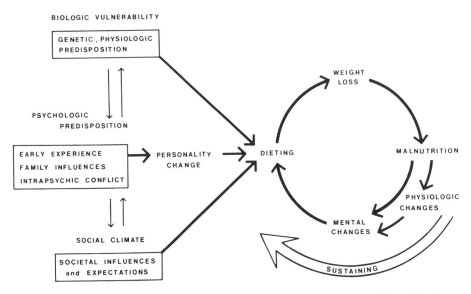

FIG. 1. Hypothetical model of pathogenesis and etiology of anorexia nervosa. (For explanation, see text.)

al. (22) and Winokur et al. (161) showed an overrepresentation of affective illness in families of anorectics. These studies should be viewed critically, since the diagnosis of depression was made from information given by relatives and not directly from psychiatric evaluation of the sick persons. Kay and Leigh (91), Halmi and Loney (75), and Kalucy et al. (88) reported an increased incidence of alcoholism in parents of anorectic patients.

There is still controversy as to the premorbid personality of the anorectic patient. Halmi et al. (74) found that the majority of their patients were "perfectionistic, competitive, achieving." Smart et al. (142) found that their patients were more neurotic, introverted, and anxious than normal controls. Garfinkel and Garner (58) have criticized these studies. They indicate that anorexia nervosa brings about secondary changes in personality, which according to their and our opinion, make it impossible to obtain correct information on the premorbid personality of the anorectic patient.

1. Influences of the Family

The disease is more common in upper- than in lower-class families (33,70,111). It is accepted that there is no single family constellation responsible for the development of the disease, and that its existence changes the attitude of parents and siblings. These secondary changes make reconstruction of the original family unit difficult. Selvini-Palazzoli (138) and Minuchin et al. (113) described certain family interactions that favor the development of anorexia nervosa. However, there are no systematic empirical studies to prove that the assumed constellations are indeed more frequently observed in the families of anorectic patients than in those of controls. Problem areas in the family relate to perceived expectations, demands for performance, and problems with communication and affective expression (60). Whether these disturbances are part of the pathogenesis of the illness cannot be stated.

2. Sociocultural Factors

The increasing frequency of the disease (47,71,86) and the preference for upper and middle classes (77,88,111) indicate the role of sociocultural factors. Thinness and dieting are related to higher social class (67,145). Garner et al. (63) studied the height and weight measurements of Miss America contestants and of women depicted in *Playboy* magazine. The average weight for age and height decreased during the last 20 years, indicating a changing ideal of female beauty. Diet articles in women's magazines increased in frequency during the same period of time (63).

Studies by Abraham et al. (3) of school and university students indicated that disordered eating and weight control behavior are common among adolescent girls. Thinness seems to represent a symbol of success and self-control for women. It is plausible, therefore, that adolescent girls seeking a way to function autonomously choose the route of dieting and starving (19).

The importance of life events that trigger the onset of the disease has been emphasized. Halmi (71), Theander (147), and Morgan and Russell (111) found precipitating events in 50 to 65% of their patients, whereas Casper and Davis (24) found such events in all their patients. Such factors as death in the family, breakup of the parental marriage, and separation from the family while attending summer school or college were the most frequently observed events.

D. Factors Sustaining the Course of the Disease

Once the patients acquire the habit of dieting and starving and using other means, such as vomiting, laxatives, and diuretics, to reduce body weight, a state of malnutrition rapidly evolves. In this state, adjustment to caloric deprivation progresses, in the course of which an abundance of somatic and mental changes are observed. Various authors (58,104,123) have stressed the importance of such factors secondary to starvation in sustaining or aggravating the disease.

The continuous preoccupation with food observed in anorexia nervosa clearly is a consequence of starvation (96). Self-selected social isolation, indecisiveness, and mood lability are consequences of starvation that impair the patient's ability to find a way out of the disease alone or with the help of psychotherapy. Changes in gastrointestinal motility occur (45,81,133), which result in delayed gastric emptying and in feeling stuffed and bloated (62). These sensations prevent consumption of full meals, despite the feeling of hunger. We believe that the psychosomatic interactions mentioned here are one of the major challenges in anorexia nervosa research today. In order to gain a better understanding we will have to answer the following questions:

1. How does food choice and the consequent qualitatively and quantitatively abnormal food consumption influence central and peripheral neurotransmitter activity in the starved anorectic patient? Some of the neurotransmitter abnormalities in anorexia nervosa have already been described (48) and are discussed later. The relationship to food choice and consumption have not yet been investigated.

2. Which mental symptoms of anorexia nervosa can be attributed to certain neurotransmitter disturbances known to occur in anorexia nervosa? This question may be answered when systematic observation of mental symptoms and neurotransmitter activities will be conducted in anorectic patients in various states of the disease and during treatment.

Besides these somatic and psychosomatic processes, there are psychological mechanisms that may sustain the disease. Loss of weight becomes an indicator of personal success and develops into the strongest reinforcer of the pathological behavior. With the development of the syndrome in the patient, the behavior of the whole family changes. The patient receives more attention, which would be lost upon normalization of eating behavior and weight. The overprotection of the family thus reinforces the patients's behavior.

E. Related Diseases

A syndrome closely related to anorexia nervosa is bulimia nervosa, which was described by Russell in 1979 (131). This syndrome is now widely recognized as a distinct entity and should be diagnosed according to the DSM-III criteria. The prevalence of this syndrome is high. Halmi et al. (73) and Pope et al. (124) observed that 13 and 10%, respectively, of their subjects fulfilled the DSM-III criteria for bulimia in female student populations:

1. Recurrent episodes of binge eating (rapid consumption of a large amount of food in a discrete period of time, usually less than 2 hr).
2. At least three of the following:
   a. consumption of high-calorie, easily ingested food during a binge;
   b. inconspicuous eating during a binge;
   c. termination of such eating episodes by abdominal pain, sleep, social interruption, or self-induced vomiting;
   d. repeated attempts to lose weight by means of severely restrictive diets, self-induced vomiting, or use of cathartics or diuretics;
   e. frequent weight fluctuations greater than 10 pounds, due to alternating binges and fasts.
3. Awareness that the eating pattern is abnormal and fear of not being able to voluntarily stop eating.
4. Depressed mood and self-deprecating thoughts following eating binges.
5. Bulimic episodes not due to anorexia nervosa or any known physical disorder.

As mentioned earlier, bulimic attacks followed by vomiting are seen in approximately half the patients with anorexia nervosa (26). Russell (131) noted that more than 50% of his patients with bulimia nervosa had a former history of anorexia nervosa. In a recent study by our group, 50% of the bulimia patients (diagnosed according to DSM-III) also had former history of anorexia nervosa (120). These observations indicate that anorexia nervosa may be converted to bulimia during the course of the disease, frequently making it difficult to distinguish between the two.

It is not clear what converts restricting anorectics into bingeing and vomiting patients and in some cases into bulimics. Russell (131) has speculated that starvation and the consequent feeling of hunger may precipitate bulimic episodes. Pirke et al. (120) have observed the metabolic and endocrine signs of starvation in at least 50% of patients with bulimia. Many bulimic patients reported an altered state of consciousness, including a feeling of weakness or extreme hunger preceding the bingeing episode. These clinical observations raise several questions: (i) Do some bulimic or anorectic patients (with bulimic attacks) experience transient states of hypoglycemia? (ii) Are the central and peripheral mechanisms regulating hunger and satiety disturbed in bulimia? Study of these questions may provide information about whether there is a state- or trait-dependent disturbance in the metabolism of anorectic and bulimic patients which facilitates the development of the disease or perpetuates it.

In recent years, an attempt has been made to interpret anorexia nervosa as a subform of endogenous depression. "Depressive mood" was described by Kay (90) in half, and by Rollins and Piazza (127) in three-fourths, of their patients. Many symptoms of depression, such as hopelessness and low self-esteem, together with vegetative symptoms, such as sleep disturbances, weight loss, and loss of appetite and sexual interest, and still other symptoms, such as social withdrawal, may also be observed in anorexia nervosa. Recent reports of increased occurrence of primary affective disorders in first-degree relatives of anorectic patients (22,161) have further stimulated discussion of the relationship between anorexia nervosa and endogenous depression. Since weight loss is a rather frequently observed symptom in the latter, weight deficit is thought to be the common source of some of the somatic, and probably also of some of the mental, symptoms observed in both syndromes.

We have demonstrated that a pathological dexamethasone suppression test (DST) is seen more frequently in patients with endogenous depression who lost more than 1 kg body weight during the week preceding the study than in those patients whose weight did not change (7). (For a detailed discussion of nutrition and depression, see Rosenthal, *this volume.*)

F. Therapeutic Considerations

It exceeds the scope of this chapter to deliver a full account of the numerous therapeutic proposals recommended and used so far in the treatment of anorexia nervosa. Crisp (34) has provided a recent review of pharmacological treatment.

Garfinkel and Garner (58) discussed in detail hospital treatment and psychotherapy. Only a brief summary of the current thought on therapy is given here. The first and most essential step is to lead the patient out of her state of starvation and emaciation. The experience of many authors (19,32,58,130) indicates that psychotherapy cannot achieve meaningful effects in an emaciated patient. This first step, and the interruption of the vicious cycle of starvation and/or bingeing/vomiting, can best be achieved in the hospital. Tube feeding and parenteral, alimentation should be reserved for the most severe cases of emaciation. General supporting nursing care with a high-calorie diet, with or without bed rest or behavioral modification techniques, has been used successfully. Psychotherapy, including individual, group, and family therapy, should then—independently of the methods used—be tailored to the personal needs and problems of the individual patient. It is important to emphasize that the vast majority of patients will not be healed of anorexia upon release from the hospital after several months of treatment. Continued psychotherapy and support must be provided for the next 1 to 4 years in order to prevent relapses and worsening of symptoms.

G. Prognosis

Catemnestic studies have been hampered greatly by the poor methodological standards used (32). Garfinkel and Garner (58) summarized 13 studies, in which there was a relatively long follow-up and in which patients of variable ages were considered. Among these 724 patients, 43% had recovered and 28% had improved, whereas 20% had not improved and 9% had died. Those patients who maintained normal body weight generally showed normalization of their psychopathology and resumption of normal menstrual cycles. This occurred in about 50% of the cases. When a pediatric sample (seven studies of 198 patients) was evaluated, the outcome was much more favorable (58). Only 2% had died and 9% had not improved, whereas 76% had recovered and 13% had improved.

II. METABOLIC AND SOMATIC CONSEQUENCES OF STARVATION

A. Metabolic Studies

When the energy consumption of the body exceeds the caloric intake, body tissue must be burned to provide energy. At the onset of starvation, glycogen reserves are depleted within the first hours. Next, muscle tissue is consumed. Amino acids provide the necessary substrate for gluconeogenesis. At the third stage, primarily fat is mobilized. Free fatty acids serve as the energy supply in many tissues, including muscular cells. Since free fatty acids do not pass the blood-brain barrier, the energy supply of the brain, which usually is provided by glucose, becomes dependent on metabolites of the free fatty acids: the ketone bodies. Under conditions of starvation, gluconeogenesis is greatly suppressed, and up to 70% of brain energy needs are supplied by ketone bodies (21).

Figure 2 indicates glucose concentrations in the blood of patients with anorexia nervosa and in normal controls. Although glucose levels are lower in anorexia nervosa, they do not drop into the hypoglycemia range.

Figure 3 shows the plasma levels of free fatty acids, β-hydroxybutryic acid (β-HBA), and acetoacetate in patients with anorexia nervosa in the first week after admission to the hospital and during treatment over a period of 12 weeks. All three parameters are greatly elevated at the time of the first blood sampling but are normalized rapidly thereafter.

Similar observations have been made in patients with bulimia (120). Elevated free fatty acids and β-HBA were found in up to 50% of this group, indicating that many of these patients, at least transiently, starved themselves in order to maintain control over their body weight.

There have been several studies on amino acid levels in the plasma of anorectic patients (31,93,164). Studies of the large neutral amino acids (LNAAs) in plasma are of special interest, since Wurtman and his co-workers (63) showed in animals and humans that the relationship of tyrosine and tryptophan to the other LNAAs determines, respectively, the transport of tyrosine, which serves as a precursor of dopamine and NE, and of tryptophan, which is the precursor of serotonin, into the brain. Brain precursor concentration then will determine, under certain conditions, the turnover of serotonin, dopamine, and NE.

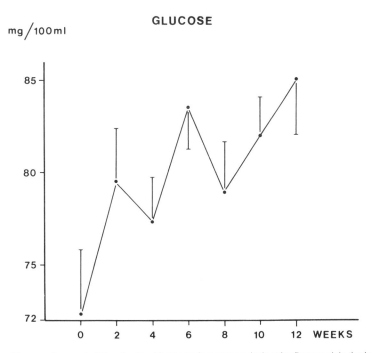

FIG. 2. Plasma glucose in 22 patients with anorexia nervosa during the first week in the hospital (0) and after 2,4,6,8,10, and 12 weeks of treatment.

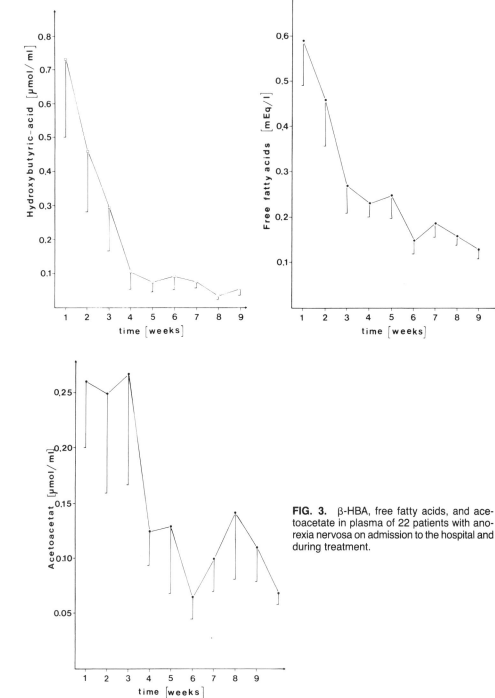

FIG. 3. β-HBA, free fatty acids, and ace-toacetate in plasma of 22 patients with ano-rexia nervosa on admission to the hospital and during treatment.

TABLE 1. *LNAAs in serum of patients with anorexia and in normal healthy controls*[a]

Amino acid	Anorexia nervosa (n = 26)		Control subjects (n = 25)	
	$\bar{x}$	S	$\bar{x}$	S
Valine	174 ± 56		177 ± 31	
Tryptophan	39 ± 11		44 ± 9	
Phenylalanine	45 ± 14		47 ± 7	
Leucine and isoleucine	148 ± 64		149 ± 26	
Tyrosine	45 ± 12		48 ± 8	
Tyrosine/LNAA	0.110 ± 0.028		0.110 ± 0.023	
Tryptophan/LNAA	0.089 ± 0.018		0.098 ± 0.014	

[a]p, NS.

Table 1 lists the concentration of the LNAAs for 26 patients with anorexia nervosa and for 25 age- and sex-matched controls. There were no significant differences between the two groups.

At the suggestion of Wurtman and Wurtman (163), the quotients of tyrosine and tryptophan to LNAAs after test meals were studied by our group (134). The test meals had 500 kcal and consisted of either carbohydrates or protein. Results are illustrated in Fig. 4. The tyrosine quotient was significantly increased following the protein meal and was slightly but not significantly decreased after the carbohydrate meal. The tryptophan quotient was significantly decreased after the protein meal. The decrease after carbohydrate ingestion was significant only 60 min after the meal. These observations indicate that the tyrosine quotient and probably the tyrosine inflow into the brain after meals is not reduced but elevated in patients with anorexia nervosa. However, the tryptophan quotient after meals is lower in anorexia nervosa, pointing to a decreased tryptophan supply to the central nervous system (CNS). In agreement with this finding, Kaye et al. (94) observed low 5-hydroxyindolacetic acid concentrations in the cerebrospinal fluid (CSF) of anorectic patients.

B. Water and Electrolyte Disturbances

Partial diabetes insipidus in anorexia nervosa has been described. Urine cannot maximally be concentrated (109,129,155), and intracellular water is reduced (132). Ebert et al. (48) reported that vasopressin secretion after a hyperosmolar challenge was inadequate or missing. It is not clear whether the disturbed vasopressin secretion reflects a nonspecific effect of chronic inanition or a process unique to anorexia nervosa. While this malfunction caused increased water loss, another mechanism was responsible for the inadequate storage of water in the body of the anorectic patient. Hypoalbuminemia, which then causes edema and even occasionally ascites, was observed in many patients (52).

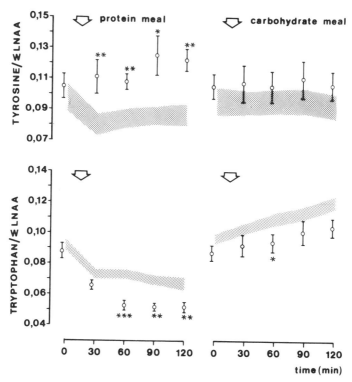

FIG. 4. Tyrosine and tryptophan ratio to the sum of LNAAs (ΣLNAA) after a carbohydrate meal (500 kcal) and after a protein meal (500 kcal). *Shaded areas,* ranges observed in 10 normal young women. The tyrosine ratio was significantly elevated and the tryptophan ratio was significantly reduced in 12 patients with anorexia nervosa during their first week in the hospital.

Patients with anorexia nervosa who vomit frequently (vomiters) exhibit a loss of potassium, which may become severe enough to endanger the life of the patient by ameliorating the already impaired cardiac function (43,68). Recently, it became apparent that a potassium loss in tissue occurs not only in vomiters but also in anorectic patients who do not vomit (restricters). Russell et al. (132) reported that total body potassium was reduced to a greater extent than total body nitrogen in six patients with anorexia nervosa (four restricters and two vomiters). Decreased potassium content of erythrocytes was observed not only in vomiters but also in restricters (119). Russell et al. (132) provided evidence that the potassium loss plays a major role in the development of muscular weakness and fatigue in anorexia nervosa.

C. Body Composition

Body composition of patients with anorexia nervosa was recently studied by measuring the total body potassium (potassium-40 technique) and/or the total body nitrogen by means of analysis (18,119,132). Both body compartments, cell mass and fat, were decreased in all studies. Russell et al. (132) followed six patients during weight gain from 63 to 76% of ideal body weight (IBW). They found a rapid increase of fat tissue from 5.5 to 8 kg on the average, while the cell mass, as judged from the total body nitrogen, increased only slowly. Pirke et al. (119) studied 16 anorectic patients with an average body weight increase from 72.8 to 91.8% IBW. These patients normalized their cell mass but still had a deficit in fat tissue when compared with normal age-matched controls (98.8% IBW).

D. Pseudoatrophy of the Brain

Pseudoatrophy of the brain was recently described by several groups (49,77,97). Computed tomography revealed enlarged inner and outer CSF space. Kohlmeyer et al. (97) found this to be reversible during hospital treatment in approximately 50% of their patients, which raises the question of whether the morphological change observed is actually a pseudoatrophy in all cases (i.e., shrinkage without loss of tissue) or whether actual atrophy also may develop. Furthermore, Kohlmeyer et al. (97) conducted concentration and memory tests in their patients and found a correlation between the severity of pseudoatrophy and the impairment revealed by these tests. This observation warrants replication.

The nature of the pseudoatrophy remains unclear. It may be a consequence of water imbalance (described above): A loss of intracellular water would bring about shrinkage of the brain, accompanied by enlargement of the ventricles. Since pseudoatrophy is also observed in Cushing's syndrome (77), the increased cortisol production observed in anorexia nervosa (see below) may also play a role.

III. AUTONOMOUS DYSREGULATION

A. Daytime Electroencephalogram and Sleep Disturbances

Abnormal daytime electroencephalogram (EEG) was found by Neil et al. (115) in 35% of anorectic patients and by Crisp et al. (36,37) in 59%. Three categories of abnormalities were described: (i) a generalized slowing of the background activity, (ii) the occurrence of 14- and 6-per-sec positive spikes (65,140), and (iii) unstable and prolonged hyperventilation responses (115). Interpretation of these observations has been controversial. Since Crisp et al. (36,37) provided convincing evidence that the EEG abnormalities reported correlated well with other clinical features of emaciation, however, it appears likely that the EEG disturbances are a consequence of metabolic and electrolyte imbalances.

Crisp et al. (36,39) examined the sleep of anorexia nervosa patients by polygraphic recording. The authors found insomnia, which was characterized primarily by early morning awakening. Lacey et al. (100) found that the total sleep time was normalized when body weight increased. Basic architecture of sleep was altered in emaciated anorexia nervosa patients (39). The time spent in states 3 and 4 and in rapid eye movement (REM) sleep was decreased, while that spent in stage 1 and wakefulness increased. Similar although less drastic changes in sleep architecture were reported by Neil et al. (115). Since sleep disturbances also occur in patients who undergo weight loss and do not suffer from anorexia nervosa, and since sleep is rapidly normalized in anorectic patients after weight gain (39), it can be concluded that the sleep disturbance observed was secondary to the weight loss.

B. Temperature Regulation

Mecklenburg et al. (109) and Vigersky et al. (154) reported alterations in temperature regulation in anorexia nervosa. The patients with reduced basal core temperature did not show the so-called paradoxical increase of core temperature that is then followed by a stabilization in normal subjects when challenged with hypothermia. Instead, anorectic patients demonstrated decreased core temperature, with missing shivering response. Hyperthermia caused an initial decrease in core temperature, which was followed by a slow increase, in control subjects. Anorectic patients did not show the initial drop in core temperature and showed a greater increase in central temperature. Luck and Wakeling (106) studied this phenomenon in greater detail and found that anorectic patients show an onset of vasodilation and thermal sweating at lower core temperature in rising room temperatures than did normal controls. The thermal response to meals was also altered, with anorectic patients showing a higher increase in core and peripheral temperatures after test meals.

Anterior hypothalamic areas are responsible for thermoregulation (76,114). Since Vigersky et al. (153) also found abnormal temperature in underweight subjects not suffering from anorexia nervosa, it is clear that the disturbed temperature regulation is not a consequence of a primary hypothalamic defect in anorexia nervsoa but a consequence of weight loss.

C. The Sympathetic Nervous System

The resting heart rate is decreased in the majority of patients with anorexia nervosa (54,137,141). Heart rates between 50 and 60/min are frequently observed. Low blood pressure is equally frequently observed (159). When the patients are challenged with exercise (54,68), increases of pulse rate and blood pressure lower than in healthy controls are seen. Both symptoms indicate impaired functioning of the sympathetic nervous system.

Various studies of the sympathetic nervous system have been conducted. Halmi et al. (72), Abraham et al. (1), Gerner and Gwirtsman (64), and Riederer et al. (126) found decreased excretion of 3-methoxy-4-hydroxyphenylethyleneglycol (MHPG) in urine. Biederman et al. (11) claimed that MHPG excretion was elevated only in those anorectic patients who also met the diagnostic criteria of major depressive disorder. This view was not shared by the other authors, however, who found that MHPG was determined mainly by weight loss and was normalized by weight gain.

Reduced plasma NE levels were reported by Gross et al. (69) and by Darby et al. (40). Baseline values in supine body position and the response to standing were significantly lowered. Nudel et al. (116) studied NE, dopamine, and epinephrine after maximal exercise and found that in anorectics, all three catecholamines were reduced in plasma, compared to normal subjects. This finding corresponded to the lower increase in heart rate and blood pressure after exercise in anorectics. Ebert et al. (48) and Kaye et al. (92) found a persistently low NE concentration in plasma and CSF of weight-recovered patients with anorexia nervosa. There is no simple interpretation for this finding. It may mean that anorexia nervosa patients have a low NE turnover as a trait-dependent variable, or it may mean that the reduced sympathetic activity is only very slowly normalized in these patients.

Recent studies (78) suggest a different interpretation. Figure 5A shows the orthostatic NE response in controls and in anorectics on hospital admission and during a follow-up study 1 year after release. The data for bulimic (not weight-deficient) patients are also given. The figure indicates that all groups had a reduced orthostatic NE response. β-HBA levels are given for these groups in Fig. 5B. Weight-recovered anorectic and bulimic patients showed, on the average, elevated plasma levels of this ketone body, indicating that despite normal weight, at least some of these patients were dieting or starving at the time of the study.

Landsberg and Young (101,102) showed that fasting reduces the activity of the peripheral sympathetic nervous system. Since catecholamines stimulate cellular metabolism, reduced noradrenergic activity may help to reduce energy consumption in the state of starvation. Pirke and Spyra (122) and Schweiger et al. (135) showed that noradrenergic activity is reduced in the CNS of acutely and chronically starved rats, which demonstrated that peripheral and central noradrenergic systems are affected equally by starvation.

As mentioned in Section I.B, different diets affect the activity of the sympathetic nervous system in a different way (41) in human subjects. Similar observations have been made in semistarved rats (135). Brain tyrosine and NE turnover were reduced to a greater extent in rats fed a protein-rich diet than in animals on a carbohydrate-rich diet. These observations in humans and rats may explain the great variability in the orthostatic NE response seen among patients with a similar extent of inanition. Future studies on NE secretion in anorexia nervosa and bulimia should take into account not only the quantitative but also the qualitative aspects of the patients' self-imposed diet.

Recently, Luck et al. (105) extended the studies on the peripheral noradrenergic system by measuring α_2-adrenoceptors on platelet membranes. Receptor capacity was significantly increased in patients with anorexia nervosa. This corresponded to the increase in α_2-receptor capacity observed in the hypothalamus of the starved rat (144). Heufelder et al. (78) studied the biochemical effect mediated by the α_2 receptors of the platelets: the inhibition of adenylate cyclase. The upper part of Fig. 6 shows the stimulation of adenylate cyclase by different doses of prostaglandin E_1; the lower part illustrates the inhibition of this effect by epinephrine. Elevated stimulation and increased inhibition by epinephrine is observed in anorectics on admission to the hospital and after a 10% weight gain in bulimics. The corresponding orthostatic effects on NE are depicted in Fig. 5a.

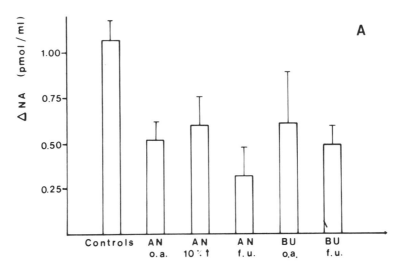

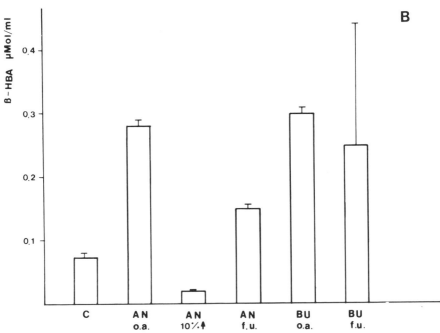

FIG. 5.   A: Orthostatic response of NE (Δ NA) in 24 control subjects and in 24 patients with anorexia nervosa (AN) on admission (o.a), after 10% weight gain (10% ↑), and on follow-up (f.u.) after 6 months to 1 year. Thirteen patients with bulimia (BU) were also studied on admission to the hospital and at follow-up.   **B:** β-HBA in the same patient and control groups as in **A**.

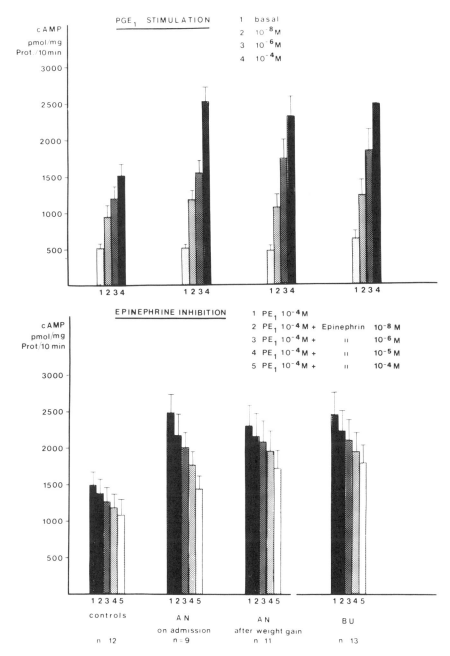

FIG. 6. Stimulation of cyclic AMP (cAMP) production by prostaglandin E_1 (PGE$_1$) and inhibition by epinephrine in platelets in anorexia nervosa (AN) on admission to the hospital and after 10% weight gain in bulimia (BU) and in healthy age- and sex-matched controls.

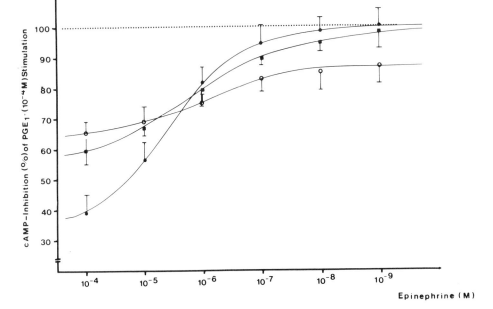

FIG. 7. Dose-response curve for the inhibition of cyclic AMP (cAMP) by epinephrine in anorexia nervosa (●), in bulimia (■), and in controls (○). Average and SEM are given for nine subjects in each group.

Figure 7 shows the dose-response curve of the epinephrine effect in controls and anorectic and bulimic patients. The figure illustrates that although the maximal effects are greater in both groups of patients, the dose necessary to elicit half the maximal effect is not different from that for normal controls.

IV. ENDOCRINE ABNORMALITIES

A. Growth Hormone, Prolactin, and Melatonin

1. Growth Hormone

The secretion of growth hormone (GH) is increased in patients with anorexia nervosa (16,25,139,154). Garfinkel et al. (57) observed that increased GH levels did not correlate with the degree of weight loss but with the actual caloric intake. As a consequence, elevated GH levles were rapidly normalized when patients resumed eating. Elevated GH values are not specific for anorexia nervosa but are also observed in other forms of malnutrition, such as kwashiorkor (117). Fichter and Pirke (53) observed elevated values throughout the 24-hr day and an especially high increase during slow-wave sleep in healthy, normal-weight controls during starvation (Fig. 8). In contrast to healthy controls, anorectic patients showed an increase of GH after a standardized glucose meal (25,151). Sherman and Halmi

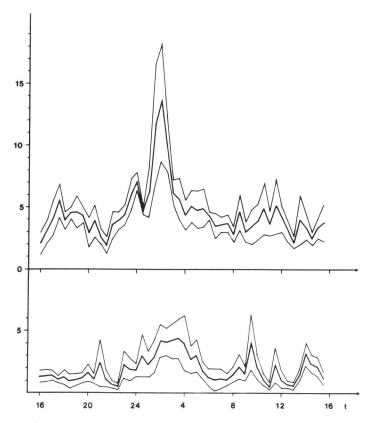

FIG. 8. GH levels during a 24-hr period sampled in 30-min intervals in five healthy normal-weight female subjects during fasting *(upper)* and after normalization of body weight *(lower)*. Average and SEM are given for five subjects.

(139) and Casper et al. (25) observed a reduced increase of GH after application of such dopamine agonists as apomorphine and L-DOPA. The authors suggested that this finding may point to an impaired functioning of dopamine receptors. Further pharmacological experiments are needed to substantiate this hypothesis.

2. Prolactin

In contrast to GH values, prolactin (PRL) resting levels were not altered in anorexia nervosa (9,109,154,157). Normal stimulation of PRL was observed after application of chlorpromazine (9). Different results were reported when the secretion of PRL provoked by thyrotropin-releasing hormone (TRH) was studied. Isaacs et al. (85) found an impaired, and Vigersky and Loriaux (154) a delayed although normal, response. Wakeling et al (157) found normal responses. The observations of GH secretion stress how important the actual state of energy consumption may be for some hormonal abnormalities. It may be, therefore, that differing results are

attributable to the different metabolic states of the patients. The controversy over
PRL response to TRH injections could probably be resolved, were measurements
conducted under strict control of the metabolic situation.

Kalucy et al. (87) and Brown et al. (17) observed a diminished nocturnal increase
of PRL. Fichter and Pirke (53) studied healthy, nonobese starving subjects and
found a significant decrease of PRL during sleep (Fig. 9). Since nocturnal PRL
secretion is sleep dependent (160), and since sleep disturbances in anorectic patients
can be assumed (see Section III.A), the most likely explanation for the reduced
nocturnal PRL values appears to be the impairment of sleep. Nutritional factors
may also be of importance, since Hill and Wynder (79) observed impaired nocturnal
PRL increases in normal healthy subjects who started a vegetarian diet.

3. Melatonin

A strong circadian rhythm governs the secretion of melatonin (152). Two studies
of anorexia nervosa noted a normal circadian melatonin rhythm in the disease
(12,17). The latter authors found a small but significant reduction of circadian
amplitude.

B. Hypothalamic–Pituitary–Adrenal Axis

A number of different disturbances of the hypothalamic–pituitary–adrenal axis
have been described in anorexia nervosa. Under physiological conditions, cortisol

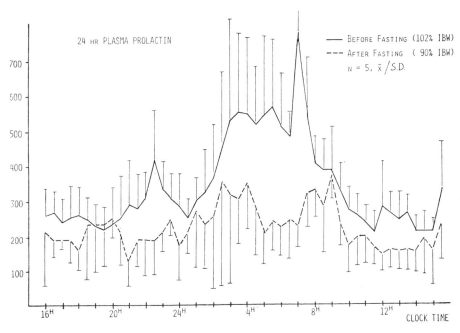

FIG. 9. PRL values during a 24-hr sleep–wake study in five healthy normal-weight women
before fasting (——) and after loss of 10% weight (-----).

production is closely related to body surface. For example, as children grow, their cortisol production increases, but it remains constant in relation to body surface (95). In patients with anorexia nervosa, cortisol production does not increase absolutely but in relation to body weight and surface (158). As a consequence, Walsh et al. (158) observed an increase of free cortisol in urine (205 μg/day in patients on the average, compared to 65 μg/day in healthy controls). The average plasma levels were also elevated. The 24-hr secretion pattern shows elevated plasma levels during the evening and the first half of the night when values are low or undetectable in healthy controls (14,42). Plasma half-life of cortisol is prolonged. Doerr et al. (42) found an average half-life of 137 min in patients during their first week in the hospital. This decreased significantly to 84 min on the average when patients had gained 10% of body weight. The sensitivity of the adrenal–pituitary–hypothalamic feedback can be tested by application of dexamethasone.

In normal subjects, 1.5 mg dexamethasone reliably suppresses cortisol secretion for the next 24 hr when given at 11 p.m. (98). Only in half the anorectic patients was the cortisol not suppressed during the morning hours. Those who had suppressed values during the morning showed an "early escape" phenomenon (23), with elevated values during the afternoon (42). This early escape is not specific for anorexia nervosa but is also observed in endogenous depression (23). Fichter and Pirke (53) studied the effect of starvation on cortisol. They observed all disturbances seen in anorectics: prolonged cortisol half-life in plasma, increased plasma levels during the evening and early night hours, and pathological dexamethasone tests.

When starving healthy subjects (53) or anorectic patients (42) resume eating, the abnormal cortisol secretion and the impaired metabolism are rapidly normalized, indicating that the increased cortisol secretion is an adaptation to starvation. It can be assumed that cortisol stimulates gluconeogenesis, which can become dangerously low in starvation.

It is remarkable that the low-protein, low-calorie malnutrition observed in many developing countries has a different effect on cortisol production than does anorexia nervosa. Leonard and McWilliam (103), Alleyne and Young (4), and Smith et al. (143) observed a decreased cortisol production rate and normal excretion of free cortisol in urine. The decreased triiodothyronine (T3) production in anorexia nervosa is responsible not only for the quantitative impairment of cortisol metabolism (13) but also for qualitative changes in steroid metabolism (14). The relationship of the cortisol metabolites tetrahydrocortisol and tetrahydrocortisone increases.

C. Hypothalamic–Pituitary–Thyroid Axis

Circulating thyroid-stimulating hormone (TSH) values are not altered in patients with anorexia nervosa (10,16,112,154,157). The TSH response to TRH is of normal amplitude (107). The response is delayed, however (154,157), a consequence of weight loss (153) that is normalized by weight gain.

Thyroxine (T4), the hormone secreted by the thyroid gland, is converted in tissue to the biologically active T3. While T4 plasma concentrations in anorexia nervosa are in the normal range, T3 values are decreased (110,112). Burman et al. (20) demonstrated that the conversion of T4 to T3 was reduced, while more biologically inactive retro-T3 was produced. Since T3 stimulates cell metabolism, the decrease of T3 has been interpreted to be a protective mechanism responsible for the reduced energy consumption of the tissue (149). The changes in T4 metabolism are not specific for anorexia nervosa but also can be observed in chronic diseases and in low-protein, low-calorie malnutrition (29,30). Obese people who fast also show reduced T3 values (125,136). Low T3 plasma concentrations are not only responsible for reduced tissue metabolism, they also bring about qualitative changes in cortisol metabolism (see Section IV.B). Testosterone metabolism is also changed. In relation to 5-α-reduced metabolites, more 5-β metabolites are formed. This effect is reversible by application of T3 (13).

Values for T3 normalize when anorectic patients gain weight. In contrast to the rapid normalization of cortisol and GH, however, T3 values increase only slowly.

D. Hypothalamic–Pituitary–Gonadal Axis

Amenorrhea is a symptom that occurs in all severely emaciated patients with anorexia nervosa. The loss of cyclic gonadal function has been studied intensively. Plasma concentrations of gonadal hormones are greatly reduced (148). In male patients, plasma testosterone diminished to subnormal concentrations. Beumont et al. (10) analyzed the relationship between weight loss and plasma estradiol. They found that estradiol values were not normalized before patients had reached at least 80% of their standard weight (normal weight for age and height). The amenorrhea in anorexia nervosa is not primarily a consequence of impaired gonadal hormone secretion but of hypothalamic dysfunction.

Boyar et al. (15) showed that the secretion pattern of luteinizing hormone (LH) reflects the following development during normal puberty in girls and boys. Before puberty, an infantile secretion pattern of LH is observed that is characterized by low average LH concentrations and by the lack of major fluctuations. In midpuberty, a pubertal pattern arises that shows still low LH values during the waking hours but a sleep-dependent increase of LH values during the night. With proceeding puberty, the sleep dependence of LH secretion is lost, and equally high values with more or less (depending on the state of the cycle) frequent fluctuations occur.

In emaciated patients with anorexia nervosa, an infantile or pubertal LH pattern is observed (89,118), which then slowly matures during weight gain. Figure 10 shows an example of the development from an infantile to a pubertal to an adult secretion pattern in a 14-year-old patient with anorexia nervosa. A pubertal LH secretion pattern also is observed in dieting women not suffering from anorexia nervosa (153).

In a recent study, Fichter and Pirke (53) showed that the total fasting and weight loss (5–8 kg) in healthy normal-weight women caused an infantile LH pattern in three of five subjects. The importance of weight was further emphasized by the observation (118) that in anorectic patients during refeeding, no pubertal LH pattern

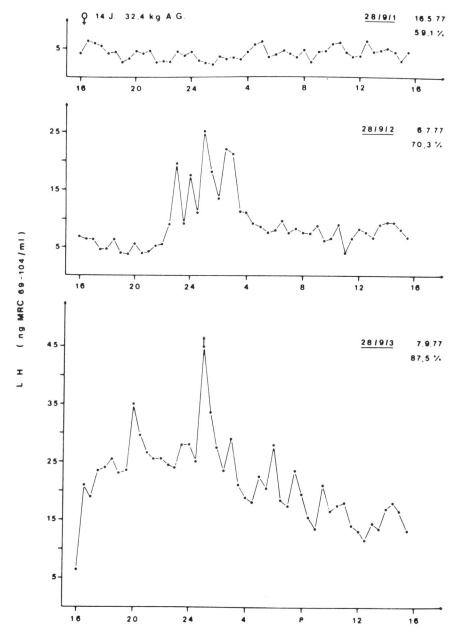

FIG. 10. A 24-hr sleep–wake pattern of plasma LH. *Upper*, "infantile" pattern observed at 59.1% of IBW; *middle*, "pubertal" and *lower*, "adult" pattern shown in the same patient after weight gain.

developed before a minimal weight of 69% of IBW was reached. No adult LH pattern was seen below 80% of IBW. The data indicated that the time needed for LH secretion patterns to return to normal increased with age of the patients and the duration of the disease. Katz et al. (89) and Falk and Halmi (50) reported that weight-recovered anorectic patients, who were otherwise still symptomatic, showed no maturation of LH patterns, while those who were essentially free of symptoms had an adult LH secretion pattern. The authors claimed that the psychological distress of ongoing anorexia nervosa may be responsible for this phenomenon.

An alternate explanation is that the ongoing disturbance of eating behavior and its metabolic consequences prevent the maturation of the LH secretion pattern. The ability of the pituitary gland to secrete gonadotropic hormones has been tested by injection of synthetic gonadotropin-releasing hormone (GNRH). The most detailed analysis was performed by Beumont et al. (10). In emaciated patients, the response of LH and follicle-stimulating hormone (FSH) was decreased and delayed.

When 70% of the standard weight is reached, an exaggerated FSH response is observed. At about 80% of standard weight, the LH response becomes greater, exceeding the normal response in adult subjects. With further weight gain, the increased sensitivity of the pituitary gland is normalized. This transient supersensitivity of gonadotropin release also occurs during normal puberty (128).

The first step in pubertal development is an increase of adrenal androgen secretion (46), a phenomenon called adrenarche. Zumoff et al. (165) reported that in emaciated patients with anorexia nervosa, subnormal dehydroepiandrosterone values were observed, which became normal during weight gain. This is the third phenomenon, in addition to the alteration in LH secretion pattern and the changes in pituitary sensitivity to GNRH, reflecting the regression of the endocrine system to a prepubertal state. The complex hormonal development of puberty appears to be repeated during recovery from anorexia nervosa.

Wakeling et al. (156) studied the function of the gonadal–pituitary–hypothalamic feedback by application of ethinyl estradiol. In healthy women, this treatment first suppressed LH values (negative feedback), later inducing a strong increase of LH (posititve feedback). The positive feedback could not be provoked in weight-deficient anorectics and was still absent in 50% of weight-recovered patients. Similar results were obtained when clomiphene, and estrogen antagonist, was given (156). This substance was used to provoke a positive feedback effect with subsequent ovulation. No effect was seen in emaciated anorectics and in approximately 50% of weight-recovered patients. Marshall and Kelch (108) treated anorectic patients with pulsatile GNRH injections. Ovulatory cycles developed, indicating that amenorrhea in anorexia nervosa is brought about by the lack of GNRH release from the hypothalamus.

Frisch (55) reported that patients with anorexia nervosa had to attain at least 87% of IBW before normal menstrual cycles resumed. Frisch interpreted this finding in the context of the theory on pubertal maturation proposed by Frisch and Revelle (56). This theory, based on demographic and anthropometric observations, postulates that the maturation of reproductive function is initiated only when a certain amount of body fat has accumulated. Although many of the above-cited observations support this assumption (10,55,118), other evidence is incompatible with the Frisch theory.

First, amenorrhea occurs very early in the course of the disease (159), frequently before a substantial weight loss has occurred. Second, amenorrhea is also observed in patients with bulimia who have no weight deficit (120). Recent studies (121) suggest a second mechanism (besides weight deficit) of disturbance of reproductive function in eating disorders. A group of nine healthy normal-weight women were observed during a 6-week diet period, in which a weight loss of 5 to 8 kg occurred. There was no change in LH secretion pattern; nevertheless, three subjects developed transient amenorrhea, and three additional subjects showed anovulatory cycles while dieting. In these six subjects, a progressive decline of plasma estradiol concentrations, without changes in LH, FSH, and progesterone, was observed.

Reproductive function is disturbed in many women who undergo intensive physical training (2,51). Whether this is a consequence of altered body composition (decrease in fat and increase in muscular tissue) or an effect of a stressful intensive training is unclear.

Physical hyperactivity is a feature in many anorectic patients that often persists after weight gain (99). The role of hyperactivity in reproductive disturbances in anorexia nervosa has not been studied systematically.

V. CONCLUSIONS AND OUTLOOK

Research on the syndrome of anorexia nervosa has revealed a great number of functional disturbances, both somatic and psychological. The psychophysiological, physiological, metabolic, and endocrine abnormalities reported thus far most likely result from the disturbed eating behavior. No convincing evidence has yet emerged to prove a primary biochemical defect in the brain function of anorectic patients. It should be kept in mind, however, that present knowledge is too scarce to finally decide the question as to whether or not there exists a predisposition, describable in biochemical or physiological terms, and important to the etiology and/or pathogenesis of anorexia nervosa.

Research on bulimia is just beginning. In the future, it may provide a way to compare a syndrome characterized by weight loss and starvation with a syndrome lacking weight loss but characterized by intermittent starvation. The different effects of weight deficit and starvation thus might be studied.

One of the challenges in exploring the hypothalamic dysfunctions in anorexia nervosa is the search for alterations in neurotransmission, which may be the common explanation of the different effects on temperature regulation, water and electrolyte disturbances, and other neuroendocrine abnormalities. Only few results have been obtained. Animal studies, in which the effects of different forms of malnutrition (deficits in basic food components, including vitamins and trace elements) are examined, are necessary to gain insight into the probably complex changes in neurotransmitter and neuromodulator function in starvation. Only when this goal has been achieved will we be able to understand the biochemical basis of the effects of starvation on complex brain functions, such as mood, cognition, and behavior.

REFERENCES

1. Abraham, S. F., Beumont, P. J. V., and Cobbin, D. M. (1981): Catecholamine metabolism and body weight in anorexia nervosa. *Br. J. Psychiatry*, 138:244–247.
2. Abraham, S. F., Beumont, P. J. V., Fraser, I. S., and Llewellyn-Jones, D. (1982): Body weight, exercise and menstrual status among ballet dancers in training. *Br. J. Obstet. Gynaecol.*, 89:507–510.
3. Abraham, S. F., Mira, M., Beumont, P. J. V., Sowerbutts, T. D., and Llewellyn-Jones, D. (1983): Eating behaviours among young women. *Med. J. Aust.*, 2:225–228.
4. Alleyne, G. A. O., and Young, V. H. (1967): Adrenocortical function in children with severe protein caloric malnutrition. *Clin. Sci.*, 33:189.
5. Anderson, A. E. (1977): Atypical anorexia nervosa. In: *Anorexia Nervosa*, edited by R. A. Vigersky, pp. 11–19. Raven Press, New York.
6. Beeley, J. M., Daley, J. J., Timperley, W. R., and Warner, J. (1973): Ectopic pinealoma: An unusual clinical presentation and a histochemical comparison with a seminoma of the testis. *J. Neurol. Neurosurg. Psychiatry*, 36;864–873.
7. Berger, M., Pirke, K. M., Doerr, P., Krieg, J. C., and von Zerssen, D. (1984): The limited utility of the dexamethasone suppression test for the diagnostic process in psychaitry. *Br. J. Psychiatry*, 145:372–382.
8. Beumont, P. J. V., Chamers, T. L., Rouse, L., and Abraham, S. F. (1981): The diet composition and nutritional knowledge of patients with anorexia nervosa. *J. Hum. Nutr.*, 35:265–273.
9. Beumont, P. J. V., Friesen, H. G., Gelder, M. G., and Kolakowska, T. (1974): Plasma prolactin and luteinizing hormone levels in anorexia nervosa. *Psychol. Med.*, 4:219–221.
10. Beumont, P. J. V., George, G. C. W., Pimstone, B. L., and Vinik, A. I. (1976): Body weight and the pituitary response to hypothalamic releasing hormones in patients with anorexia nervosa. *J. Clin. Endocrinal. Metab.*, 43:487–496.
11. Biederman, J., Herzog, D. B., Rivinus, T. M., Ferber, R. A., Harper, G. P., Orsulak, P. J., Harmatz, J. S., and Schildkraut, J. J. (1984): Urinary MHPG in anorexia nervosa patients with and without a concomitant major depressive disorder. *J. Psychiatr. Res.*, 18(2):149–160.
12. Birau, N., Alexander, D., Bertholdt, S., and Meyer, C. (1984): Low nocturnal melatonin serum concentration in anorexia nervosa—further evidence for body weight influence. *IRCS Med. Sci.*, 12:477.
13. Boyar, R. M., and Bradlow, H. L. (1977): Studies of testosterone metabolism in anorexia nervosa. In: *Anorexia Nervosa*, edited by R. A. Vigersky, pp. 271–276. Raven Press, New York.
14. Boyar, R. M., Hellman, L., Raffwarg, H. P., Katz, J., Zumoff, B., O'Connor, J., Bradlow, H. L., and Fukushima, D. K. (1977): Cortisol secretion and metabolism in anorexia nervosa. *N. Engl. J. Med.*, 296:190–193.
15. Boyar, R. M., Katz, J., Finkelstein, J. W., Kapen, S., Weiner, H., Weitzman, E. D., and Hellman, L. (1974): Anorexia nervosa: Immaturity of the 24-hour luteinizing hormone secretory pattern. *N. Engl. J. Med.*, 291:861–865.
16. Brown, G. M., Garfinkel, P. E., Jeuniewic, N., Modolfsky, H., and Stancer, H. C. (1977): Endocrine profile in anorexia nervosa. In: *Anorexia Nervosa*, edited by R. A.Vigersky, pp. 123–135. Raven Press, New York.
17. Brown, G. M., Kirwan, P., Garfinkel, P., and Moldofsky, H. (1979): Overnight patterning of prolactin and melatonin in anorexia nervosa (Abstr.). 2nd International Symposium on Clinical Psycho-Neuro-Endocrinology in Reproduction. Venice, Italy.
18. Bruce, V., Crosby, L. O., Reicheck, N., Perschuk, M., Lusk, E., and Mullen, J. L. (1984): Energy expenditure in primary malnutrition during standardized exercise. *Am. J. Phys. Med.*, 63(4):165–174.
19. Bruch, H. (1973): *Eating Disorders*. Basic Books, New York.
20. Burman, K. D., Vigersky, R. A., Loriaux, D. L., Djuh, Y. Y., Wright, E. D., and Martofsky, L. (1977): Investigations concerning thyroxine deiodinative pathways in patients with anorexia nervosa. In: *Anorexia Nervosa*, edited by R. A. Vigersky, pp. 255–261. Raven Press, New York.

21. Cahill, G. F., Herrera, M. G., Morgan, A. P., Soeldner, J. S., Steinke, J., Levy, P. L., Reichard, G. A., and Kipnis, D. M. (1966): Hormone-fuel interrelationships during fasting. *J. Clin. Invest.*, 45(11):1751–1768.

22. Cantwell, D. P., Sturzenberger, S., Burroughs, J., Salkin, B., and Green, J. K. (1977): Anorexia nervosa; an affective disorder? *Arch. Gen. Psychiatry*, 34:1087–1093.

23. Carroll, B. J., Curtis, G. C., and Mendels, J. (1976): Neuroendocrine regulation in depression. I. Limbic system-adrenocortical dysfunction. *Arch. Gen. Psychiatry*, 33:1039–1044.

24. Casper, R. C., and Davis, J. A. (1977): On the course of anorexia nervosa. *Am. J. Psychiatry*, 134:974–978.

25. Casper, R. C., Davis, J. M., and Pandey, G. N. (1977): The effect of the nutritional status and weight changes of hypothalamic function tests in anorexia nervosa. In: *Anorexia Nervosa*, edited by R. A. Vigersky, pp. 137–147. Raven Press, New York.

26. Casper, R. C., Eckert, E. D., Halmi, K. A., Goldberg, S. C., and Davis, J. M. (1980): Bulimia. Its incidence and clinical importance in patients with anorexia nervosa. *Arch. Gen. Psychiatry*, 37:1030–1034.

27. Casper, R. C., Halmi, K. A., Goldberg, S. C., Eckert, E. D., and Davis, J. M. (1979): Disturbances in body image estimation as related to other characteristics and outcome in anorexia nervosa. *Br. J. Psychiatry*, 134:60–66.

28. Casper, R. C., Kirschner, B., Sandstead, H. H., and Jacob, R. A. (1980): An evaluation of trace metals, vitamins, and taste function in anorexia nervosa. *Am. J. Clin. Nutr.*, 33:1801–1808.

29. Chopra, I. J., Chopra, U., Smith, S. R., Reza, M., and Solomon, D. H. (1975): Reciprocal changes in serum concentrations of 3,3′,5′-triiodothyronine (reverse T3) and 3,3′5-triiodothyronine(T3) in systemic illness. *J. Clin. Endocrinol. Metab.*, 41:1043–1049.

30. Chopra, I. J., and Smith, S. R. (1975): Circulating thyroid hormones and thyrotropin in adult patients with protein caloric malnutrition. *J. Clin. Endocrinol. Metab.*, 40:221–227.

31. Coppen, A. J., Gupta, R. K., Eccleston, E. G., Wood, K. M., Wakeling, A., and De Sousa, V. F. (1976): Plasma-tryptophan in anorexia nervosa. *Lancet*, I:961.

32. Crisp, A. H. (1965): Clinical and therapeutic aspects of anorexia nervosa—a study of thirty cases. *J. Psychosom. Res.*, 9:67–78.

33. Crisp, A. H. (1980): *Anorexia Nervosa: Let Me Be*. Grune & Stratton, New York.

34. Crisp, A. H. (1984): Treatment of anorexia nervosa: What can be the role of psychopharmacological agents? In: *The Psychobiology of Anorexia Nervosa*, edited by K. M. Pirke and D. Ploog, pp. 148–169. Springer-Verlag, Berlin.

35. Crisp, A. H., Blendis, L. M., and Pawan, G. L. S. (1968): Aspects of fat metabolism in anorexia nervosa. *Metabolism*, 17:1109–1118.

36. Crisp, A. H., Fenton, G. W., and Scotton, L. (1967): A controlled study of the EEG in anorexia nervosa. *Br.. J. Psychiatry*, 114:1149–1160.

37. Crisp, A. H., Fenton, G. W., and Scotton, L. (1967): The electroencephalogram in anorexia nervosa. *EEG Clin. Neurophysiol.*, 23:490.

38. Crisp, A. H., Palmer, R. L., and Kalucy, R. S. (1976): How common is anorexia nervosa? A prevalence study. *Br. J. Psychiatry*, 128:549–554.

39. Crisp, A. H., Stonehill, E., and Fenton, G. W. (1970): An aspect of the biological basis of the mind-body apparatus: The relationship between sleep, nutritional state and mood in disorders of weight. *Psychother. Psychosom.*, 18:161–175.

40. Darby, P., VanLoon, G., Garfinkel, P. E., Brown, G. M., and Kirwan, P. (1980): LH growth hormone, prolactin and catecholamine responses to LHRF and bromocryptine in anorexia nervosa. Presented at the American Psychosomatic Society, New York.

41. DeHaven, J., Sherwin, R., Hendler, R., and Felig, P. (1980): Nitrogen and sodium balance and sympathetic-nervous-system activity in obese subjects treated with a low-calorie protein or mixed diet. *N. Engl. J. Med.*, 302:477–482.

42. Doerr, P., Fichter, M., Pirke, K. M., and Lund, R. (1980): Relationship between weight gain and hypothalamic pituitary adrenal function in patients with anorexia nervosa. *J. Steroid Biochem.*, 13:529–537.

43. Drossman, D. A., Ontjes, D. A., and Heizer, W. D. (1979): Clinical conference. Anorexia nervosa. *Gastroenterology*, 77:1115–1131.

44. DSM-III (1980): Infancy, childhood, or adolescence disorders. Diagnostic criteria for identity disorder, pp. 67–71. The American Psychiatric Association, Washington, D. C.

45. Dubois, A., Gross, H. A., Ebert, M. H., and Castell, D. O. (1979): Altered gastric emptying and secretion in primary anorexia nervosa. *Gastroenterology*, 77:319–323.
46. Ducharme, J. R., Forest, M. G., De Peretti, E., Sempe, M., Collu, R., and Bertrand, J. (1976): Plasma adrenal and gonadal sex steroids in human pubertal development. *J. Clin. Endocrinol. Metab.*, 42:468–476.
47. Duddle, M. (1973): An increase of anorexia nervosa in a university population. *Br. J. Psychiatry*, 123:711–712.
48. Ebert, M. H., Kaye, W. K., and Gold, P. W. (1984): Neurotransmitter metabolism in anorexia nervosa. In: *The Psychobiology of Anorexia Nervosa*, edited by K. M. Pirke and D. Ploog, pp. 58–72. Springer-Verlag, Berlin.
49. Enzmann, D. R., and Lane, B. (1977): Cranial computed tomography findings in anorexia nervosa. *J. Comput. Assist. Tomog.*, 1:410–413.
50. Falk, J. R., and Halmi, K. A. (1982): Amenorrhea in anorexia nervosa: Examination of the critical body weight hypothesis. *Biol. Psychiatry*, 17(7):799–806.
51. Fears, W. B., Glass, A. R., and Vigersky, R. A. (1983): Role of exercise in the pathogenesis of the amenorrhea associated with anorexia nervosa. *J. Adolesc. Health Care*, 4:22–24.
52. Fichter, M. M., and Pirke, K. M. (1982): Somatische Befunde bei Anorexia nervosa und ihre differentialdiagnostische Wertigkeit. *Nervenarzt*, 53:635–643.
53. Fichter, M. M., and Pirke, K. M. (1984): Hypothalamic pituitary function in starving healthy subjects. In: *The Psychobiology of Anorexia Nervosa*, edited by K. M. Pirke and D. Ploog, pp. 124–135. Springer Verlag, Berlin.
54. Fohlin, L. (1977): Body composition, cardiovascular and renal function in adolescent patients with anorexia nervosa. *Acta. Paediatr. Scand. [Suppl.]*, 268:1–20.
55. Frisch, R. E. (1977): Food intake, fatness and reproductive ability. In: *Anorexia Nervosa*, edited by R. A. Vigersky, pp. 149–162. Raven Press, New York.
56. Frisch, R. E., and Revelle, R. (1970): Height and weight at menarche and a hypothesis of critical body weights and adolescent events. *Science*, 169:397–398.
57. Garfinkel, P. E., Brown, G. M., Stancer, H. C., and Moldofsky, H. (1975): Hypothalamic pituitary function in anorexia nervosa. *Arch. Gen. Psychiatry*, 32:739–744.
58. Garfinkel, P. E., and Garner, D. M. (1982): *Anorexia Nervosa—A Multidimensional Perspective.* Brunner/Mazel, New York.
59. Garfinkel, P. E., and Garner, D. M. (1984): Perceptions of the body in anorexia nervosa. In: *The Psychobiology of Anorexia Nervosa*, edited by K. M. Pirke and D. Ploog, pp. 136–147. Springer Verlag, Berlin.
60. Garfinkel, P. E., Garner, D. M., Rose, J., Darby, P. L., Brandes, J. S., O'Hanlon, J., and Walsh, N. (1983): A comparison of characteristics in the families of patients with anorexia nervosa and normal controls. *Psychol. Med.*, 13:821–828.
61. Garfinkel, P. E., Moldofsky, H., and Garner, D. M. (1979): The stability of perceptual disturbances in anorexia nervosa. *Psychol. Med.*, 9:703–713.
62. Garfinkel, P. E., Moldofsky, H., Garner, D. M., Stancer, H. C., and Coscina, D. V. (1978): Body awareness in anorexia nervosa: Disturbances in "body image" and "satiety." *Psychosom. Med.*, 40:487–498.
63. Garner, D. M., Garfinkel, P. E., Schwartz, D., and Thompson, M. (1980): Cultural expectation of thinness in women. *Psychol. Rep.*, 47:483–491.
64. Gerner, R. H., and Gwirtsman, H. E. (1981): Abnormalities of dexamethasone suppression test and urinary MHPG in anorexia nervosa. *Am. J. Psychiatry*, 138(5):650–653.
65. Gibbs, F. A., and Gibbs, E. (1964): *Atlas of electroencephalography, Vol. III.* Addison-Wesley, London.
66. Goldberg, S. C., Halmi, K. A., Casper, R., Eckert, E., and Davis, J. M. (1977): Pretreatment predictors of weight change in anorexia nervosa. In: *Anorexia Nervosa*, edited by R. A. Vigersky, pp. 31–42. Raven Press, New York.
67. Goldblatt, P. B., Moore, M. E., and Stunkard, A. J. (1965): Social factors in obesity. *JAMA*, 192:97–102.
68. Gottdiener, J. S., Gross, H. A., Henry, W. L., Borer, J. S., and Ebert, M. H. (1978): Effects of self-induced starvation on cardiac size and function in anorexia nervosa. *Circulation*, 58:425–433.
69. Gross, H. A., Lake, C. R., Ebert, M. H., Ziegler, M. G., and Kopin, I. J. (1979): Catecholamine metabolism in primary anorexia nervosa. *J. Clin. Endocrinol. Metab.*, 49:805–809.

70. Hall, A. (1978): Family structure and relationships of 50 female anorexia nervosa patients. *NZ J. Psychiatry*, 12:263–268.
71. Halmi, K. A. (1974): Anorexia nervosa: Demographic and clinical features in 94 cases. *Psychosom. Med.*, 36:18–25.
72. Halmi, K. A., Dekirmenjian, H., Davis, J. M., Casper, R., and Goldberg, S. (1978): Catecholamine metabolism in anorexia nervosa. *Arch. Gen. Psychiatry*, 35:458–460.
73. Halmi, K. A., Falk, J. R., and Schwartz, E. (1981): Binge-eating and vomiting: A survey of a college population. *Psychol. Med.* 11:697–706.
74. Halmi, K. A., Goldberg, S. C., Eckert, E., Casper, R., and Davis, J. M. (1977): Pretreatment evaluation in anorexia nervosa. In: *Anorexia Nervosa*, edited by R. A. Vigersky, pp. 43–54. Raven Press, New York.
75. Halmi, K. A., and Loney, J. (1973): Familial alcoholism in anorexia nervosa. *Br. J. Psychiatry*, 123:53–54.
76. Hardy, J. D., Hellon, R. F., and Sutherland, K. (1964): Temperature-sensitive neurones in dog's hypothalamus. *J. Physiol.*, 174:242.
77. Heinz, E. R., Martinez, J., and Haenggeli, A. (1977): Reversibility of cerebral atrophy in anorexia nervosa and cushing's syndrome. *J. Comput. Assist. Tomogr.*, 1(4):415–418.
78. Heufelder, A., Warnhoff, M., and Pirke, K. M. (1984): Alpha-adrenergic receptors and adenylate cyclase in patients with anorexia nervosa and bulimia. *J. Clin. Endocrinol. Metab.* (in press).
79. Hill, P., and Wynder, F. (1976): Diet and prolactin release. *Lancet*, 2:806–807.
80. Holland, A. J., Hall, A., Murray, R., Russell, G. F. M., and Crisp, A. H. (1984): Anorexia nervosa: A study of 34 twin pairs and one set of triplets. *Br. J. Psychiatry*, 145:414–419.
81. Hölzl, R., and Lautenbacher, S. (1984): Psychophysiological indices of the feeding response in anorexia nervosa patients. In: *The Psychobiology of Anorexia Nervosa*, edited by K. M. Pirke and D. Ploog, pp. 93–113. Springer Verlag, Berlin.
82. Hsu, L. K. G., Crisp, A. H., and Harding, B. (1979): Outcome of anorexia nervosa. *The Lancet*, 1:61–65.
83. Hurst, P. S., Lacey, J. H., and Crisp, A. H. (1977): Teeth, vomiting and diet: A study of the dental characteristics of seventeen anorexia nervosa patients. *Postgrad. Med. J.*, 53:298–305.
84. Huse, D. M., and Lucas, A. R. (1984): Dietary patterns in anorexia nervosa. *Am. J. Clin. Nutr.*, 40:251–254.
85. Isaacs, A. J., Leslie, R. D. G., Gomez, J., and Bayliss, R. (1980): The effect of weight gain on gonadotrophins and prolactin in anorexia nervosa. *Acta Endocrinol.*, 94:145–150.
86. Jones, D. J., Fox, M. M., Babigan, H. M., and Hutton, H. E. (1980): Epidemiology of anorexia nervosa in Monroe County, New York: 1960–1967. *Psychosom. Med.*, 42:551–558.
87. Kalucy, R. C., Crisp, A. H., Chard, T., McNeilly, A., Chen, C. N., and Lacey, J. H. (1976): Nocturnal hormonal profiles in massive obesity, anorexia nervosa and normal females. *J. Psychosom. Res.*, 20:595–604.
88. Kalucy, R. S., Crisp, A. H., and Harding, B. (1977): A study of 56 families with anorexia nervosa. *Br. J. Med. Psychol.*, 50:381–395.
89. Katz, J. L., Boyar, R., Raffwarg, H., Hellman, L., and Weiner, H. (1978): Weight and circadian luteinizing hormone secretory pattern in anorexia nervosa. *Psychosom. Med.*, 40:549.
90. Kay, D. W. K. (1953): Anorexia nervosa: Study in prognosis. *Proc. R. Soc. Med.*, 46:669–674.
91. Kay, D. W. K., and Leigh, D. (1954): The natural history, treatment and prognosis of anorexia nervosa, based on a study of 38 patients. *J. Ment. Sci.*, 100:411–431.
92. Kaye, W. H., Ebert, M. H., Gwirtsman, H. E., and Weiss, S. R. (1984): Brain serotonergic metabolism differentiates between patients with anorexia nervosa that fast or binge. *Am. J. Psychiatry (in press)*.
93. Kaye, W. H., Ebert, M. H., Raleigh, M., and Lake, R. (1984): Abnormalities in CNS monoamine metabolism in anorexia nervosa. *Arch. Gen. Psychiatry*, 41:350–355.
94. Kaye, W. H., Jimerson, D. C., Lake, C. R., and Ebert, M. H. (1985): Altered norepinephrine metabolism follwoing long term weight recovery in patients with anorexia nervosa. *Psychiatry Res.*, 14:333–342.
95. Kenny, F. M., Preeaysombat, C., and Migeon, C. J. (1966): Cortisol production rate in normal infants, children and adults. *Pediatrics*, 37:34
96. Keys, A., Brozek, J., Henschel, A., Mickelson, O., and Taylor, H. L. (1950): *The Biology of Human Starvation*. University of Minnesota Press, Minneapolis.

97. Kohlmeyer, K., Lehmkuhl, G., and Poutska, F. (1983): Computed tomography of anorexia nervosa. *AJNR*, 4:437–438.
98. Krieger, D. T., Allen, W., Rizzo, F., and Krieger, H. P. (1971): Characterization of the normal temporal pattern of plasma corticosteroid levels. *J. Clin. Endocrinol.*, 32:266–289.
99. Kron, L., Katz, J. L., Gorzynski, G., and Weiner, H. (1978): Hyporeactivity in anorexia nervosa: A fundamental clinical feature. *Compr. Psychiatry*, 19(5):433–440.
100. Lacey, J. H., Crisp, A. H., Kalucy, R. S., Hartmann, M. K., and Chen, C. N. (1975): Weight gain and the sleep electroencephalogram: A study of ten patients with anorexia nervosa. *Br. Med. J.*, 4:556–558.
101. Landsberg, L., and Young, J. B. (1978): Fasting, feeding and regulation of the sympathetic nervous system. *N. Engl. J. Med.*, 298(23):1295–1301.
102. Landsberg, L., and Young, B. (1982): Effects of nutritional status on autonomic nervous system function. *Am. J. Clin. Nutr.*, 35:1234–1240.
103. Leonard, P. J., and McWilliam, K. M. (1964): Cortisol binding in the serum in Kwashiorkor. *J. Endocrinol.*, 29:273.
104. Lucas, A. R. (1981): Towards the understanding of anorexia nervosa as a disease entity. *Mayo Clin.Proc.*, 56:254–264.
105. Luck, P., Mikhailidis, D. P., Dashwood, M. R., Barradas, M. A., Sever, P. S., Dandona, P., and Wakeling, A. (1983): Platelet hypoeraggregability and increased α-adrenoceptor density in anorexia nervosa. *Clin. Endocrinol. Metab.*, 57:911–914.
106. Luck, P., and Wakeling, A. (1980): Altered thresholds for thermoregulatory sweating and vasodilatation in anorexia nervosa. *Br. Med. J.*, 281:906–908.
107. Lundberg, P. O., Walinder, J., Werner, I., and Wide, L. (1972): Effects of thyrotropin-releasing hormone on plasma levels of TSH, FSH, LH, and GH in anorexia nervosa. *Eur. J. Clin. Invest.*, 2:150–153.
108. Marshall, J. C., and Kelch, R. P. (1979): Low dose pulsatile gonadotropin-releasing hormone in anorexia nervosa: A model of human pubertal development. *J. Clin. Endocrinol. Metab.*, 49:712–718.
109. Mecklenburg, R. S., Loriaux, D. L., Thompson, R. H., Andersen, A. E., and Lipsett, M. B. (1974): Hypothalamic dysfunction in patients with anorexia nervosa. *Medicine*, 53(2):147–159.
110. Miayi, K. T., Yamamoto, M., Zukizawa, M., Ishibashi, K., and Kumahara, Y. (1975): Serum thyroid hormones and thyrotropin in anorexia nervosa. *J. Clin. Endocrinol.*, 40:334–338.
111. Morgan, H. G., and Russell, G. F. M. (1975): Value of family background and clinical features as predictors of long-term outcome in anorexia nervosa: Four year follow-up study of 42 patients. *Psychol. Med.*, 5:355–371.
112. Moshang, T., Parks, J. S., Baker, L., Vaidya, V., Utiger, R., Bongiovanni, A. M., and Snyder, P. J. (1975): Low serum triiodothyronin in patients with anorexia nervosa. *J. Clin. Endocrinol.*, 40:470–473.
113. Minuchin, S., Rosman, B. L., and Baker, L. (1978): *Psychosomatic Families: Anorexia Nervosa in Context.* Harvard University Press, Cambridge, Massachusetts.
114. Nakayama, T., Eisenman, J. S., and Hardy, J. D. (1961): Single unit activity of anterior hypothalamus during local heating. *Science*, 134:560–561.
115. Neil, J. F., Merikangas, J. R., Forster, F. G., Merikangas, K. R., Spiker, D. G., and Kupfer, D. J. (1980): Waking and all-night sleep EEG's in anorexia nervosa. *Clin. Electroencephalogr.*, 11:9–15.
116. Nudel, D. B., Gootman, N., Nussbaum, M. P., and Shenker, I. R. (1984): Altered exercise performance and abnormal sympathetic responses to exercise in patients with anorexia nervosa. *J. Pediatr.*, 105:34–37.
117. Pimstone, B. L., Barbezat, G., and Hansen, J. P. L. (1968): Studies on growth hormone secretion in protein caloric malnutrition. *Am. J. Clin. Nutr.*, 21:482.
118. Pirke, K. M., Fichter, M. M., Lund, R., and Doerr, P. (1979): Twenty-four hour sleep-wake pattern of plasma LH in patients with anorexia nervosa. *Acta Endocrinol.*, 92:193–204.
119. Pirke, K. M., Pahl, J., Schweiger, U., Münzing, W., Lang, P., and Büll, U. (1985): Total body potassium, intracellular potassium and body composition in patients with anorexia nervosa during refeeding. *Int. J. Eating Disord.* (in press).
120. Pirke, K. M., Pahl, J., Schweiger, U., and Warnhoff, M. (1985): Metabolic and endocrine indices of starvation in bulimia: A comparison with anorexia nervosa. *Psychiatry Res.*, 15:33–39.
121. Pirke, K. M., Schweiger, U., Lemmel, W., Krieg, J. C., and Berger, M. (1985): The influence of

dieting on the menstrual cycle of healthy young women. *J. Clin. Endocrinol. Metab.*, 60:1174–1179.

122. Pirke, K. M., and Spyra, B. (1982): Catecholamine turnover in the brain and the regulation of luteinizing hormone and corticosterone in starved male rats. *Acta Endocrinol.*, 100:168–176.

123. Ploog, D. (1984): The importance of physiologic, metabolic, and endocrine studies for the understanding of anorexia nervosa. In: *The Psychobiology of Anorexia Nervosa*, edited by K. M. Pirke and D. Ploog, pp. 1–3. Springer-Verlag, Berlin.

124. Pope, H. G., Hudson, J. I., and Yurgelun-Todd, D. (1984): Anorexia nervosa and bulimia among 300 suburban women shoppers. *Am. J. Psychiatry*, 141:292–294.

125. Portnay, G. I., O'Brian, J. T., Vagenakis, A. G., Rudolph, M., Arky, R., Ingbar, S. H., and Braverman, L. E. (1974): Abnormalities in triiodothyronine metabolism induced by starvation in man. *J. Clin. Invest.*, 53;191–194.

126. Riederer, P., Toifl, K., and Kruzik, P. (1982): Excretion of biogenic amine metabolites in anorexia nervosa. *Clin. Chim. Acta*, 123:27–32.

127. Rollins, N., and Piazza, E. (1978): Diagnosis of anorexia nervosa. A critical reappraisal. *J. Am. Acad. Child Psychiatry*, 17:126–137.

128. Roth, J. C., Kelch, R. P., Kaplan, S. L., and Grumbach, M. M. (1972): FSH and LH response to luteinizing hormone-releasing factor in prepubertal and pubertal children. *J. Clin. Endocrinol.*, 35:926–930.

129. Russell, G. F. M. (1965): Metabolic aspects of anorexia nervosa. *Proc. R. Soc. Med.*, 58:811–814.

130. Russell, G. F. M. (1967): The nutritional disorder in anorexia nervosa. *J. Psychosom. Res.*, 11:141–149.

131. Russell, G. F. M. (1979): Bulimia nervosa: An ominous variant of anorexia nervosa. *Psychol. Med.*, 9:429–448.

132. Russell, G. M., Prendergast, P. J., Darby, P. L., Garfinkel, P. E., Whitwell, J., and Jeejeebhoy, K. M. (1983): A comparison between muscle function and body composition in anorexia nervosa: The effect of refeeding. *Am. J. Clin. Nutr.*, 38:229–237.

133. Saleh, J. W., and Lebwohl, P. (1980): Metoclopramide-induced gastric emptying in patients with anorexia nervosa. *Am. J. Gastreonterol.*, 74:127–132.

134. Schweiger, U., Warnhoff, M., and Pirke, K. M. (1984): Large neutral amino acid ratios after carbohydrate and protein test meals in anorectic patients. *Metabolism* (in press).

135. Schweiger, U., Warnhoff, M., and Pirke, K. M. (1985): Noradrenergic turnover in the hypothalamus of adult male rats: Alteration of circadian pattern by semistarvation. *J. Neurochem.*, 45:706–709.

136. Scriba, P. C., Bauer, M., Emmert, D., Fateh-Moghadam, A., Hofmann, G. G., Horn, K., and Pickardt, C. R. (1979): Effects of obesity, total fasting and re-alimentation on L-thyroxine (T4), 3,5,3'-L-triiodothyronine (T3), 3,3'5'-L-triiodothyronine (rT3), thyroxine binding globulin (CBG), transferrin, α2-haptaglobin and complement C'3 in serum. *Acta Endocrinol.*, 91:629–643.

137. Seidensticker, J. F., and Tzagournis, M. (1968): Anorexia nervosa—clinical features and long term follow-up. *J. Chronic Dis.*, 21:361–367.

138. Selvini-Palazzoli, M. (1974): *Self-Starvation*. Chancer Publishing, London.

139. Sherman, B. M., and Halmi, K. A. (1977): Effect of nutritional rehabilitation on hypothalamic-pituitary function in anorexia nervosa. In: *Anorexia Nervosa*, edited by R. A. Vigersky, pp. 211–223. Raven Press, New York.

140. Shimoda, Y., and Kitagawa, T. (1973): Clinical and EEG studies on the emaciation (anorexia nervosa) due to disturbed function of the brain stem. *J. Neural. Transm.*, 34:195–204.

141. Silverman, J. A. (1977): Anorexia nervosa: Clinical and metabolic observations in a successful treatment plan. In: *Anorexia Nervosa*, edited by R. A. Vigersky, pp. 331–339. Raven Press, New York.

142. Smart, D. E., Beumont, P. J. V., and George, G. C. W. (1976): Some personality characteristics of patients with anorexia nervosa. *Br. J. Psychiatry*, 128:57–60.

143. Smith, S. R., Belsoe, T., and Chatri, M. K. (1975): Cortisol metabolism and the pituitary adrenal axis in adults with protein caloric malnutrition. *J. Clin. Endocrinol.*, 40:43–52.

144. Spyra, B., and Pirke, K. M. (1982): Binding of (^{3}H) clonidine and (^{3}H)WB4101 to the pre-and postsynaptic alpha-adrenoceptors of the basal hypothalamus of the starved male rat. *Brain Res.*, 245:179–182.

145. Stunkard, A. J. (1975): From explanation to action in psychosomatic medicine. The case of obesity. Presidential address. *Psychosom. Med.*, 37:195–236.
146. Swann, I. (1977): Anorexia nervosa—a difficult diagnosis in boys. Illustrated by three cases. *Practioner*, 218:424–427.
147. Theander, S. (1970): Anorexia nervosa: A psychiatric investigation of 94 female cases. *Acta Psychiatr. Scand. [Suppl.]*, 214:1–194.
148. Travaglini, P., Beck-Peccoz, P., Ferrari, C., Ambrosi, B., Paracchi, A., Severgnini, A., Spade, A., and Faglia, G. (1976): Some aspects of hypothalamic-pituitary function in patients with anorexia nervosa. *Acta Endocrinol.*, 81:252–262.
149. Vagenakis, A. G. (1977): Thyroid hormone metabolism in prolonged experimental starvation in man. In: *Anorexia Nervosa*, edited by R. A. Vigersky, pp. 243–253. Raven Press, New York.
150. Vandereycken, W., and Meermann, R. (1984): *Anorexia Nervosa: A Clinician's Guide to Treament.* Walter de Gruyter, Berlin.
151. Vanderlaan, W. P., Parker, D. C., Roseman, L. G., and Vanderlaan, E. F. (1970): Implication of growth hormone release in sleep. *Metabolism*, 19:891.
152. Vaughan, G. M., Pelham, R. W., Pang, S. F., Loughlin, L. L., Wilson, K. M., Sandock, K. L., Vaughan, M. K., Koslow, S. H., and Reiter, R. J. (1976): Nocturnal elevation of plasma melatonin and urinary 5-hydroxyindoleacetic acid in young men: Attempts at modification by brief changes in environmental lighting and sleep and by autonomic drugs. *J. Clin. Endocrinol. Metab.*, 42:752–764.
153. Vigersky, R. A., Andersen, A. E., Thompson, R. H., and Loriaux, D. L. (1977): Hypothalamic dysfunction in secondary amenorrhea associated with simple weight loss. *N. Engl. J. Med.*, 297:1141–1145.
154. Vigersky, R. A., and Loriaux, D. L. (1977): Anorexia nervosa as a model of hypothalamic dysfunction. In: *Anorexia Nervosa*, edited by R. A. Vigersky, pp. 109–122. Raven Press, New York.
155. Vigersky, R. A., Loriaux, D. L., Andersen, A. E., Mecklenburg, R. S., and Vaitukaitis, J. L. (1976): Delayed pituitary hormone response to LRF and TRF in patients with anorexia nervosa and with secondary amenorrhea associated with simple weight loss. *J. Clin. Endocrinol. Metab.*, 43:893–900.
156. Wakeling, A., DeSouza, V. A., and Beardwood, C. J. (1977): Assessment of the negative and positive feedback effects of administered oestrogen on gonadotrophin release in patients with anorexia nervosa. *Psychol. Med.*, 7:397–405.
157. Wakeling, A., DeSouza, V. A., Gore, M. B. R., Sabur, M., Longstone, D., and Boss, A. M. B. (1979): Amenorrhea, body weight and serum hormone concentration, with particular reference to prolactin and thyroid hormones in anorexia nervosa. *Psychol. Med.*, 9:265–272.
158. Walsh, B. T., Katz, J. K., Levin, J., Kream, J., Fukushima, D. K., Hellman, L. D., Weiner, H., and Zumoff, B. (1978): Adrenal activity in anorexia nervosa. *Psychosom. Med.*, 40:499.
159. Warren, M. P., and Vande Wiele, R. L. (1973): Clinical and metabolic features of anorexia nervosa. *Am. J. Obstet. Gynecol.*, 117:435–449.
160. Weitzman, E. D. (1976): Circadian rhythms and episodic hormone secretion. *Annu. Rev. Med.*, 27:225–243.
161. Winokur, A., March, V., and Mendels, J. (1980): Primary affective disorder in relatives of patients with anorexia nervosa. *Am. J. Psychiatry*, 137(6):695–698.
162. White, J. H., Kelly, P., and Dorman, K. (1977): Clinical picture of atypical anorexia nervosa associated with hypothalamic tumor. *Am. J. Psychiatry*, 134:323–325.
163. Wurtman, R. J., and Wurtman, J. J. (1984): Nutritional control of central neurotransmitters. In: *The Psychobiology of Anorexia Nervosa*, edited by K. M. Pirke and D. Ploog, pp. 4–11. Springer Verlag, Berlin.
164. Yap, S. H., Hafkenscheid, J. C. M., and van Tongeren, J. H. M. (1975): Important role of tryptophan on albumin synthesis in patients suffering from anorexia nervosa and hypoalbuminemia. *Am. J. Clin. Nutr.*, 28:1356–1363.
165. Zumoff, B., Walsh, B. T., Katz, J. L., Levin, J., Rosenfeld, R. S., Kream, J., and Weiner, H. (1983): Subnormal plasma dehydroisoandrosterone to cortisol ratio in anorexia nervosa: A second hormonal parameter of ontogenic regression. *J. Clin. Endocrinol. Metab.*, 56(4):668–672.

Nutrition and the Brain, Vol. 7, edited by
R. J. Wurtman and J. J. Wurtman. Raven Press,
New York © 1986.

Potential Effects of the Dipeptide Sweetener Aspartame on the Brain

William M. Pardridge

Department of Medicine, UCLA School of Medicine, Los Angeles, California 90024

I. INTRODUCTION

Aspartame (L-aspartyl-L-phenylalanine methyl ester) is a new, nonnutritive sweetener introduced into the diet in 1981 as a constituent of dry foods and, in 1983, in carbonated beverages (Fig. 1). The use of this agent has engendered considerable enthusiasm owing to the high palatability of foods that contain it, and to the fact that aspartame is composed only of substances normally found in the diet and the body, i.e., the amino acids aspartic acid and phenylalanine, and the alcohol methanol (68). Since aspartame is composed of such substances, it had been anticipated that even high doses would be associated with relatively few, if any, side effects. However, this seems not to have been the case: the Center for Disease Control (CDC) recently published results of a study based on passive surveillance of consumer-initiated complaints associated with aspartame-containing food products (136). Among the 517 subjects who completed the CDC's questionnaires, purported side effects fell, in general, into three general categories (Table 1) primarily involving the central nervous system (CNS); the gastrointestinal tract; or gynecologic symptoms. The CNS symptoms, analyzed further by the CDC, were found to be related primarily to either mood changes or insomnia. In addition,

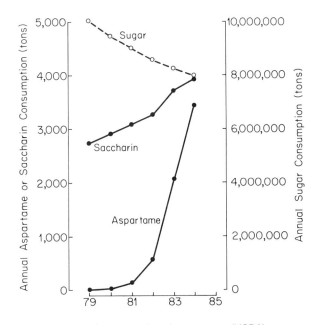

FIG. 1. Annual consumption of sweeteners (USDA).

nine cases of seizures occurring in relation to high-dose aspartame ingestion were reviewed by the CDC (Table 1). On the basis of these findings, the CDC report concluded that the "highest priority for any future investigation might be in the neurologic–behavioral area" (136). In keeping with this recommendation, the purpose of this chapter is to review the possible ways by which high doses of aspartame, or metabolites of aspartame produced in the course of digestion, might have neurochemical effects that could underlie its neurologic or behavioral side effects. Since the products of aspartame metabolism are more likely to produce CNS effects than the parent compound, this chapter examines five such metabolites: (i) methanol, (ii) aspartic acid, (iii) the dipeptide, either aspartame or the aspartylphen-

TABLE 1. *CDC evaluation of consumer complaints related to aspartame use*

System	Complaint
CNS	Mood changes
	Insomnia
	Seizures
Gastrointestinal	Abdominal pain
	Nausea
	Diarrhea
Gynecologic	Irregular menses

From ref. 136.

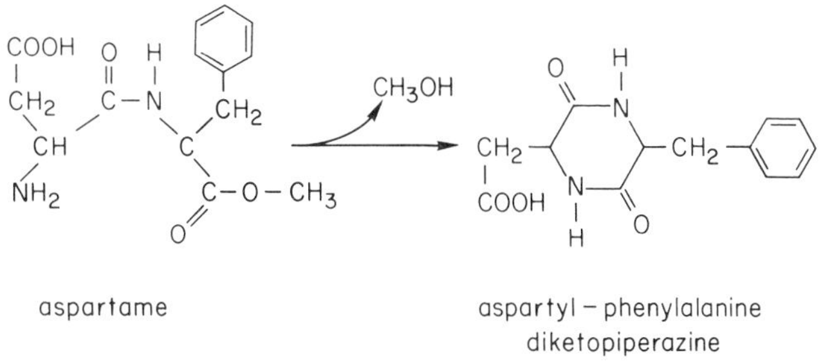

FIG. 2. Structures of the two aspartame dipeptides: aspartame (L-aspartyl-L-phenylalanine methyl ester) and the aspartyl phenylalanine DKP, which is formed upon hydrolysis of the methyl ester followed by condensation of the dipeptide to form the cyclic compound.

ylalanine diketopiperazine (DKP) (Fig. 2), (iv) phenylalanine, and (v) phenethylamine. Prior to discussion of these individual compounds, the important matter of projections of daily aspartame intake is reviewed.

II. PROJECTIONS OF DAILY ASPARTAME INTAKE

A central principle in attempting to relate the ingestion of aspartame to possible neurologic–behavioral sequelae is that the dosage of aspartame in milligrams per kilogram per day must be sufficiently high to cause significant elevations in the blood levels of its possibly active metabolites. Accordingly, the following discussion considers the likely daily dosages of aspartame that have been projected by the Food and Drug Administration (FDA) (36) and by sources in the literature (115).

A hypothetical individual weighing 70 kg might consume 2,500 calories per day, 17% of which are in the form of sucrose (or 425 calories per day). Since 1 g sucrose is equivalent to 4 calories, then 106 g sucrose are consumed per day (or 1.5 g/kg). Since aspartame is 180 times more potent than sucrose as a sweetener, its expected daily intake would be 8 mg/kg. Other estimates have assumed that 25% of the daily calories are in the form of sucrose; this assumption would imply a daily aspartame intake of 12 mg/kg (105). The 99th percentile of aspartame ingestion has been set at 34 mg/kg/day (36), which would be equivalent to a 70-kg individual consuming 70% of the daily 2,500 calories in the form of sucrose. The advisable daily intake (ADI) has been established by the Joint Expert Committee on Food Additives (JEC/FA) of the Food and Agricultural Organization of the United Nations and the World Health Organization (FAO/WHO) at 40 mg/kg/day (73). This dosage of aspartame is 1% of the no-observed-effect dose (4 g/kg/day) used in preclinical studies on rats (73). The safety factor of 100 is somewhat arbitrary and is believed to provide a safe and realistic distance between the ADI and the minimal toxic dose of aspartame or of aspartame products.

The above expected daily dosages of aspartame intake were established on the basis of a norm of a 70-kg individual. Thus in children who weigh approximately 20 to 40 kg, the expected daily dosage of aspartame intake will be considerably

TABLE 2. *Dosage of aspartame in food products*

Product	Amount	Aspartame dose (mg)
Table top sweetener	2 packets	80
Dry beverage mix	12 oz	180
Gelatin or pudding	8 oz	64
Whipped topping	2 tablespoons	10
Breakfast cereal	2 oz	180
Chewing gum	5 sticks	40
Soft drink	12 oz	200

From ref. 138.

higher and will exceed the expected 99th percentile of 34 mg/kg/day. For example, 7- to 12-year-old-children with access to aspartame-containing products consumed up to 77 mg/kg/day aspartame (30). Even adults, when admitted to a clinical research center wherein aspartame-containing products were used liberally in the diet, consumed up to 36 mg/kg/day, with a mean daily intake of 20 mg/kg (99). The main point to be emphasized in this analysis is that children, owing to their low body weight, will consume daily dosages of aspartame that are large relative to FDA predicted standards for either the 99th percentile or the ADI. Indeed, a 20-kg child who consumes a quart of an aspartame-flavored beverage (such as diet cola) will achieve an acute dosage of more than 25 mg/kg, without having to consume any other aspartame-containing products (Table 2).

A second point to be emphasized in estimating daily aspartame intakes relates to the extrapolation of acute aspartame intakes in humans to experimental animals for the purposes of evaluating product toxicity in animals. In general, the metabolism of aspartame or its constituent amino acids, aspartate or phenylalanine, is inversely related to the size of the animal. For example, the acute administration of 34 mg/kg aspartame to humans doubles plasma phenylalanine levels approximately 60 min after the dosage (118). In rats, however, the doubling of the sum of plasma phenylalanine plus tyrosine[1] is not observed until the aspartame dose is increased to 200 mg/kg (27,132). Thus rats metabolize phenylalanine approximately six times faster than does a human. Moreover, Reynolds et al. (104) observed that monkeys metabolize phenylalanine considerably faster than humans, and this is consistent with the higher daily protein requirement of these smaller-sized primates in terms of grams of protein per kilogram per day. The inverse relationship between body size and metabolic rate is well known and is embodied in the concept of metabolically active mass (13). In general terms, the relationship among mammalian

---

[1]Rats convert about half of an oral dose of phenylalanine into tyrosine, and the plasma tyrosine level increases markedly after aspartame intake in rats (27,132). In contrast, plasma tyrosine elevations in humans after aspartame ingestion are relatively small (115). Therefore, the aspartame-induced inhibition of brain uptake of tryptophan and other large neutral amino acids (LNAAs) (other than phenylalanine or tyrosine) in rats is a function of the sum of plasma phenylalanine and tyrosine concentrations.

species between metabolic rate (M, in calories per day) and body mass (B, in kilograms) is given by the following expression (13):

$$M = 70 \times B^{0.75}$$

Insight into the need for scaling of aspartame daily dosages among species, e.g., from rat to human, is critical to the quantitative analysis of aspartame toxicity studies in animals. For example, if one were to attempt to administer to humans an aspartame dose equal to the 200 mg/kg used in rats, this would require giving 14,000 mg aspartame to a 70-kg man, an amount equal to that in 78 12-oz cans of diet cola. The direct extrapolation to humans of dosages administered to rats would be fallacious, however, since it ignores the need for pharmacokinetic scaling among species of different body mass. Taking into consideration the concepts of metabolically active mass and of scaling between species (13), and the increases in plasma phenylalanine observed after aspartame administration to rats or humans, it is apparent that an aspartame dose of 200 mg/kg for rats (132) is equivalent to a dose of 34 mg/kg for humans (118). Although the dosage of 34 mg/kg is the putative 99th percentile of aspartame ingestion (36), the preceding analysis indicates that this dosage is a likely approximation of acute aspartame intake for a typical 7- to 12-year-old child (30). Thus these considerations suggest that a dosage of 200 mg/kg aspartame in rats (132) is reasonable for simulating possible neurochemical changes in humans, particularly in children.

III. METHANOL METABOLISM

Methyl alcohol (methanol) is a normal constituent of the diet and a normal intermediate in cellular metabolic pathways (Fig. 3). Since aspartame is 10% by weight methanol (Fig. 2), a liter of an aspartame-sweetened beverage containing approximately 500 mg aspartame (Table 2) provides 50 mg of the methanol moiety of aspartame. This dosage of methanol is comparable to that found in canned fruit juices (63), where methanol levels are typically 70 mg/liter. Methanol levels in fresh fruit juice are only one-tenth as great (63), and it appears that the methanol is produced by nonspecific hydrolysis of methyl esters in the fruit constituents. In contrast to aspartame-sweetened beverages, canned or fresh fruit juices also contain acetaldehyde (about 80 mg/liter) and ethyl alcohol (about 500 mg/liter). Thus there is about a fivefold molar excess of ethanol over methanol in canned fruit juice (63). The coexistence of ethanol in the food product may cause important differences between the abilities of the methanol derived from aspartame versus canned fruit juice to be toxic. It is hypothesized that the formation of toxic metabolites of methanol is slowed by the ethanol in fruit juice, and that this protective effect is lacking when the source of the methanol is aspartame. However, quantitative analyses suggest that the methanol from fruit juice or aspartame beverages is metabolized at the same rate in humans, independent of the small quantities of ethanol in fruit juice.

In the rat (Fig. 3), methanol is converted to formaldehyde by a combined peroxidase–catalase reaction (120). In the primate, however, methanol is converted

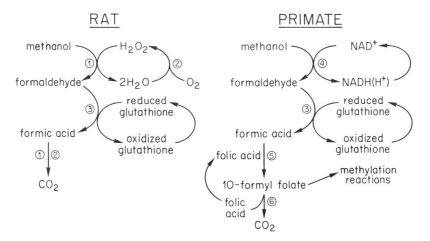

FIG. 3. Pathways of methanol metabolism in the rat *(left)* and in primates *(right)*. There are two major differences in methanol metabolism in these two groups: (a) oxidation of methanol by peroxidase-catalase in the rat, which is weakly inhibited by ethanol, as opposed to the oxidation of methanol in primates by alcohol dehydrogenase, which is strongly inhibited by ethanol; and (b) the folate-dependent oxidation of formic acid in the primate. The enzymes involved in these pathways are: 1, peroxidase; 2, catalase; 3, formaldehyde dehydrogenase; 4, alcohol dehydrogenase; 5, formylfolate synthetase; 6, formylfolate dehydrogenase. (These pathways are from ref. 120.)

to formaldehyde by alcohol dehydrogenase (120). Both the catalase–peroxidase and the alcohol dehydrogenase reactions also metabolize ethanol. Ethanol and methanol have equal avidities for the peroxidase–catalase reaction in the rat, but ethanol has a sixfold greater affinity for the alcohol dehydrogenase reaction in primates (49). Therefore, in species, e.g., primates, wherein alcohol dehydrogenase is the major first step in methanol clearance, the coadministration of large amounts (>10 g) of ethanol can greatly slow the metabolism of methanol and slow the formation of such methanol metabolites as formaldehyde or formic acid (120). However, the K_m of alcohol dehydrogenase for ethanol is 3 mM (49). As discussed in subsequent sections (see Eq. 1), competition effects are not significant until the concentration of the inhibitor approximates the K_m. The amounts of ethanol in fruit juice would be expected to produce only micromolar concentrations of ethanol *in vivo*, and these concentrations are $<<K_m$ of 3 mM. Thus there is no reason to expect a delay in the formation of methanol metabolites after the consumption of aspartame products as compared to fruit juice.

Formaldehyde is converted to formic acid by formaldehyde dehydrogenase, a glutathione-dependent pathway, in both rats and primates (120) (Fig. 2). In the rat, however, formic acid is converted to carbon dioxide primarily by the peroxidase–catalase reaction, whereas in primates, formic acid is cleared primarily by a folic-acid-dependent formylfolate synthetase reaction, which leads to the formation of 10-formylfolate (120). This substance is an intermediate in biosynthetic pathways that involve methylation reactions in the synthesis of pyrimidines and amino acids, such as methionine. Alternatively, 10-formylfolate can be cleared by formation of carbon dioxide by another enzyme, formylfolate dehydrogenase (Fig. 3).

These considerations illustrate a second major species difference in the metabolism of methanol by the rat and the primate: The primate relies on the normal availability of folic acid stores for formic acid clearance, whereas the rat is able to clear formic acid primarily by folate-independent pathways (120). In primates, folate deficiency does not inhibit the rate of clearance of methanol from blood, but the metabolic acidosis after methanol intoxication is worsened by folate deficiency (120).

A third difference between methanol metabolism in rats and primates is the clinical manifestations of methanol intoxication. In primates, methanol toxicity occurs after ingestion of an acute single load of 2 g/kg methanol, which results in ocular toxicity and in metabolic acidosis secondary to the formation of formic acid (120). Conversely, in rats, there is little ocular toxicity, and significant metabolic acidosis does not generally develop. The major effects of methanol intoxication in rats are depression of the CNS and ataxia (120). The etiology of the ocular toxicity associated with methanol intoxication in primates is poorly understood but may be due to the *in situ* generation of either formaldehyde or formic acid in the eye owing to the presence of the necessary enzymes (Fig. 3) in the ocular tissue.

Biochemical studies on methanol metabolism after aspartame ingestion have been described by Stegink (115). In the normal individual, methanol levels in plasma are lower than the limits of detection. Methanol levels rise in proportion to the acute aspartame dose. For example, peak methanol levels in humans are 0.34 mg/dl after 50 mg/kg aspartame and 2.6 mg/dl after 200 mg/kg aspartame. There is no increase in plasma formic acid even after an extremely high acute dose of aspartame (200 mg/kg) in adult humans (115). However, urinary formate clearance increases with large doses of aspartame (115), indicating that hepatic production of formic acid from ingested ethanol is slow compared with renal clearance of the acid under normal conditions. Concentrations of plasma formaldehyde after acute aspartame ingestion have apparently not been measured. These data would be of interest, since plasma acetaldehyde levels are elevated in ethanol toxicity and may mediate many of the toxic phenomena of ethanol ingestion (51).

Such studies would appear to be only of academic interest, since there is, at present, no basis for anticipating that the sequelae that follow the consumption of toxic doses of methanol (e.g., >1 g/kg) will also be associated with the much smaller amounts (e.g., <0.01 g/kg) that enter the body with even large doses of aspartame. The effects, if any, of consuming the small amounts of methanol in aspartame and in canned fruit juice appear to be comparable.

IV. ASPARTIC ACID METABOLISM

Aspartic acid (aspartate) and glutamic acid (glutamate) are acidic amino acids that are normally found in high concentrations in dietary protein and to a lesser extent as free amino acids. The monosodium salt of glutamate (monosodium glutamate, MSG) has enjoyed a long and widespread use as a food additive, particularly in Chinese cooking. Olney (81) has advocated that the use of amino acids, such as glutamate or aspartate, as elective food additives be restricted because of their cytotoxic effects on the brain. Both glutamate and aspartate are putative excitatory neurotransmitters in brain, and high concentrations of these amino acids may lead to excessive neuronal stimulation and cell death in laboratory animals. A dose as low as 0.5 g/kg, given subcutaneously to neonatal mice, can produce neuronal cell death in some regions, particularly those around the circumventricular organs (CVOs) of brain (100), i.e., areas that lack a blood-brain barrier (BBB) (see below). Since aspartame is 40% aspartic acid (Fig. 2), an acute dose of 50 mg/kg aspartame would be equivalent to an acute dose of 0.02 g/kg aspartic acid, or about $\frac{1}{25}$ the dose that causes brain lesions in neonatal mice. This apparent 25-fold safety factor is somewhat small, considering that a 100-fold factor is usually invoked to establish the safety of a compound (73).

On the basis of this kind of superficial analysis, one would have to consider the possibility that the aspartate moiety in aspartame (81) could cause harmful effects on the brains of humans. This line of reasoning is unwarranted, however; as Stegink (115) has cogently argued, it is not the comparative dosage among species that is important in evaluating the safety of a food additive, but the peak blood level in each species that a given dosage produces. Moreover, within the background of a physiologic-based analysis of aspartate or glutamate metabolism in mammals, it becomes apparent that the aspartate moiety in aspartame is relatively harmless to humans. Three areas should be considered in a physiologic-based analysis of the safety of dietary aspartate for humans: (i) splanchnic barriers to aspartate, (ii) BBB, and (iii) CVOs.

Two splanchnic barriers, the intestinal epithelia and the hepatocytes, separate the gut lumen from the systemic circulation. The acidic amino acids, aspartate and glutamate, are transported through the intestinal mucosal membrane. Once within the intestinal epithelial cell, they can be either transported through the basolateral membrane to the portal circulation or metabolized within the epithelial cell.

Metabolism of the acidic amino acids occurs via transamination (114). In the case of glutamate, the nitrogen moiety is transferred directly to alanine; in the case of aspartate, the nitrogen group is transferred to alanine via a glutamate intermediate (Fig. 4). The 3-carbon skeleton, pyruvate, which acts as the nitrogen acceptor, may be donated from the carbon skeletons of aspartate or glutamate, directly via the decarboxylation pathway, involving either malic enzyme or phosphoenolpyruvate carboxykinase (Fig. 4). The decarboxylation or anaplerotic pathways are important routes by which the carbon skeletons of acidic amino acids may be degraded completely to CO_2 via the Krebs cycle (58); only carbon entering the Krebs cycle in the form of pyruvate can be completely oxidized, whereas carbon entering the Krebs cycle in the form of the 4-carbon skeletons, oxalacetate or malate, undergo no net oxidation. However, the rates of the decarboxylation pathways are slow compared to the rates through the transamination pathways. Thus the metabolism of the acidic amino acids in the intestinal epithelia to alanine is

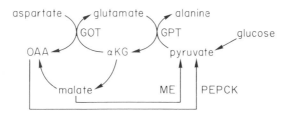

FIG. 4. Pyruvate limitation of gut aspartate metabolism. Aspartate is readily metabolized in intestinal epithelia to alanine, which is released to the portal circulation. The conversion of aspartate to alanine occurs via sequential transamination reactions involving glutamate. The limiting compound in the conversion of aspartate to alanine is the availability of pyruvate, which acts as the nitrogen acceptor. Pyruvate can be formed from the carbon skeleton of aspartate, oxalacetate (OAA), via anaplerotic pathways, i.e., the conversion of 4-carbon compounds to the 3-carbon pyruvate skeleton, via either malic enzyme (ME) or phosphoenolpyruvate carboxykinase (PEPCK). However, the formation of pyruvate via these anaplerotic pathways is relatively slow compared to the formation of pyruvate derived via glucose metabolism. Thus the coavailability of glucose in intestinal epithelia allows for rapid conversion of aspartate to alanine via the transaminase pathways, glutamate oxalacetate transaminase (GOT), and glutamate pyruvate transaminase (GPT). (Data are from refs. 58 and 114.)

slow in the absence of carbohydrate-derived pyruvic acid. In the presence of carbohydrate, the availability of pyruvate in the intestinal epithelia is not limiting; hence the acidic amino acids can be rapidly metabolized, via transamination, to form alanine (114).

The metabolic relationships in Fig. 4 and the key role of pyruvate availability are well illustrated in a study by Stegink (114), in which peak plasma glutamate levels were 0.7 mM in adults ingesting 0.15 g/kg MSG in water[2] but only 0.1 mM after a comparable MSG dose was administered with carbohydrate. When aspartame was administered at a dose of 0.1 g/kg to adults (in orange juice) or to infants (in water), essentially no changes in plasma aspartate levels were observed (114,115). The entry of glutamate, and possibly of aspartate, into the systemic circulation after the acute ingestion of large doses is largely aborted by the coadministration of carbohydrate. The peak aspartate level after the acute ingestion of 0.1 g/kg aspartame in the absence of coadministered carbohydrate has apparently not been measured for adults. Based on the studies with MSG, an acute dose of 0.05 to 0.1 g/kg aspartame, which would be equivalent to a dose of 0.02 to 0.04 g/kg aspartate, would be expected to produce only a modest increase in blood aspartate, e.g., increasing it to 0.1 mM, when administered in the absence of carbohydrate.

Subsequent to the parenteral administration of large doses of the acidic amino acids or the oral administration of abuse dosages in the absence of carbohydrate, their blood levels may achieve values on the order of 2 to 3 mM (4). However, brain levels of the acidic amino acids do not increase at all (100), even in the

[2]A dose of 0.15 g/kg of MSG is the ADI of the WHO. This dose is more than double the 99th percentile of expected MSG ingestion of 61 mg/kg/day (135) Since some soups contain up to 0.72% MSG (137), however, the acute dosage of MSG by a 20-kg child who consumes 2 cups of soup is 0.17 g/kg.

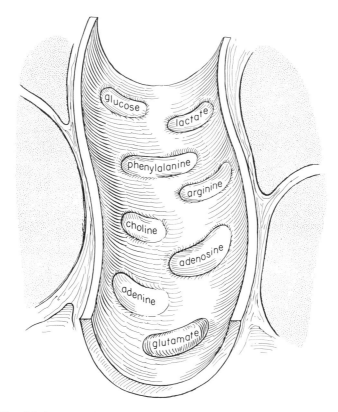

FIG. 5. The eight known nutrient transport systems situated in the brain capillary, i.e., the BBB, are depicted in this sketch of the capillary (87). The eight different carriers transport classes of nutrients, and a representative substrate is given for each system. The glutamate carrier is believed to act as an active efflux system, which actively pumps glutamate and aspartate, two putative excitatory neurotransmitters, from brain interstitial space to plasma (85). Conversely, the other seven transport systems are believed to mediate the bidirectional movement of these essential nutrients between plasma and brain interstitial space. The biochemical identity of these eight carrier systems is yet to be described, but they are believed to be specific enzyme-like proteins that are under genetic regulation.

presence of such high plasma concentrations, owing to the presence of the BBB. Unlike those of any other organ, the capillaries of brain in virtually all vertebrates are endowed with specialized morphologic features, such as high-resistance tight junctions and minimal pinocytosis (15). The tight junctions literally cement together all the capillary endothelial cells of the brain, forming an epithelium-like high-resistance diffusion barrier, which separates the circulating blood from the interstitial space of the brain. Circulating nutrients gain access to this interstitial space only by virtue of their affinity for one of the specific nutrient transport systems localized in the BBB (87) (Fig. 5).

Unlike the transport systems that mediate the BBB flux of the other seven classes of nutrients, the acidic amino acid carrier in the capillaries of the brain is an active

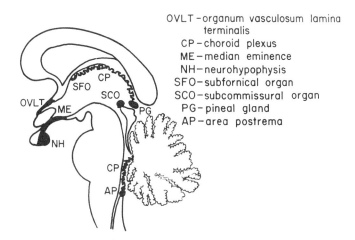

OVLT – organum vasculosum lamina
terminalis
CP – choroid plexus
ME – median eminence
NH – neurohypophysis
SFO – subfornical organ
SCO – subcommissural organ
PG – pineal gland
AP – area postrema

FIG. 6. The CVOs are tiny areas surrounding the ventricles that lack a BBB (see Fig. 7). Areas of brain immediately contiguous with the CVOs (e.g., the hypothalamic arcuate nucleus is immediately adjacent to the median eminence) are sensitive to the development of cytotoxic lesions when plasma glutamate or aspartate is artificially elevated by the acute administration of toxicologic amounts of these acidic amino acids. (From ref. 125, with permission.)

efflux system (85). Thus the glutamate–aspartate carrier actively transports the excitatory amino acids out of the interstitial space of the brain and into the blood. The large flux of acidic amino acids in the direction of brain to blood prevents the net movement of these amino acids from blood into brain. Little information is available about the macromolecule that constitutes the BBB glutamate–aspartate carrier, and this is clearly an area in need of additional study. The ability of this carrier to produce active efflux has been inferred by comparing the rates of influx of glutamate into the brain and its net rate of output from brain to blood (85). The movement of glutamate and aspartate through the BBB is most restricted compared with the movements of all other classes of nutrients (87), and the relative impermeability of the BBB to acidic amino acids is consistent with the observation that the brain levels of these compounds are not increased even when there are large elevations in their plasma levels (100).

The generalization that brain glutamate or aspartate levels cannot be changed by elevating plasma levels of these compounds is not true for the CVOs. These tiny areas of brain surrounding the ventricles lack a BBB and have porous, fenestrated capillaries (125). The concentrations of glutamate or aspartate in the CVOs can be increased when plasma levels of these amino acids are greatly elevated (100). Moreover, the areas of brain that are most sensitive to the toxic effects of exogenous MSG are those areas that are directly contiguous to one of the CVOs (Fig. 6). For example, the arcuate nucleus, which is the area most widely examined in studies on MSG neurotoxicity (81), is adjacent to the median eminence, which is one of the CVOs (125). The arcuate nucleus is also the site at which a number of hypothalamic releasing factors, e.g., gonadotropin-releasing hormone (GNRH) (50), are synthesized. The prominent role played by the arcuate nucleus in various neuroendocrine mechanisms underlies the syndrome seen in adult rodents after neonatal administration of large doses of MSG; its neuroendocrine manifestations include hypogonadism, short stature, and obesity (80). Indeed, the MSG syndrome has proved to be a useful neuroendocrine paradigm for studying the role of the arcuate nucleus in neuroendocrine function. However, the probability of developing a similar syndrome in humans after aspartame ingestion appears near zero: the syndrome has not been consistently demonstrable in primates (33), and a plasma threshold level of approximately 2 mM of acidic amino acid must be achieved in order to develop the brain lesion in rodents (4).

As discussed above, plasma aspartate levels are essentially unchanged, even after abuse doses, when the sweetener is coadministered with carbohydrate (115). Plasma aspartate levels after ingestion of such doses without dietary carbohydrate apparently have not been determined in adults. However, extrapolating the results of MSG administration in water, it is likely that acute ingestion of even 0.1 g/kg aspartame would not elevate plasma aspartate above 0.1 mM, and this concentration would be expected to have no effects on the brain either behind the BBB or at the CVOs. (It should be noted, as discussed below, that consuming aspartame along with a carbohydrate both protects against the brain effects of aspartate and potentiates the brain effects of the aspartame's phenylalanine.)

V. ASPARTAME DIPEPTIDES

The aspartame-related peptides are aspartylphenylalanine methyl ester (aspartame), aspartylphenylalanine, and aspartylphenylalanine DKP (Fig. 2). Aspartame is converted to aspartylphenylalanine by enzymes with esterase activity, such as chymotrypsin (82). Essentially all the esterase hydrolysis of aspartame into aspartylphenylalanine occurs in the small intestinal lumen and not in the stomach (82). In addition, it is believed that intestinal peptidases hydrolyze aspartylphenylalanine into the constituent free amino acids, aspartate and phenylalanine (82). The conversion of aspartame into the DKP occurs via a nonenzymatic process that involves the release of methanol and the cyclization of the dipeptide (38). The formation of the DKP is enhanced rapidly at temperatures above 120° C and by extreme pHs, particularly acid pH<2. The catalysis of the DKP formation from aspartame by acid pH is of interest since many carbonated beverages are acid pH (e.g., pH = 2.4–4.4) (39). Despite the relatively low pH of carbonated beverages, the formation of the DKP is still quite slow under normal conditions, and aspartame is stable over a period of several weeks of storage (39). If aspartame liquid products are stored for prolonged periods and DKP is formed, there is a release of methanol into the beverage (Fig. 2). However, since free methanol is liberated in the intestinal lumen by esterases, the dietary intake of methanol is the same whether aspartame is consumed in the native form or as the aspartylphenylalanine DKP plus free methanol.

There is no reason to expect that the aspartame dipeptides will have effects on the brain unless there is a measurable distribution of the aspartame dipeptides into the general circulation. With regard to aspartame, studies to date indicate there is no measurable transport of unmetabolized aspartame from the gut lumen to the general circulation (82). That is, the hydrolysis of aspartame by intestinal esterases and peptidases is much faster than the transport of the dipeptide through the mucosal barrier.

The evidence for the lack of distribution of aspartame into the general circulation comes from studies wherein ^{14}C-labeled aspartame was adminstered to dogs, and plasma extracts were analyzed by thin-layer chromatography (TLC) (82). Under these conditions no radioactivity comigrated with the aspartame standard. However, these studies should be repeated with techniques more sensitive than TLC. For example, the uptake of only 0.1% of the ingested aspartame dosage could result in an aspartame concentration in the portal circulation in the high nanomolar range that is not detectable by TLC. Moreover, an analog of aspartame, aspartylphenylalanine amide, is a weak cholecystokinin (CCK) antagonist (43). The C-terminal dipeptide of the CCK–gastrin family of peptides is aspartylphenylalanine amide (102). Indeed, aspartame was discovered in the 1960s by Searle Research Laboratories in an investigation involving the development of gastrin inhibitors (67). Although aspartylphenylalanine amide is known to be a weak antagonist of the CCK–gastrin peptide family (43), it is not clear whether aspartame, i.e., aspartylphenylalanine methyl ester, has properties similar to the dipeptide amide.

Studies in this area need to define the following: (i) the binding constant of aspartame to the CCK or gastrin receptors, and (ii) the portal concentration of aspartame using sensitive technologies. Since CCK antagonists promote satiety (3), presumably through a peripheral action, aspartame taken up into the portal circulation in nanomolar concentrations may have indirect effects on the brain and satiety control through actions in the intestinal–portal system. However, it must be shown that intestinal–portal concentrations of aspartame in the regions of the CCK receptor do approximate the binding constant (K_D) of the receptor for aspartame. Otherwise, the distribution of a small amount of aspartame into the region of CCK receptors would not be expected to exert any meaningful biological effect. In this regard, the K_D of aspartylphenylalanine amide at the splanchnic CCK receptor is in the high micromolar range (102). Thus portal concentrations of dipeptide of nanomolar concentrations would not exert any significant competitive inhibition (see Eq. 1).

Assuming either aspartame or aspartylphenylalanine does enter the systemic circulation, it is unlikely that these compounds will have any major effect on the brain owing to their high polarity and the very low transport of dipeptides through the BBB. Although free amino acids are rapidly transported through the BBB by specific carrier systems (Fig. 5), previous studies have shown that dipeptides such as glycylphenylalanine are not transported through the BBB (134). This is in marked contrast to the intestinal epithelial barrier, where approximately one-third to one-half of dietary protein is absorbed in the form of di- and tripeptides rather than as free amino acids (1).

The possibility of the aspartylphenylalanine DKP having effects on the brain is less remote than that of the aspartylphenylalanine dipeptide or native aspartame. Unlike uncyclized dipeptides, the cyclized moieties, i.e., the DKPs, are readily transported through the BBB when there is an absence of polar side groups on the DKP (88). The cyclization process results in a log order drop in the polarity of the dipeptide owing to the release of several hydrogen bonds formed with water upon formation of the DKP bond. For example, the leucine-glycine DKP (38) or the histidine-proline DKP (96), which are fragments of oxytocin and thyrotropin-releasing hormones (TRH), respectively, are readily transported through the BBB and exert important effects on brain (96). The transport properties of the aspartylphenylalanine DKP at the BBB have not yet been studied. There is reason to believe that it would be less transportable than the leucine-glycine or histidine-proline DKPs owing to the highly charged carboxyl group on the aspartate phenylalanine DKP (Fig. 2). Nevertheless, the comparative transport properties of the various dipeptide DKPs are of interest and comprise an area in need of additional study in regard to the possible effects of aspartylphenylalanine DKP on the brain.

A patient was recently described in whom aspartame consumption was clearly associated with a recurring clinical syndrome *(granulomatous Panniculitis)* associated with the formation of numerous bilateral, nontender nodular lesions on both legs (74a). Since it can be presumed that this condition was not caused by the breakdown products of aspartame, phenylalanine, aspartic acid, and methanol, all of which would also enter the bloodstream from natural foods, it is possible that the actual etiologic agent was a dipeptide metabolite of the sweetener.

VI. PHENYLALANINE

Unlike blood levels of aspartic acid, blood phenylalanine levels can rise markedly after ingestion of aspartame, and peak blood phenylalanine levels are linearly related to the dose of aspartame (115). While the absence of any substantial increase in plasma aspartate precludes aspartame's affecting the brain via its acidic amino acid constituent, the rise in blood phenylalanine after aspartame intake does provide a mechanism by which the sweetener can affect the CNS. Moreover, the peak increase in blood phenylalanine occurring after aspartame ingestion provides an objective criterion for evaluating possible adverse effects on the brain that might result from high-dosage aspartame usage. The corollary of this view is that if a given aspartame dose causes no substantial increase in blood phenylalanine, it is then unlikely that it will affect the brain (unless, as discussed above, it acts via a dipeptide) (115). Within this context, the crucial question becomes: What is a substantial increase in blood phenylalanine?

Blood phenylalanine also rises after consumption of protein-containing foods; thus it has been argued that an increase produced by ingesting aspartame is a normal metabolic event, with possible brain effects equivalent to those that might

TABLE 3. *Kinetic parameters for neutral amino acid transport in conscious rats*

Amino acid	Plasma concentrations (μM)	K_m (μM)	V_{max} (nmole/min^{-1}/g^{-1})	K_D (μl/min^{-1}/g^{-1})	K_m^a (μM)	Influx (nmole/min^{-1}/g^{-1})
Phenylalanine	50	32 ± 9	14 ± 4	44 ± 14	213	4.9
Tryptophan	70	52 ± 14	18 ± 5	41 ± 15	356	5.9
Methionine	40	83 ± 16	18 ± 5	45 ± 7	642	2.9
Tyrosine	90	86 ± 17	25 ± 5	39 ± 7	615	6.7
Leucine	100	87 ± 11	23 ± 4	45 ± 13	614	7.7
Isoleucine	70	145 ± 29	36 ± 9	31 ± 9	1120	4.3
Histidine	50	164 ± 28	30 ± 7	33 ± 6	1296	2.7
Valine	140	168 ± 72	14 ± 5	37 ± 7	1239	6.6

From ref. 72, except plasma concentrations, which are from ref. 6. The total tryptophan concentration reported by Baños et al. (6), 100 μM, has been normalized to reflect the transport of albumin-bound tryptophan. Tryptophan, the only amino acid bound by albumin, is only 15 to 20% free *in vitro* (87), but owing to the availability to brain of albumin-bound tryptophan, 70% of plasma tryptophan is exchangeable *in vivo* in brain capillaries (87).

follow a minor increase in dietary protein intake. However, the aspartame–protein analogy is fallacious insofar as it predicts effects on brain phenylalanine. A phenylalanine imbalance is created when the blood level of phenylalanine is selectively raised relative to the other LNAAs in blood. After a protein meal, blood phenylalanine increases, but so do blood levels of the other LNAAs, e.g., tryptophan, tyrosine, leucine, isoleucine, valine, histidine, and methionine (Table 3). After aspartame ingestion, blood phenylalanine selectively rises, whereas the blood levels of the other LNAAs may remain the same, or may actually decrease, if the meal or snack includes significant amounts of carbohydrates. The carbohydrate elicits insulin secretion, thus causing amino acids (especially some of the LNAAs) to leave the bloodstream by being taken up into skeletal muscle (28).

The phenylalanine imbalance paradigm gains particular significance when it is recognized that the brain may be selectively vulnerable to aspartame-induced imbalances in blood phenylalanine, among the various organs of the body (84). In short, the selective vulnerability of the brain to blood phenylalanine imbalances comes about by virtue of the very high affinity (very low K_m) of the neutral amino acid transport in the BBB for its circulating ligands (Tables 4 and 6). In order to more fully understand the unique effects of blood phenylalanine imbalances on the brain, the following sections review BBB transport and, in particular, the movement of neutral amino acids through the BBB.

A. BBB Versus Blood-CSF Barrier

There are two barrier systems in brain, and since these systems are often lumped together, but are vastly different from a quantitative point of view, it is important to explain them briefly. The BBB separates circulating compounds in capillaries from more than 99% of the brain; the remaining 0.5% of possible interface occurs

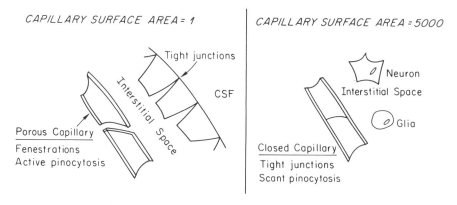

FIG. 7. The BBB *(right)* and the blood-CSF barrier *(left)* comprise two major membrane systems separating brain extracellular space (ECS) from the systemic ECS. The blood-CSF barrier is found at the CVOs (Fig. 6). The capillaries in the CVOs are porous and allow for the rapid distribution of proteins and small molecules into the immediate interstitial space. The presence of low-resistance tight junctions on the ventricular side of the ependymal cells prevents further distribution of circulating substances into the CSF. The ependymal junctions are porous in non-CVO areas wherein brain capillaries possess tight junctions; therefore, a reciprocal relationship exists between the anatomical distribution of the BBB and the blood-CSF barrier. Since the surface area of the BBB is 5,000-fold greater than the surface area of the blood-CSF barrier (26), the rapid distribution of circulating nutrients into the brain interstitial space is dependent on the diffusibility of the substance through the BBB via either lipid or carrier mediation (Fig. 5). (From ref. 93, with permission.)

at a blood-CSF barrier, present in the capillaries perfusing the choroid plexus and the other CVOs (Fig. 7) (126). Thus the major diffusion barrier separating blood from brain's interstitial space is the BBB, and not the blood-CSF barrier. Capillaries in brain of virtually all vertebrate organisms are endowed with unique morphologic characteristics, which include epithelium-like high-resistance tight junctions which literally cement together all of the endothelia in brain capillaries, and a scarcity of fenestrations or signs of pinocytosis, i.e., a scarcity of transendothelial channels (15).

Conversely, in capillaries perfusing the CVOs, there are no tight junctions, and the capillaries are widely fenestrated (15). Thus circulating substances may readily gain access to the small amount of brain interstitial space surrounding these capillaries in the CVOs. From here, substances may move into brain ventricular spaces. By virtue of the presence of the BBB, circulating substances may gain access to 99 + % of the brain's interstitial space only via lipid mediation [e.g., for steroid hormones or lipid-soluble drugs (86)] or carrier-mediation, [e.g., for water-soluble nutrients that have affinity for specific transport systems located on the lumenal and antilumenal membranes of brain capillaries (87)].

Thus far, transport systems have been identified for eight different classes of nutrients (Fig. 5). In addition, transport systems have also been characterized for thyroid hormones (86) and for water-soluble vitamins, such as thiamine (34). The half-saturation constants (K_m) and the maximal transport rates (V_{max}) for repre-

TABLE 4. *Kinetic constants[a] of BBB nutrient transport systems*

Transport system	Representative substrate	K_m (mM)	V_{max} (nmole/min^{-1}/g^{-1})	K_D (ml/min^{-1}/g^{-1})
Hexose	Glucose	11.0 ± 1.4	$1,420 \pm 140$	0.017 ± 0.003
Monocarboxylic acid	Lactate	1.8 ± 0.6	91 ± 35	0.019 ± 0.009
Neutral amino acid	Phenylalanine	0.11 ± 0.01	28 ± 7	0.014 ± 0.008
Basic amino acid	Arginine	0.088 ± 0.011	7.8 ± 0.9	0.0044 ± 0.0016
Amine	Choline	0.34 ± 0.07	11.3 ± 0.7	0.0069 ± 0.0059
Nucleoside	Adenosine	0.025 ± 0.003	0.75 ± 0.08	0.0066 ± 0.0003
Purine base	Adenine	0.011 ± 0.003	0.50 ± 0.09	0.0024 ± 0.0010

[a]Determined by nonlinear regression analysis of transport data previously reported for anesthetized rats (87).

sentative substrates for seven of the nutrient transport systems are shown in Table 4. Unlike those seven systems, the acidic amino acid carrier is, as discussed above, an active efflux system (85) and actively pumps aspartate and glutamate from brain interstitial space back to blood. The seven systems are believed to mediate the bidirectional movement of essential nutrients between blood and brain (87).

B. Overview of BBB Nutrient Transport

The hexose carrier transports glucose, which the brain needs on a second-to-second basis, as well as other sugars, such as mannose or galactose, or the glucose analogs, 2-deoxyglucose, 2-fluorodeoxyglucose, or 3-*O*-methylglucose (87). The transport of glucose analogs, such as deoxyglucose or 2-fluorodeoxyglucose, by the BBB hexose carrier has important implications for the analysis of regional brain metabolism with such imaging techniques as positron emission tomography.

The monocarboxylic acid transport system transports lactate and pyruvate as well as the ketone bodies, β-hydroxybutyrate and acetoacetate (23). Under normal conditions, lactate and pyruvate are not essential fuels for brain metabolism; however, lactate may be utilized as a fuel in states of chronic hypoglycemia, such as the neonatal period (74). In states of hyperketonemia, such as fasting, a high-fat diet, or the neonatal period, the blood level of the ketone bodies rises; under this condition, the brain readily oxidizes these nutrients (74). Indeed, the rate-limiting step in brain ketone body oxidation is BBB transport of these substances (71). The monocarboxylic acid carrier also transports the α-ketoacids of several amino acids (23). However, the α-ketoacid of phenylalanine, phenylpyruvate, is essentially not transported by the BBB monocarboxylic acid system (23). Thus elevated blood levels of phenylpyruvate, which occur in phenylketonuria (PKU) or possibly after high-dose aspartame usage, would not be expected to affect the availability to brain of key nutrients, such as lactate or the ketone bodies.

The basic amino acid system transports arginine, lysine, and ornithine (87). Arginine and lysine are essential amino acids required on a minute-to-minute basis for brain protein synthesis. Ornithine is not incorporated into brain proteins but may be an important essential nutrient for brain under conditions where polyamine metabolism is accelerated, such as during the period of brain development. Ornithine is an important precursor of brain polyamines, which are transported poorly, if at all, from blood into brain (87).

The choline carrier transports choline (87), an important precursor for brain lecithin or acetylcholine. The choline carrier only transports free choline in blood and not lipid-bound choline, such as lecithin or lysolecithin. These latter two compounds have been shown not to cross the BBB to a measurable extent (91). Thus the observation that the brain releases a net amount of choline on a single pass (5) suggests that the brain is capable of substantial *de novo* synthesis of choline, e.g., by stepwise methylation of lipid-bound ethanolamine (133).

No pyrimidine-base system has been identified in the BBB, which is consistent with the ability of the brain to synthesize pyrimidine compounds at rates commensurate with its needs (95). Circulating purine bases and nucleosides are essential nutrients for the brain, and transport systems for these nutrients exist in the BBB (24). Adenosine is a putative neuromodulator (126) and also has been shown to increase cerebral blood flow when applied topically to pial vessels (8). However, the infusion of adenosine via the carotid artery does not result in any increase in cerebral blood flow (8). This suggests that an enzymatic barrier exists beyond the capillary transport system and prevents the movement of the circulating adenosine into brain interstitial space. Studies of isolated capillaries show that adenosine is rapidly phosphorylated within the endothelial cytoplasma subsequent to uptake (128).

C. BBB Neutral Amino Acid Transport

The above review indicates that all the BBB nutrient transport systems play vital roles in the minute-to-minute regulation of brain intermediary metabolism (87). The BBB neutral amino acid transport system is no exception. This system is a sodium-independent, insulin-insensitive, leucine-preferring or L-system that mediates the bidirectional movement of neutral amino acids between blood and brain (84). The BBB neutral amino acid carrier has a preferential affinity for the LNAAs but also transports the small, nonessential amino acids, such as alanine, serine, cysteine, glutamine, or others (79).

The alanine-preferring system, or A-system, which concentrates amino acids against a gradient and is sodium dependent (20), is apparently absent on the lumenal surface of the BBB (94). Studies of isolated capillaries provide data consistent with the presence of the A-system on brain capillaries (11), and this carrier has been tentatively localized to the antilumenal membrane. The A-system and the alanine–serine–cysteine system (ASC-system) are localized on brain cell membranes (109).

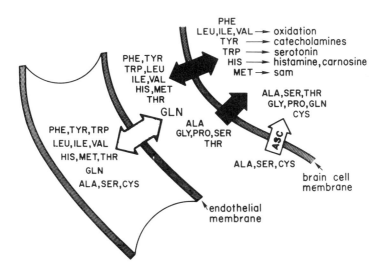

FIG. 8. Neutral amino acids in the bloodstream are transported into brain cells through two membranes in series: the endothelial membrane, which makes up the BBB (Fig. 7), and the brain cell membrane, found on either neurons or glia. There is only one transport system in the BBB for neutral amino acids (87). However, there are at least three different transport systems at brain cell membranes: the leucine-preferring (L), the alanine-preferring (A), and the alanine-, serine-, cysteine-preferring (ASC) transport systems (109). The L-system at the brain cell membrane and at the BBB mediates the bidirectional movement of amino acids across the brain cell membrane. The A- and ASC-systems on brain cell membranes mediate the concentrative uptake of neutral amino acids against a concentration gradient (20). Once inside brain cells, the LNAAs are all precursors to a variety of substrate-limited pathways of brain metabolism (Table 7). Thus brain availability of neutral amino acids as controlled by BBB transport may influence the rate of a number of important pathways of brain amino acid metabolism. (From ref. 87, with permission.)

As shown in Fig. 8, approximately 14 neutral amino acids circulating in the blood are transported into the interstitial space of the brain via a single BBB neutral amino acid transport system, which has a preferential affinity for phenylalanine, tryptophan, and the other large, neutral, or essential amino acids. Once inside brain interstitial space, these amino acids are rapidly taken up by brain cell membranes owing to two major properties of amino acid transport at brain cell membranes. First, the surface area of brain cell membranes is many times greater than the surface area of brain capillaries. Thus, on this basis alone, transport of amino acids between blood and brain intracellular space is limited by the movement of amino acids through the BBB, not through the brain cell membranes. Second, the presence of the A- and ASC-systems allows for concentrative uptake of amino acids by brain cells. Both these properties likely lead to the maintenance of very low concentrations of neutral amino acids in brain interstitial space (84). Indeed, the concentration of the neutral amino acids in CSF is only on the order of approximately 10% of the corresponding levels in plasma (69). Assuming CSF levels are in near equilibrium with brain interstitial space concentrations of amino acids, these considerations indicate the brain side of the BBB is normally unsaturated with neutral amino acids (87).

The idea that the concentration of phenylalanine and other LNAAs in brain interstitial space is only approximately 10% that of the corresponding plasma levels is supported by an analysis of the rate of efflux of a nonmetabolizable amino acid, cycloleucine, from brain back to blood (87). However, the idea that the concentration of phenylalanine and other LNAAs in brain interstitial space is only approximately 10% of plasma levels presents an apparent conflict with the picture of bidirectional movement of amino acids across the BBB in the steady state.

On the basis of arteriovenous difference measurements across the brain (9), it has been concluded that the net utilization of phenylalanine and other LNAAs by brain is immeasurably low, with the exception of the branched chain amino acids, such as leucine or isoleucine (84,87). For these latter two amino acids, the rates of net uptake are approximately 20 to 25% of the rates of amino acid influx from blood to brain. The low net uptake of the nonbranched chain LNAAs by brain is consistent with the model that the major pathway of amino acid utilization in brain is protein turnover (84). Thus for every amino acid that influxes into brain and is incorporated into protein, another amino acid is released via proteolysis for efflux back to blood. Of course, there is net utilization of neutral amino acids, such as tyrosine or tryptophan, in their irreversible conversion to brain neurotransmitters. However, the rates at which these conversions occur are on the order of 10 to 50 pM/min/g, or only about 5% of the influx rates, and thus are too low to be detected by measurements of arteriovenous differences in amino acid levels (84).

If one incorporates these two general observations (i.e., low interstitial concentration of neutral amino acids in brain and a near balance of amino acid influx and efflux rates across the BBB), then the conflict becomes apparent. That is, in order for the efflux of amino acids from brain to blood to balance the influx of amino acids from blood to brain, the permeability on the brain side of the BBB to the neutral amino acids must be severalfold greater than the permeability of the BBB on the blood side of the barrier. In other words, the neutral amino acid transport system must act in a manner analogous to an active efflux system. However, the evidence is that the carrier is a bidirectional, equilibrative system (84).

The resolution of this paradox comes from the recognition that the increase in neutral amino acid permeability on the brain side of the BBB is only an apparent increase. It is due to the relatively unsaturated state of the carrier and the much lower apparent K_m values on the brain side as opposed to the blood side of the barrier (87), which is heavily saturated and characterized by high apparent K_m values. The distinction between the absolute and the apparent K_m's of BBB transport processes is vital to the quantitative understanding of BBB neutral amino acid transport. The relationship between the absolute and the apparent K_m's is shown in Eq. 1,

$$K_{m_1}^a = K_{m_1} [1 + \Sigma \frac{(AA)}{K_m^i}] \tag{1}$$

where K_{m1} equals the absolute K_m of the amino acid in question; K_{m1}^a equals the apparent K_m of the amino acid; (AA) equals the concentration of each competing amino acid; and K_m^i equals the absolute K_m of the other competing amino acid. The values for V_{max} and absolute K_m, and also the constant of nonsaturable transport (K_D), are given in Table 3, as are the apparent K_m values. The plasma levels of the individual amino acids in fasting rats are also given in Table 3. The data in Table 3 show that the BBB neutral amino acid transport system has the highest affinity for phenylalanine (77). Thus the carrier is most easily saturated by phenylalanine among the various LNAAs.

The physiologic basis for saturation of a transport site is given in Eq. 1. If the K_m of the transport process is large relative to the concentration in plasma of the competing amino acid, then it follows that there is no deviation of the apparent K_m from the absolute K_m. In other words, there would be little or no competition among the amino acids *in vivo* under physiologic conditions. The higher the ratio, $(AA)/K_m^i$, the greater the sensitivity of the transport process to competition effects. On the basis of this important principle, one can predict the sensitivity of a given organ or a given species to amino acid competition effects, i.e., the sensitivity to the development of dietary phenylalanine imbalances.

The analysis by K_m indicates that species such as rabbit are much less prone to the development of diet-induced imbalances in brain phenylalanine than species such as rat. For example, the K_m of BBB tryptophan transport in the rabbit is approximately eightfold greater than the BBB transport K_m in the rat (Table 5). Thus the rabbit would be expected to be eight times less sensitive to competition effects and, specifically, to plasma phenylalanine imbalances. Studies in the dog have shown that this species is not sensitive to competition effects in the physiologic range (40). The K_m of neutral amino acid transport through the BBB in the dog (10) must be as high or higher than the K_m values seen in the rabbit (Table 5). In addition to explaining species differences in the susceptibility to BBB competition effects, the analysis by K_m also explains the selective vulnerability of the brain to hyperaminoacidemias compared to other organs of the body (84).

Table 6 shows a survey of K_m values for LNAAs in the rat. The K_m values for the BBB of the rat are 10-fold higher, or more, than those for peripheral tissues. Many years ago, Guroff and Udenfriend (35) showed that the brain was acutely sensitive to competition effects *in vivo*, whereas skeletal muscle examined under similar conditions was essentially independent of any competition effects on neutral amino acid transport. Inspection of Eq. 1 shows that there will be relatively little deviation from the absolute K_m if the K_m value of the competing amino acid is much higher than the existing plasma amino acid concentrations. Of course, competition effects can be shown in peripheral tissues *in vitro*, wherein the muscle is removed from the animal, and large concentrations (e.g., 10 mM or higher) are placed in the extracellular media *in vitro*. These experiments provide the basis for sorting out which amino acids are transported by a common system. However, they have relatively little physiologic significance in terms of predicting the sensitivity of the tissue to competition effects *in vivo*, because plasma amino acid

TABLE 5. *Comparison of BBB tryptophan transport in rats[a] and rabbits[b]*

Species	K_D (μl/min^{-1}/g^{-1})	V_{max} (nmole/min^{-1}/g^{-1})	K_m (μM)
Rabbit	14 ± 10	47 ± 20	440 ± 170
Rat	41 ± 15	18 ± 5	52 ± 14

[a]Data from ref. 72.
[b]Data from Pardridge and Fierer (*unpublished data*).

concentrations of the neutral amino acids are on the order of 50 to 200 μM, not 10 to 20 mM.

D. BBB Phenylalanine Transport in Humans

The kinetics of phenylalanine transport through the human BBB have not been studied in the same detail as those of laboratory animals. Indeed, the K_m of phenylalanine transport through the human BBB has not been measured. Given the marked species differences among rats, rabbits, and dogs in terms of BBB transport K_m values, and the presumptive difference in sensitivity of these species to the effects on brain of dietary phenylalanine balances, it is of utmost importance to characterize the kinetics of BBB neutral amino acid transport in humans. Indirect observations reported several years ago by Oldendorf et al. (78) suggest that the human BBB may be as sensitive to competition effects as that of the rat.

As shown in Fig. 9, the uptake of methionine by human brain is lowered by increases in phenylalanine concentrations in the high physiologic range. Similarly, studies with positron emission tomography indicate that, when plasma phenylalanine is greater than 0.3 mM, the brain's uptake of methionine [another LNAA transported into brain on the same phenylalanine carrier (Table 3)] is also inhibited (22).

TABLE 6. *Tissue survey of neutral amino acid transport K_m (mM)*

Amino acid	Intestinal epithelia[a]	Renal tubule[b]	Exocrine pancreas[c]	Red blood cell[d]	Liver[e]
Phenylalanine	1			4	4
Leucine	2			2	6
Tryptophan		4			
Methionine	5		3	5	
Histidine	6	5			
Valine	3		7	7	

[a]From ref. 55.
[b]From refs. 62 and 18.
[c]From ref. 7.
[d]From ref. 127.
[e]From ref. 57.

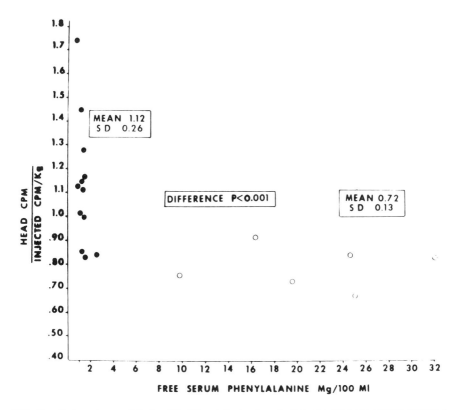

FIG. 9. Brain selenomethionine (Se 75) uptake in phenylketonurics (○) and mentally retarded control subjects (●) plotted as a function of serum phenylalanine. The mean uptake of Se 75 for the PKU and control subjects is shown in the boxes. The difference is highly significant. Substantial inhibition of brain neutral amino acid uptake is shown at a serum phenylalanine level of 10 mg/100 ml, or 0.6 mM. (From ref. 78.)

With the introduction of the isolated human brain capillary as a model system for investigating BBB transport (92), the kinetics of phenylalanine transport through the human BBB may soon be clarified. Previous studies have shown that neutral amino acid K_m values determined with isolated brain capillaries approximate the K_m values determined *in vivo* in the rat (37). Thus there is reason to believe that K_m values determined with the isolated capillary preparation may predict the sensitivity of the human brain to competition effects *in vivo* and to dietary phenylalanine imbalances. A photomicrograph of the isolated human brain capillary is shown in Fig. 10. This preparation has been shown to be positive for human factor 8, γ-glutamyl transpeptidase, alkaline phosphatase, and the insulin receptor (92).

E. Neutral Amino Acid Metabolism in Brain

The preceding section emphasized the view that owing to the low K_m of BBB neutral amino acid transport, selective elevations in plasma phenylalanine may

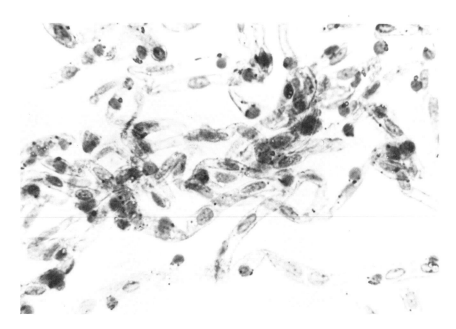

FIG. 10. Light micrograph of freshly isolated human brain capillaries. Capillaries are isolated in high yield from autopsy brain obtained within 24 hr of death. The capillaries are positive for endothelial markers, such as factor 8, for BBB-specific enzyme markers, such as γ-glutamyl transpeptidase or alkaline phosphatase, and for insulin receptor activity. (From ref. 92, with permission.)

decrease the availability of other LNAAs to the brain. Phenylalanine-induced alterations in brain amino acid availability can, in turn, lead to changes in brain amino acid and neurotransmitter metabolism (28).

The connection between amino acid availability and amino acid metabolism in brain comes from the fact that many pathways of amino acid metabolism in cerebral tissues are influenced by precursor availability (129). Owing to the desaturation of the rate-limiting enzymes in a number of important metabolic pathways in brain (Table 7), the flux through these pathways may rise or fall in proportion to changes in precursor availability. For example, serotonin or catecholamine synthesis rates

TABLE 7. *Substrate-limited pathways of brain amino acid metabolism*

Precursor	Brain level (μmole/g^{-1})	Rate-limiting enzyme	Substrate (K_m, mM)	Product
Tryptophan	0.05	Tryptophan hydroxylase	0.05	Serotonin
Tyrosine	0.09	Tyrosine hydroxylase	0.14	Catecholamines
Methionine	0.02	Methionine adenosyltransferase	0.09	S-adenosylmethionine
Histidine	0.06	Histidine decarboxylase	0.40	Histamine
Histidine	0.06	Carnosine synthetase		Carnosine

Data from refs. 6, 21, 25, 31, 66, and 107.

can depend on tryptophan or tyrosine availability, respectively (28,32). The rate-limiting enzymes, tryptophan and tyrosine hydroxylase, are normally desaturated by precursor amino acids, owing to the K_m/precursor concentration relationships (Table 7). When the K_m is large relative to the existing precursor concentration, as is the case for the pathways shown in Table 7, then substrate availability may exert an important influence on pathway regulation. Although in the normal state tyrosine hydroxylase may be close to saturation with its precursor tyrosine, the enzyme apparently becomes unsaturated with substrate in conditions when noradrenergic or dopaminergic neurons are rapidly firing (32).

Other monoamines that may act as putative neurotransmitters in brain are histamine and carnosine, which are products of histidine metabolism (21,107). In addition, the rate-limiting enzyme in these pathways is normally desaturated by intracellular histidine concentrations (21,107). The metabolism of some monoamines involves methylation at the postsynaptic membrane, and the methyl donor is S-adenosylmethionine. This compound is formed from methionine in proportion to methionine availability in brain (106).

Another important pathway of neutral amino acid metabolism in brain is branched chain amino acid oxidation. Subsequent to transamination, the branched chain α-ketoacids are oxidized by an α-ketoacid dehydrogenase (89). This enzyme is normally unsaturated by existing concentrations of the precursor α-ketoacid (110). Brain levels of the α-ketoacids are, in turn, a function of brain levels of the branched chain amino acid precursors. The oxidation of the branched chain amino acids provides only a trivial amount of energy for the brain. Nevertheless, the ongoing oxidation of these amino acids in brain approximates amino acid incorporation into proteins (84); thus this pathway may have an unknown function, perhaps related to the regulation of protein synthesis in brain. Whatever the exact function of branched chain amino acid oxidation in the brain may be, it is clear that this pathway is strongly influenced by changes in the availability of the amino acids.

A pathway of neutral amino acid metabolism in brain that is of vital importance is protein turnover. Although it is strongly influenced by amino acid availability in such peripheral tissues as liver or skeletal muscle (42), it is apparent that, under normal conditions, this pathway in brain is independent of precursor amino acid availability (130). That is, the rate-limiting step in protein synthesis, e.g., either amino acid acylation with transfer RNA (tRNA) or chain initiation, is mediated by enzymes that normally are fully saturated with their substrates. The K_m's of these rate-limiting enzymes are low compared to the normal concentrations of precursor amino acids in brain (84). However, in experimental model systems using phenylalanine imbalance, a number of investigators have shown that brain protein synthesis can be impaired under conditions of hyperphenylalaninemia. For example, Hughes and Johnson (41) have shown that hyperphenylalaninemia causes a reduction in methionine availability in brain. Since methionine acylation of tRNA in brain leads to the formation of formylated tRNA–methionine, and this compound mediates chain initiation, the hyperphenylalaninemia, by reducing the availability of methionine, blocks chain initiation (41). Binek-Singer and Johnson (12) have also shown that the inhibition of brain protein synthesis caused by hyperphenylalaninemia can be reversed by coadministration of other LNAAs that compete with phenylalanine at BBB transport sites.

F. Comments on PKU

The transport K_m analysis discussed in the previous section emphasized the view that the brain is unique among the organs of the body in the rat (84), and possibly in humans, owing to the markedly reduced K_m of BBB neutral amino acid transport compared to comparable values in other tissues. Thus the brain is uniquely susceptible to the effects of competition for transport sites within the physiologic range (28).

The predictions of this model are strengthened by the clinical presentation of PKU, wherein the brain is virtually the only organ affected in patients with this congenital hyperphenylalaninemia (2). A curious phenomenon in PKU research is the apparent lack of appreciation of the unique susceptibility of the brain to selective hyperaminoacidemias. Indeed, authorities in the PKU field have written that "the central problem in PKU is the cause of the brain defect" (108). Yet the paradigm elaborated above and in previous studies, going back to the work of Udenfriend (121), emphasizes that the brain is uniquely susceptible to hyperaminoacidemia due to transport competition effects. Moreover, the metabolic lesion may be potentially reversed by the administration of other LNAAs that enter the brain on the same transport system as the amino acid that is elevated (2,12).

A further apparent lack of appreciation for the unique role of hyperaminoacidemia in regulating brain metabolism is the idea that other hyperaminoacidemias, such as histidinemia, are benign conditions (59). Histidinemia is as potentially devastating as PKU. In practice, however, the usual case of histidinemia presents with much less CNS damage, probably for two major reasons: First, the blood histidine level is typically about 0.85 mM (59), or only about one-half the blood level of phenylalanine in the usual case of PKU. Second, and more important, the affinity of the BBB neutral amino acid transport system for phenylalanine is about fivefold greater than for histidine (Table 4). Thus blood histidine must actually be fivefold greater than blood phenylalanine in order to cause a comparable effect on amino acid availability in brain. Within this context, it becomes clear that histidinemia is qualitatively similar to PKU in its potential effects on the brain but is quantitatively much less significant. Although histidinemic patients lack the same severe mental retardation as patients with PKU, it is possible that subtle changes in brain development that are not readily perceptible by routine clinical examination are present in individuals not given special dietary treatment.

Finally, an important confirmation of the predictions of the analysis by K_m as applied to PKU are the observations of McKean (70), showing that in autopsied brains of patients with PKU, phenylalanine levels were increased fivefold. Moreover, this elevation was associated with the anticipated decreases in brain tyrosine

TABLE 8. *Potential effects of hyperphenylalaninemia on the brain*

Effect	References
Reduction in I.Q.	60
Seizures	44, 108
Behavioral change: hyperactivity, response to pain	16, 61, 64
Insomnia	19, 98
Neuroendocrine function	
Growth hormone secretion	54
Prolactin secretion	54
Gonadotropin secretion	46
Cardiovascular: blood pressure	119
Blockade of CNS drug therapy	
L-DOPA	75
α-Methyldopa	65
Melphalan	*a*
α-Methyl-*p*-tyrosine	83
5-Hydroxytryptophan	123

[a]Pardridge (*unpublished observations*).

and tryptophan levels owing to the expected impairment of their transport through the BBB. In addition, brain serotonin, dopamine, and norepinephrine levels were decreased substantially in the PKU brain (70), findings also expected given the known influence of precursor availability on their syntheses (Table 7).

G. Potential Effects of Hyperphenylalaninemia on the Brain

Table 8 lists a spectrum of potential effects of hyperphenylalaninemia on the human brain. Prior to discussion of these effects individually, it is important to emphasize the following caveat. Most workers agree that hyperphenylalaninemia of a severe nature, e.g., plasma phenylalanine levels greater than 0.6 to 1.0 mM, may have profound effects that, if present in the developing brain, are potentially irreversible. The caveat is this: *it is not clear whether the effects of hyperphenyl-alaninemia on the brain follow a threshold versus a linear relationship.* That is, increases in plasma phenylalanine between 0.1 and 0.6 mM may have no effects on the brain if a threshold relationship exists, and increases above a 0.6 mM threshold may then be found to cause marked derangements in brain function. On the other hand, if the relationship between plasma phenylalanine and abnormalities in brain is linear, then increases in plasma phenylalanine between 0.1 and 0.6 mM would also have small but definite effects on brain function, which may not be perceptible unless specifically examined. Increases in plasma phenylalanine above 0.6 mM may then have relatively large effects, so that even a routine clinical examination could discern abnormalities, e.g., frank mental retardation, seizures, or spasticity.

The linear-versus-threshold dialogue is especially germane in regard to intellectual function. Figure 11 shows the work of Levy and Waisbren (60), wherein the I.Q. (or developmental quotient) of newborns born of mothers with mild to severe

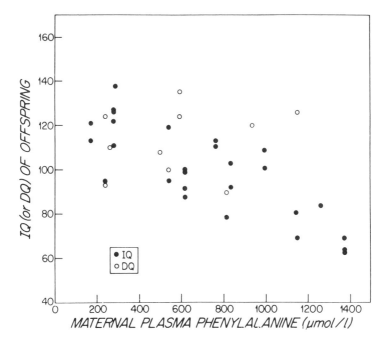

FIG. 11. Relationship between intelligence quotient (I.Q., •) or developmental quotient (DQ., ○) in offspring and the maternal blood phenylalanine level in women with PKU or hyperphenylalaninemia. The relationship between the offspring I.Q. and the maternal blood phenylalanine follows a linear relationship ($r = 0.82$) that is highly significant ($p < 0.001$). (Data from ref. 60, with permission.)

hyperphenylalaninemia is plotted versus the mother's existing plasma phenylalanine level. If one criterion for assessing the effects on brain of hyperphenylalaninemia is mental retardation, then it is clear that one can view this as a threshold relationship, and any plasma phenylalanine above 1 mM will lead to the development of an I.Q. in the range of mental retardation. However, the relationship between the I.Q. of the baby and the mother's phenylalanine level follows a linear correlation pattern that is highly statistically significant (Fig. 11). On this basis, one would predict a linear relationship between intellectual development and hyperphenylalaninemia. An increase in plasma phenylalanine from a normal level of 0.1 mM to 0.3 mM would not be expected to cause mental retardation in the fetus but might cause a 10-point drop in I.Q. that is clinically imperceptible.

Additional evidence supporting a linear relationship between plasma phenylalanine and brain function in humans has recently been reported by Krause et al. (53). As shown in Fig. 12, there is an inverse and linear relationship between neuropsychologic performance (choice reaction time) and incremental increases in plasma phenylalanine. Thus it appears that when quantitative criteria are applied to clinical testing, hyperphenylalaninemia effects on the human brain may prove to adhere to a linear, not a threshold, relationship.

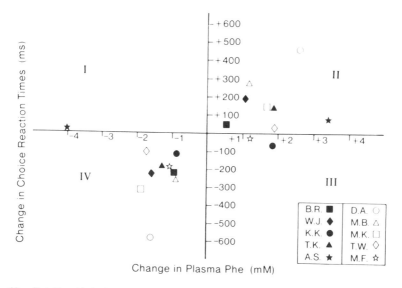

FIG. 12. Relationship between neuropsychological performance (choice reaction time) and incremental changes in plasma phenylalanine in 10 phenylketonuric subjects on low or normal phenylalanine diets. Each patient is represented by a symbol which appears twice on the graph, indicating the difference in mean choice reaction time between first and second week (high- to low-phenylalanine diet) and the second and third week (low- to high-phenylalanine diet) plotted against the parallel change in plasma phenylalanine. (From ref. 53, with permission.)

The observation that PKU is also associated with seizures (108) is consistent with the postmortem examination of brain chemistry in PKU, wherein the levels of the putative inhibitory neurotransmitters, e.g., serotonin and the catecholamines, are decreased (70). Moreover, in an animal model system of spontaneous seizures, brain levels of the inhibitory monoamine neurotransmitters are decreased (44). Thus a mild to moderate depression in brain levels of the inhibitory neurotransmitter monoamines might be expected to lower the seizure threshold in a given individual. In this regard, it is of interest that the CDC report describes nine case reports of previously healthy individuals experiencing seizure activity after aspartame ingestion (Table 1). Clearly, clinical studies in this area are needed to define quantitatively subtle changes in seizure thresholds in individuals experiencing aspartame-induced hyperphenylalaninemia (52).

Behavioral changes are also expected in conditions in which brain levels of monoamine neurotransmitters are decreased. For example, rats become hyperactive when brain levels of serotonin are depleted by special diets that are deficient in tryptophan (16,64). Rats fed a corn- or maize-based diet developed a serotonin-depletion state, since these foodstuffs are both deficient in tryptophan and enriched in branched chain amino acids (84). This dual metabolic alteration leads to a great decrease in the ratio of the plasma tryptophan concentration to the summed concentrations of its neutral amino acid competitors (i.e., the "plasma tryptophan ratio") in rats fed these diets (16,64), Moreover, the behavioral changes are reversed simply by the restoration of adequate tryptophan in the diet (64).

Insomnia is a further manifestation that would be expected in conditions in which the putative inhibitory monoamine neurotransmitters are decreased in brain. Indeed, tryptophan has been shown to be a useful adjunct for the therapy of insomniacs, possibly acting by increasing brain serotonin levels (19,98). In addition, Yogman and Zeisel (131) have shown that the administration of a sugar formula enriched in tryptophan enhances sleep in newborns, whereas valine added to the formula depresses sleep in the neonates. These observations are also consistent with the abundant evidence that serotonin levels in brain are a function of tryptophan availability (129), which can be either increased by the administration of tryptophan or decreased by the administration of another amino acid (e.g., valine or phenylalanine, which compete for tryptophan for uptake at BBB transport sites).

Blockade of the therapeutic effects of some drugs would also be a complication associated with hyperphenylalaninemia. The on–off effects seen in L-DOPA therapy of Parkinson patients have been attributed to the effects of the amino acids in dietary protein on L-DOPA uptake into the brain (75). Since L-DOPA, a neutral amino acid, is transported into brain on the same phenylalanine transport system (124), it would be expected that L-DOPA levels in brain are inversely related to plasma neutral amino acid levels.

Similarly, the effects of α-methyldopa in decreasing blood pressure in spontaneously hypertensive rats are inversely related to the existing plasma levels of LNAAs (65). Both α-methyldopa and its related compound, α-methylparatyrosine, a substance used in the treatment of pheochromocytoma (112), are LNAAs that enter brain via the transport system common to phenylalanine (65,83). Another neutral amino acid drug, phenylalanine mustard, or melphalan, has been shown to enter the brain on the same phenylalanine transport system (Pardridge, *unpublished observations*). Melphalan is useful in the treatment of brain tumors (56), and it would be expected that hyperaminoacidemia would inhibit the uptake of melphalan by brain similar to that shown for L-DOPA or α-methyldopa. Finally, 5-hydroxytryptophan and tryptophan have been used for the treatment of postanoxic myoclonus. This therapy would also be expected to be inhibited by selective elevations of amino acids, particularly phenylalanine (17,123).

The brain monoamines have been shown to be intimately involved in neuroendocrine functions and, in particular, pituitary hormone secretion. For example, serotonin has been shown to facilitate GNRH secretion (46). Thus changes in brain serotonin would be expected to influence gonadotropin secretion. This is of interest since the CDC report on aspartame describes eight case reports of menstrual irregularities in premenopausal women (Table 1). Serotonin also facilitates growth hormone and prolactin secretion in humans (54).

Monoamine release within the brain is also believed to be linked to such cardiovascular functions as maintenance of sympathetic tone and regulation of blood pressure. Tyrosine has been shown to lower elevated blood pressure in rats by increasing central α-adrenergic tone (119). Since hyperphenylalaninemia would be expected to lower brain tyrosine in humans, a hypertensive response may be one side effect of the reduction of central α-adrenergic tone caused by hyperphenyl-alaninemia. In this regard, the rat is probably a poor model system for investigating phenylalanine metabolism after aspartame ingestion. Unlike the human's liver, which converts a relatively small portion of dietary phenylalanine to tyrosine (115), the rat's rapidly converts approximately half the dietary phenylalanine into tyrosine (27), owing to a much more active phenylalanine hydroxylase. Both phenylalanine and tyrosine rise substantially in the plasma of rats after aspartame ingestion (27), whereas in humans, marked increases occur only in plasma phenylalanine (115). Thus there will be an increase in tyrosine availability in the rat brain after aspartame ingestion but a decrease in tyrosine (and a major increase in phenylalanine) in the human brain (70).

Two published studies (27,132) have described the effects on the rat's brain of a single dose of 200 mg/kg aspartame. [As discussed in Section II, a single dose of 200 mg/kg aspartame to rats is equivalent to a dose of approximately 30 to 40 mg/kg aspartame in humans because of species differences in metabolically active body mass (13). For example, a dose of 34 mg/kg in humans results in an approximate doubling of phenylalanine in plasma (118), whereas a dose of 200 mg/kg is required to double the plasma phenylalanine plus tyrosine in rats (27,132).] Fernstrom et al. (27) showed that 200 mg/kg aspartame in rats results in no change in brain content or turnover of serotonin and minimal, if any, reduction in brain tryptophan. If brain tryptophan is not reduced by a given dose of aspartame, then it is unlikely that any changes in its monoamine product will ensue. Conversely, Yokogoshi et al. (132) showed that 200 mg/kg aspartame blunted the usual rise in brain tryptophan and serotonin caused by eating carbohydrate-containing foods.

The contrasting results of the studies of Fernstrom et al. (27) and Yokogoshi et al. (132) illustrate an important caveat. If hyperphenylalaninemia in the high physiologic range (e.g., plasma phenylalanine <0.3 mM) exerts any effects on the brain, then the biochemical and neurophysiologic or neuropathologic effects will be subtle and will not be detected without the use of a sensitive experimental paradigm. The study of brain tryptophan/serotonin levels after carbohydrate admin-istration constitutes a more sensitive experimental approach than the use of brain tryptophan/serotonin levels in the basal state.

H. Plasma Phenylalanine in Humans After Aspartame Ingestion

Unlike blood aspartic acid levels, those of phenylalanine rise acutely after as-partame ingestion, peak plasma phenylalanine being proportional to the aspartame dose (115). Moreover, since plasma phenylalanine is cleared with a half-time of approximately 60 to 90 min in humans (115), it would be expected that only postprandial and not fasting levels of phenylalanine would be increased in individ-uals who undergo long-term, sustained aspartame ingestion. For example, in one study on 7- to 12-year-old children consuming up to 77 mg/kg/day aspartame (30), fasting plasma levels of phenylalanine, although not given, were reported to be

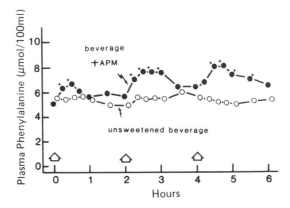

FIG. 13. Mean plasma phenylalanine concentration in normal adults ingesting three repeated servings of either unsweetened beverage (○) or beverage containing 10 mg/kg body weight aspartame (APM) (●). Values designated with a " + " differ significantly ($p < 0.05$) from baseline values. (Data from ref. 115, with permission.)

normal (30). Owing to the relatively short half-time of phenylalanine in humans, fasting levels of phenylalanine would provide very little information, in contrast to the postprandial measurements of phenylalanine obtained 30 to 120 min after aspartame ingestion.

The study of Steginik and co-workers (115) shows that the plasma phenylalanine increases in a stepwise fashion in a single day in which individuals consume three sequential doses (10 mg/kg) of an aspartame-flavored beverage (Fig. 13). Presumably, the dosage of 10 mg/kg per serving was chosen since the expected 99th percentile of aspartame ingestion was 34 mg/kg/day (36). However, as discussed in Section II, this figure should be revised upward, particularly for children in the 7- to 12-year old range, in whom a daily dose may reach approximately 80 mg/kg (30). An acute dosage of 25 mg/kg per serving of aspartame administered at three sequential intervals in a single day might approximate aspartame consumption in 7- to 12-year olds.

The form in which the aspartame is ingested may have a profound effect on the gastrointestinal absorption of phenylalanine and on the peak blood level of phenylalanine achieved. For example, Steginik and co-workers (116) have shown that when an aspartame-flavored beverage is administered as a slurry as opposed to liquid form, the absorption of the phenylalanine in some individuals is markedly enhanced. Individuals taking an acute dose of 100 mg/kg experience a mean peak plasma phenylalanine of 0.26 ± 0.19 mM. The large standard deviation in this study of a small number of individuals is due to the fact that two individuals achieved peak plasma levels of 0.46 and 0.51 mM (116). Given these relatively high levels of plasma phenylalanine, one wonders what the ultimate peak phenylalanine level would be in humans drinking 25 mg/kg of an aspartame-flavored beverage three times per day in slurry form. Those individuals with rapid gastric emptying after administration of a slurry may achieve unusually high levels of phenylalanine.

TABLE 9. *Factors predisposing to hyperphenylalaninemia*

Factor	Reference
PKU heterozygosity	60
Liver disease	122
Renal disease	45
Pregnancy	47
Biopterin cofactor deficiency	113

With the exception of the single study of Stegink and co-workers shown in Fig. 13, there have been no measurements of peak phenylalanine levels in individuals providing blood samples throughout the course of the day when aspartame is administered at doses of 25 mg/kg given three times a day and administered in a variety of forms, including slurries. Considering that a typical daily dosage for 7- to-12-year olds may be as high as 77 mg/kg, or more than twice the anticipated 99th percentile dose of 34 mg/kg, it is clear that more studies on the order of those in Fig. 13, but with higher aspartame doses, are needed to provide a rational basis for predicting the peak plasma phenylalanine levels in children.

In addition to the form in which aspartame is given, other factors may predispose certain individuals to higher-than-average peak phenylalanine levels after ingestion of aspartame-containing products. Table 9 lists a variety of factors that may cause delayed metabolism of phenylalanine in certain individuals. The most common factor is likely to be PKU heterozygosity. It is estimated that 2% of the population, or 4 million individuals, are heterozygous for the PKU lesion (117) and possess only half the normal levels of liver phenylalanine hydroxylase. These individuals metabolize ingested phenylalanine at approximately half the usual rate. Figure 14 (115) shows that peak plasma phenylalanine levels in PKU heterozygotes are approximately twice that of normal individuals throughout a range of doses of ingested aspartame. The issue of PKU heterozygosity gains added importance when it is recognized that some PKU authorities believe the heterozygous trait may be much more prevalent than just 2% of the population; it may be as high as 10% of the population, involving 20 million Americans (60). Moreover, such individuals are unaware of the fact that they are heterozygous for the PKU trait (unless they happen to have produced offspring who are homozygous for PKU).

Liver disease is an obvious cause of impaired phenylalanine metabolism, and it has been advocated that aspartame ingestion be curtailed in patients with liver disease (122). Renal disease is another example in which aspartame ingestion might be restricted. Owing to the release of putative uremic toxins and the effects of these substances on hepatic phenylalanine hydroxylase, liver clearance of phenylalanine is impaired in subjects with chronic renal failure (45). Although conclusive studies have not been performed to date, pregnancy and perhaps estrogen treatment in general may impair the ability of the liver to clear phenylalanine. Studies have

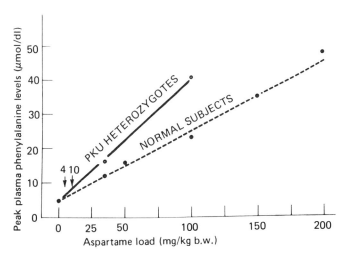

FIG. 14. Correlation of mean peak plasma phenylalanine concentration with aspartame dosage in either normal subjects or in individuals with PKU heterozygosity. (Data from ref. 115, with permission.)

shown that plasma phenylalanine levels in pregnant PKU heterozygotes are higher than in the nonpregnant heterozygotes (47).

Biopterin cofactor deficiency is another cause of impaired phenylalanine hydroxylase activity in the liver, but presumably a deficiency in this vitamin is relatively rare in the population. On the other hand, an inherited need for increased amounts of biopterin in the diet (113) may be prevalent in a large number of heterozygotes, if one considers that PKU variants are subjects with normal levels of phenylalanine hyroxylase but increased requirements for the biopterin cofactor of the enzyme.

Studies by Filer and associates (29) have shown that 1-year-old, 9-kg infants consuming aspartame in acute dosages of 34 to 100 mg/kg develop peak phenylalanine levels that are two to five times their basal levels. However, it is unlikely that 1-year olds consume large doses of aspartame. It would seem that the two segments of the population most likely to be exposed to relatively large doses of aspartame are 7- to 12-year olds (30) and developing fetuses. Mothers who go on high-dose aspartame usage in an effort to restrict weight gain during pregnancy, and who happen to be heterozygous for the PKU trait, may develop substantial increases in plasma phenylalanine in their fetuses. Clearly, detailed studies on the peak phenylalanine levels in primates, and possibly human fetuses, are needed to investigate the effects of high-dose aspartame usage during pregnancy.

One study by Ranney et al. (101) measured fetal phenylalanine levels in developing rabbits (Table 10). The use of the rabbit as an aspartame model system is not optimal in two respects. First, rabbits, like rats, convert a substantial amount of ingested phenylalanine into tyrosine (101). This blunts the peak increase in plasma phenylalanine. However, this problem can be normalized by using mea-

TABLE 10. *Fetal hyperphenylalaninemia*

Diet	Gestation age (days)	Plasma Phe + Tyr (mM)		
		Maternal	Fetal	Fetal/maternal
Aspartame	9	0.85	—	—
	16	0.57	—	—
	20	0.30	0.54	1.8
Control	16	0.20	0.38	1.9

From ref. 101.

surements of phenylalanine plus tyrosine plasma concentrations. Second, the rabbit, like the dog, has an at least eightfold higher K_m for its BBB neutral amino acid transport system (Table 5); thus the brain of the rabbit is much less susceptible to dietary phenylalanine imbalances than the brain of the rat and, possibly, human.

Nevertheless, the study by Ranney et al. (101) illustrates some general principles that may help to guide clinical studies in pregnant women ingesting aspartame on a daily basis. First, the rise in fetal phenylalanine concentration is proportional to the increase in maternal levels (101). Moreover, the fetal/maternal gradient is generally on the order of 2:1, owing to the ability of the placenta to concentrate amino acids against a gradient (14,101). That is, a rough index of fetal phenylalanine levels in developing humans may be approximated as twice the corresponding maternal phenylalanine levels. Second, the rise in phenylalanine/tyrosine in pregnant rabbits is apparently much greater in the first half of the gestational period (101). For example, the plasma level of phenylalanine plus tyrosine in the ninth day of gestation is nearly threefold greater than the corresponding levels at the near term of gestation at 20 days (101). Thus it would be important to monitor plasma phenylalanine levels in mothers throughout the course of pregnancy or, at least, to compare first, second, and third trimesters.

A study by Reynolds and co-workers (103) showed no discernible developmental effects in macaca infant monkeys after ingestion of 1, 2, and 3 g/kg aspartame per day over a prolonged period. The criteria for deleterious effects of the aspartame diet were intake of formula, growth, blood count, and serum electrolyte levels. There were no observed seizures, and electroencephalograms (EEGs) were stated to be normal, although the exact details of the EEG analyses are not given.

Although these studies clearly buttress the case for the safety of aspartame ingestion in newborns, two points should be emphasized. First, studies on the effects of aspartame ingestion during the prenatal period are much more critical than studies of aspartame ingestion in the postnatal period. This is because peak plasma phenylalanine levels are likely to be much higher in developing fetuses of mothers who ingest a large dose of aspartame (101). Second, the absence of seizures is too imprecise a criterion for assessing possible deleterious effects of hyperphenylalaninemia on the brain. Given the putative linear relationship between plasma phenylalanine levels and adverse effects on the brain (Figs. 11 and 12), it is important to develop criteria that allow for an examination of quantitative dose-response effects. For example, a quantitative analysis of the EEG in individuals with dietary phenylalanine imbalance may be more sensitive than a qualitative inspection of the EEG (52).

VII. β-PHENETHYLAMINE

β-Phenethylamine is a product of phenylalanine metabolism involving aromatic amino acid decarboxylase. This enzyme, which is widely distributed in the gut and the brain as well as other peripheral organs, converts phenylalanine into β-phenethylamine (76). The amine is subsequently metabolized to phenylacetic acid by monoamine oxidase type B (MAO-B) (97). Normally, MAO-B activity is much greater than aromatic amino acid decarboxylase, and the urinary excretion of β-phenethylamine and, presumably, the peak blood level are unlikely to increase substantially in the face of dietary phenylalanine imbalances. However, subjects with PKU who undergo treatment with MAO inhibitors (MAOIs) show log order increases in urinary phenethylamine excretion and, presumably, large increases in plasma β-phenethylamine as well (76). Owing to the renewed increase in the use of inhibitors of MAO-B to treat depression (97), the common usage of these drugs for psychiatric illnesses may increase and may predispose drug-treated individuals to increases in β-phenethylamine during periods of dietary phenylalanine imbalance. These conjectures are purely speculative at this time but do provide the basis for studies of β-phenethylamine levels in plasma in individuals undergoing high-dosage aspartame intake concomitantly with usage of inhibitors of MAO-B. (Recently (26a), a patient was described who, while taking an MAOI, developed severe headaches each time she ate aspartame-containing foods and carbohydrates concurrently.)

Phenethylamine is readily transported through the BBB, since this monoamine is not hydroxylated (77,90). Phenethylamine levels in brain are normally detectable at 1 to 5% of the levels of other monoamines (48). Moreover, β-phenethylamine administration to animals produces many of the effects of amphetamine usage, such as stereotyped behavior or increased locomotor activity (111). Perhaps the major point to be emphasized with respect to β-phenethylamine formation as a consequence of aspartame ingestion is the extremely rapid rate of clearance of this amine from the blood. In dogs, the phenethylamine half-time is approximately 6 min (111). Thus it is unlikely that even with high dosages of aspartame intake, plasma phenethylamine levels will increase substantially in humans, except when MAO-B inhibitors are administered concurrently.

VIII. SUMMARY

Although no studies to date have reported objective evidence for effects of aspartame on the brain in humans, the CDC (136) recently concluded that "the highest priority for any future investigation might be in the neurologic–behavioral area." On this basis, this chapter has attempted to provide a physiologic basis for possible future studies that evaluate the potential effects of aspartame on the brain. The main conclusions are as follows:

1. If high-dose aspartame usage does have effects on the brain, the effects are likely to be mediated via phenylalanine and not via the dipeptide itself or via the aspartate or methanol moieties of aspartame.

2. Any potential effects on the brain of aspartame-derived phenylalanine will occur only when the average daily intake in milligrams per kilogram of aspartame is sufficiently high so as to cause a substantial increase in phenylalanine concentrations in plasma, relative to the concentrations of other LNAAs.

3. The two groups of individuals most at risk for developing aspartame-induced hyperphenylalaninemia are developing fetuses, owing to the ability of the placenta to concentrate amino acids in fetal plasma approximately twofold over the maternal plasma (101); and 7- to 12-year-old children, due to their reduced body mass and, thus, increased daily dosage of aspartame in milligrams per kilogram (30).

4. Present projections of daily aspartame intakes of 8 to 10 mg/kg (36) appear to be gross underestimates of aspartame consumption; 7- to 12-year-old children consume up to 77 mg/kg/day (30).

5. A dose of 77 mg/kg/day aspartame given in three equal amounts (e.g., 25 mg/kg) during the course of a day to a PKU heterozygote will probably result (Figs. 13 and 14) in at least a fourfold increase in postprandial plasma phenylalanine, e.g., from 0.05 to 0.2 mM. Higher peak plasma phenylalanine concentrations may be achieved if the aspartame is administered as a slurry and rapid gastric emptying ensues (116).

6. A peak plasma phenylalanine concentration on the order of 0.2 to 0.3 mM would be expected to have no PKU-like effects on the brain if the relationship between hyperphenylalaninemia and brain effects is a threshold relationship, e.g., if brain effects occur only when plasma phenylalanine exceeds a threshold of 0.6 to 1.0 mM. Conversely, if the relationship between hyperphenylalaninemia and brain effects is a linear function, then increases in plasma phenylalanine up to 0.2 to 0.3 mM may have subtle but definite effects on the brain that may not be seen clinically without sensitive detection methods. Effects on brain monoamine neurotransmitters are likely to occur at considerably lower plasma phenylalanine levels.

7. Intakes of aspartame at doses of 8 to 10 mg/kg/day will result in physiologic increases in plasma phenylalanine that probably lack pathologic effects on the brain.

ACKNOWLEDGMENTS

This work was supported by NIH grant RO1-NS-19271 and by RCDA AM-00783. Dawn Brown skillfully prepared the manuscript. The author is indebted to Gary Fierer, Jody Eisenberg, Jing Yang, and Tom Choi for invaluable technical assistance.

REFERENCES

1. Adibi, S. A., Morse, W. L., Masilamani, S. S., and Amin, P. M. (1975): Evidence for two different modes of tripeptide disappearance in human intestine. *J. Clin. Invest.*, 56:1355–1363.
2. Andersen, A. E., and Avins, L. (1976): Lowering brain phenylalanine levels by giving other large neutral amino acids. *Arch. Neurol.*, 33:684–686.
3. Anika, S. M., Houpt, T. R., and Houpt, K. A. (1981): Cholecystokinin and satiety in pigs. *Am. J. Physiol.*, 240:R310–R318.
4. Applebaum, A. E., Daabees, T. T., and Stegink, L. D. (1984): Aspartate-induced neurotoxicity in infant mice. In: *Aspartame Physiology and Biochemistry*, edited by L. D. Stegink and L. J. Filer, Jr., p. 349, Marcel Dekker, New York.
5. Aquilonius, S.-M., Ceder, G., Lying-Tunell, U., Malmlund, H. O., and Schuberth, J. (1975): The arteriovenous difference of choline across the brain of man. *Brain Res.*, 99:430–433.
6. Baños, G., Daniel, P. M., Moorhouse, S. R., and Pratt, O. E. (1973): The influx of amino acids into the brain of the rat in vivo: The essential compared with some nonessential amino acids. *Proc. R. Soc. Lond. [Biol.]*, 183:59–70.
7. Begin, N., and Scholefield, P. G. (1965): The uptake of amino acids by mouse pancreas in vitro. II. The specificity of the carrier systems. *J. Biol. Chem.*, 240:332–338.
8. Berne, R. M., Knabb, R. M., Ely, S. W., and Rubio, R. (1983): Adenosine in the local regulation of blood flow: A brief overview. *Fed. Proc.*, 42:3136–3142.
9. Betz, A. L., and Gilboe, D. D. (1973): Effect of pentobarbital on amino acid and urea flux in the isolated dog brain. *Am. J. Physiol.*, 224:580–587.
10. Betz, A. L., Gilboe, D. D., and Drewes, L. R. (1975): Kinetics of unidirectional leucine transport into brain: Effects of isoleucine, valine, and anoxia. *Am. J. Physiol.*, 228:895–900.
11. Betz, A. L., and Goldstein, G. W. (1978): Polarity of the blood-brain barrier: Neutral amino acid transport into isolated brain capillaries. *Science*, 202:225–227.
12. Binek-Singer, P., and Johnson, T. C. (1982): The effects of chronic hyperphenylalaninaemia on mouse brain protein synthesis can be prevented by other amino acids. *Biochem. J.*, 206:407–414.
13. Boxenbaum, H., and Ronfeld, R. (1983): Interspecies pharmacokinetic scaling and the Dedrick plots. *Am. J. Physiol.*, 245:R768–R774.
14. Brass, C. A., Isaacs, C. E., McChesney, R., and Greengard, O. (1982): The effects of hyperphenylalaninemia on fetal development: A new animal model of maternal phenylketonuria. *Pediatr. Res.*, 16:388–394.
15. Brightman, M. W. (1977): Morphology of blood-brain interfaces. *Exp. Eye Res. [Suppl.]*, 25:1–25.
16. Carruba, M. O., Picotti, G. B., Genovese, E., and Mategazza, P. (1977): Stimulatory effect of a maize diet on sexual behaviour of male rats. *Life Sci.*, 20:159–164.
17. Chadwick, D., Harris, R., Jenner, P., Reynolds, E. H., and Marsden, C. D. (1975): Manipulation of brain serotonin in the treatment of myoclonus. *Lancet*, II:434–435.
18. Chan, Y. Z., and Huang, K. C. (1971): Microperfusion studies on renal tubular transport of tryptophan derivatives in rats. *Am. J. Physiol.*, 221:575–579.
19. Chen, C. M., Kalucy, R. S., Hartmann, M. K., Lacey, J. H., Crisp, A. H., Bailey, J. E., Eccleston, E. G., and Coppen, A. (1974): Plasma tryptophan and sleep. *Br. Med. J.*, 4:564–566.
20. Christensen, H. M. (1973): On the development of amino acid transport systems. *Fed. Proc.*, 32:19–28.
21. Chung-Hwang, E., Khurana, H., and Fisher, H. (1976): The effect of dietary histidine levels on the carnosine concentration of rat olfactory bulbs. *J. Neurochem.*, 26:1087–1091.
22. Comar, D., Saudubray, J. M., Duthilleul, A., Delforge, J., Maziere, M., Berger, G., Charpentier, C., Todd-Pokropek, A., with Crouze, M., and Depondt, E. (1981): Brain uptake of ¹¹C-methionine in phenylketonuria. *Eur. J. Pediatr.*, 136:13–19.
23. Conn, A. R., and Steele, R. D. (1982): Transport of α-keto analogues of amino acids across blood-brain barrier in rats. *Am. J. Physiol.*, 243:E272–E277.
24. Cornford, E. M., and Oldendorf, W. H. (1975): Independent blood-brain barrier transport systems for nucleic acid precursors. *Biochim. Biophys. Acta*, 394:211–219.
25. Coyle, J. J. (1972): Tyrosine hydroxylase in rat brain–cofactor requirements, regional and subcellular distribution. *Biochem. Pharmacol.*, 21:1935–1942.
26. Crone, C. (1971): The blood-brain barrier—facts and questions. In: *Ion Homeostasis of the Brain*, edited by B. K. Siesjö and S. C. Sorensen, pp. 52–62. Munksgaard, Copenhagen.

26a. Ferguson, J. M. (1985): Interaction of aspartame and carbohydrates in an eating-disordered patient. *Am. J. Psychiatry*, 142:271.

27. Fernstrom, J. D., Fernstrom, M. H., and Gillis, M. A. (1983): Acute effects of aspartame on large neutral amino acids and monoamines in rat brain. *Life Sci.*, 32:1651–1658.

28. Fernstrom, J. D., and Wurtman, R. J. (1972): Brain serotonin content: Physiological regulation by plasma neutral amino acids. *Science*, 178:414–416.

29. Filer, L. J., Jr., Baker, G. L., and Stegink, L. D. (1983): Effect of aspartame loading on plasma and erythrocyte free amino acid concentrations in one-year-old infants. *J. Nutr.*, 113:1591–1599.

30. Frey, G. H. (1976): Use of aspartame by apparently healthy children and adolescents. *J. Toxicol. Environ. Health*, 2:401–415.

31. Friedman, P. A., Kappelman, A. H., and Kaufman, S. (1972): Partial purification and characterization of tryptophan hydroxylase from rabbit hindbrain. *J. Biol. Chem.*, 247:4165–4173.

32. Gibson, C. J., and Wurtman, R. J. (1978): Physiological control of brain norepinephrine synthesis by brain tyrosine concentration. *Life Sci.*, 22:1399–1406.

33. Goldberg, L., Abraham, R., and Coulston, F. (1974): When is glutamate neurotoxic? *N. Engl. J. Med.*, 290:1326–1327.

34. Greenwood, J., Love, E. R., and Pratt, O. E. (1982): Kinetics of thiamine transport across the blood-brain barrier in the rat. *J. Physiol.*, 327:95–103.

35. Guroff, G., and Udenfriend, S. (1962): Studies on aromatic amino acid uptake by rat brain in vivo. *J. Biol. Chem.*, 237:803–811.

36. Hattan, D. G., Henry, S. H., Montgomery, S. B., Bleiberg, M. J., Rulis, A. M., and Bolger, P. M. (1983): Role of the Food and Drug Administration in regulation of neuroeffective food additives. In: *Nutrition and the Brain, Vol. 6*, edited by R. J. Wurtman and J. J. Wurtman, pp. 31–99. Raven Press, New York.

37. Hjelle, J. T., Baird-Lambert, J., Cardinale, G., Spector, S., and Udenfriend, S. (1978): Isolated microvessels: The blood-brain barrier in vitro. *Proc. Natl. Acad. Sci. USA*, 75:4544–4548.

38. Hoffman, P. L., Walter, R., and Bulat, M. (1977): An enzymatically stable peptide with activity in the central nervous system: Its penetration through the blood-CSF barrier. *Brain Res.*, 122:87–94.

39. Homler, B. E. (1984): Aspartame: Implications for the food scientist. In: *Aspartame Physiology and Biochemistry*, edited by L. D. Stegink and L. J. Filer, Jr., p. 247. Marcel Dekker, New York.

40. Huet, P.-M., Pomier-Layrargues, G., Duguay, L., and Du Souich, P. (1981): Blood-brain transport of tryptophan and phenylalanine: Effect of portacaval shunt in dogs. *Am. J. Physiol.*, 241:G163–G169.

41. Hughes, J. V., and Johnson, T. C. (1977): The effects of hyperphenylalaninaemia on the concentrations of aminoacyl-transfer ribonucleic acid in vivo. *Biochem. J.*, 162:527–537.

42. Jefferson, L. S. (1980): Role of insulin in the regulation of protein synthesis. *Diabetes*, 29:487–496.

43. Jensen, R. T., Jones, S. W., and Gardner, J. D. (1982): C-terminal fragments of cholecystokinin (CCK): A new class of CCK receptor antagonists. *Gastroenterology*, 82:1094.

44. Jobe, P. C., Ko, K. H., and Dailey, J. W. (1984): Abnormalities in norepinephrine turnover rate in the central nervous system of the genetically epilepsy-prone rat. *Brain Res.*, 290:357–360.

45. Jones, M. R., Kopple, J. D., and Swendseid, M. E. (1978): Phenylalanine metabolism in uremic and normal man. *Kidney Int.*, 14:169–179.

46. Kalra, S. P., and Kalra, P. S. (1983): Neural regulation of luteinizing hormone secretion in the rat. *Endocrine Rev.*, 4:311–350.

47. Kang, E., and Paine, R. S. (1963): Elevation of plasma phenylalanine levels during pregnancies of women heterozygous for phenylketonuria. *J. Pediatr.*, 63:283–289.

48. Karoum, F., Speciale, S. G., Jr., Chuang, L.-W., and Wyatt, R. J. (1982): Selective effects of phenylethylamine on central catecholamines: A comparative study with amphetamine. *J. Pharmacol. Exp. Ther.*, 22:432–439.

49. Kini, M. M., and Cooper, J. R. (1961): Biochemistry of methanol poisoning III. The enzymatic pathway for the conversion of methanol to formaldehyde. *Biochem. Pharmacol.*, 8:207–215.

50. Knigge, K. M., Joseph, S. A., and Hoffman, G. E. (1978): Organization of LRF- and SRIF-neurons in the endocrine hypothalamus. In: *The Hypothalamus*, edited by S. Reichlin, R. J. Baldessarini, and J. B. Martin, pp. 49–67. Raven Press, New York.

51. Korsten, M. A., Matsuzaki, S., Feinman, L., and Lieber, C. S. (1975): High blood acetaldehyde levels after ethanol administration. *N. Engl. J. Med.*, 292:386–389.

52. Krause, W., Averbook, A., Epstein, C., and Elsas, L. (1983): Changes in EEG and L-DOPA in treated patients with phenylketonuria (PKU) during a phenylalanine challenge. *Clin. Res.*, 31:898A.

53. Krause, W., Halminski, M., McDonald, L., Dembure, P., Salvo, R., Freides, D., and Elsas, L. (1985): Biochemical and neuropsychological effects of elevated plasma phenylalanine in patients with treated phenylketonuria. *J. Clin. Invest.*, 75:40–48.

54. Lancranjan, I., Wirz-Justice, A., Pühringer, W., and Del Pozo, E. (1976): Effect of L-5 hydroxytryptophan infusion on growth hormone and prolactin secretion in man. *J. Clin. Endocrinol. Metab.*, 45:588–593.

55. Larsen, P. R., Ross, J. E., and Tapley, D. F. (1964): Transport of neutral, dibasic and N-methyl substituted amino acids by rat intestine. *Biochim. Biophys. Acta*, 88:570–577.

56. Lazarus, H. M., Herzig, R. G., Graham-Pole, J., et al. (1983): Intensive melphalan chemotherapy and cryopreserved autologous bone marrow transplantation for the treatment of refractory cancer. *J. Clin. Oncol.*, 1:359–367.

57. Le Cam, A., and Freychet, P. (1977): Neutral amino acid transport. Characterization of the A and L system in isolated rat hepatocytes. *J. Biol. Chem.*, 252:148–156.

58. Lee, S. H., and Davis, E. J. (1979): Carboxylation and decarboxylation reactions. Anaplerotic flux and removal of citrate cycle intermediates in skeletal muscle. *J. Biol. Chem.*, 254:420–430.

59. Levy, H. L., Shih, V. E., and Madigan, P. M. (1974): Routine newborn screening for histidinemia. Clinical and biochemical results. *N. Engl. J. Med.*, 291:1214–1219.

60. Levy, H. L., and Waisbren, S. E. (1983): Effects of untreated maternal pheylketonuria and hyperphenylalaninemia on the fetus. *N. Engl. J. Med.*, 309:1269–1274.

61. Lieberman, H. R., Corkin, S., Spring, B. J., Growdon, J. H., and Wurtman, R. J. (1982/83): Mood, performance, and pain sensitivity: Changes induced by food constituents. *J. Psychiatr. Res.*, 17:135–146.

62. Lingard, J., Rumrich, G., and Young, J. A. (1973): Kinetics of L-histidine transport in the proximal convolution of rat nephron studied using the stationary microperfusion technique. *Pfluegers Arch.*, 342:13–28.

63. Lund, E. D., Kirkland, C. L., and Shaw, P. E. (1981): Methanol, ethanol, and acetaldehyde contents of citrus products. *J. Agric. Food Chem.*, 29:361–366.

64. Lytle, L. D., Messing, R. B., Fisher, L., and Phebus, L. (1975): Effects of long-term corn consumption on brain serotonin and the response to electric shock. *Science*, 190:692–694.

65. Markovitz, D. C., and Fernstrom, J. D. (1977): Diet and uptake of aldomet by the brain: Competition with natural large neutral amino acids. *Science*, 197:1014–1015.

66. Matthyse, S., Baldessarini, R. J., and Vogt, M. (1972): Methionine adenosyltransferase: A double-isotope derivative, enzymatic assay. *Anal. Biochem.*, 48:410–421.

67. Mazur, R. H. (1984): Discovery of aspartame. In: *Aspartame Physiology and Biochemistry*, edited by L. D. Steginck and L. J. Filer, Jr., pp. 3–9. Marcel Dekker, New York.

68. Mazur, R. H., Schlatter, J. M., and Goldkamp, A. H. (1969): Structure-taste relationships of some dipeptides. *J. Am. Chem. Soc.*, 91:2684.

69. McGale, E. H. F., Pye, I. F., Stonier, C., Hutchinson, E. C., and Aber, G. M. (1977): Studies of the interrelationship between cerebrospinal fluid and plasma amino acid concentrations in normal individuals. *J. Neurochem.*, 29:291–297.

70. McKean, C. M. (1972): The effects of high phenylalanine concentrations on serotonin and catecholamine metabolism in the human brain. *Brain Res.*, 47:469–476.

71. Miller, A. L., Hawkins, R. A., and Veech, R. L. (1973): The mitochondrial redox state of rat brain. *J. Neurochem.*, 20:1393–1400.

72. Miller, L., Braun, L. D., Pardridge, W. M., and Oldendorf, W. H. (1985): Kinetic constants for blood-brain barrier amino acid transport in conscious rats. *J. Neurochem.*, 45:1427–1432.

73. Molinary, S. V. (1984): Preclinical studies of aspartame in nonprimate animals. In: *Aspartame Physiology and Biochemistry*, edited by L. D. Steginck and L. J. Filer, Jr., pp. 289–306. Marcel Dekker, New York.

74. Moore, T. J., Lione, A. P., Sugden, M. C., and Regen, D. M. (1976): β-Hydroxybutyrate transport in rat brain: Developmental and dietary modulations. *Am. J. Physiol.*, 230:619–630.

74a. Novick, N. L. (1985): Aspartame-induced granulomatous panniculitis. *Ann. Intern. Med.*, 102:206–207.

75. Nutt, J. G., Woodward, W. R., Hammerstad, J. P., Carter, J. H., and Anderson, J. L. (1984): The "on-off" phenomenon in Parkinson's disease. Relation to levodopa absorption and transport. *N. Engl. J. Med.*, 310:483–488.

76. Oates, J. A., Nirenberg, P. Z., Jepson, J. B., Sjoerdsma, A., and Udenfriend, S. (1963): Conversion of phenylalanine to phenethylamine in patients with phenylketonuria. *Proc. Soc. Exp. Biol. Med.*, 112:1078–1081.

77. Oldendorf, W. H. (1971): Brain uptake of radiolabeled amino acids, amines, and hexoses after arterial injection. *Am. J. Physiol.*, 221:1629–1639.

78. Oldendorf, W. H., Sisson, W. B., and Silverstein, A. (1971): Brain uptake of selenomethionine Se 75. II. Reduced brain uptake of selenomethionine Se 75 in phenylketonuria. *Arch. Neurol.*, 24:524–528.

79. Oldendorf, W. H., and Szabo, J. (1976): Amino acid assignment to one of three blood-brain barrier amino acid carriers. *Am. J. Physiol.*, 230:94–98.

80. Olney, J. W. (1969): Brain lesions, obesity, and other disturbances in mice treated with monosodium glutamate. *Science*, 164:719–721.

81. Olney, J. W. (1976): Brain damage and oral intake of certain amino acids. *Adv. Exp. Biol. Med.*, 69:497–506.

82. Oppermann, J. A. (1984): Aspartame metabolism in animals. In: *Aspartame Physiology and Biochemistry*, edited by L. D. Stegink and L. J. Filer, Jr., p. 141. Marcel Dekker, New York.

83. Pardridge, W. M. (1977): Kinetics of competitive inhibition of neutral amino acid transport across the blood-brain barrier. *J. Neurochem.*, 28:103–108.

84. Pardridge, W. M. (1977): Regulation of amino acid availability to the brain. In: *Nutrition and the Brain, Vol. 1*, edited by R. J. Wurtman and J. J. Wurtman, pp. 141–204. Raven Press, New York.

85. Pardridge, W. M. (1979): Regulation of amino acid availability to brain: Selective control mechanisms for glutamate. In: *Glutamic Acid: Advances in Biochemistry and Physiology*, edited by L. J. Filer, Jr., et al., pp. 125–137. Raven Press, New York.

86. Pardridge, W. M. (1981): Transport of protein-bound hormones into tissues in vivo. *Endocr. Rev.*, 2:103–123.

87. Pardridge, W. M. (1983): Brain metabolism: A perspective from the blood-brain barrier. *Physiol. Rev.*, 63:1481–1535.

88. Pardridge, W. M. (1983): Neuropeptides and the blood-brain barrier. *Annu. Rev. Physiol.*, 45:73–82.

89. Pardridge, W. M., Casanello-Ertl, D., and Duducgian-Vartavarian, L. (1980): Branched chain amino acid oxidation in cultured rat skeletal muscle cells. *J. Clin. Invest.*, 66:88–93.

90. Pardridge, W. M., and Connor, J. D. (1973): Saturable transport of amphetamine across the blood-brain barrier. *Experientia*, 29:302–304.

91. Pardridge, W. M., Cornford, E. M., Braun, L. D., and Oldendorf, W. H. (1979): Transport of choline and choline analogues through the blood-brain barrier. In: *Nutrition and the Brain, Vol. 5*, edited by A. Barbeau, J. H. Growdon, and R. J. Wurtman, pp. 25–34. Raven Press, New York.

92. Pardridge, W. M., Eisenberg, J., and Yang, J. (1985): Human blood-brain barrier insulin receptor. *J. Neurochem.*, 44:1771–1778.

93. Pardridge, W. M., Frank, H. J. L., Cornford, E. M., Braun, L. D., Crane, P. D., and Oldendorf, W. H. (1981): Neuropeptides and the blood-brain barrier. In: *Neurosecretion and Brain Peptides*, edited by J. B. Martin, S. Reichlin, and K. L. Bick, pp. 321–328. Raven Press, New York.

94. Pardridge, W. M., and Mietus, L. J. (1982): Kinetics of neutral amino acid transport through the blood-brain barrier of the newborn rabbit. *J. Neurochem.*, 38:955–962.

95. Pardridge, W. M., and Oldendorf, W. H. (1977): Transport of metabolic substrates through the blood-brain barrier. *J. Neurochem.*, 28:5–12.

96. Peterson, J. S., Kalivas, P. W., and Prasad, C. (1984): Cyclo (HIS-PRO) (cHP) regulates striatal dopaminergic function. *Soc. Neurosci. Abstr.*, 10:1123.

97. Philips, S. R. (1981): Amphetamine, p-hydroxyamphetamine and β-phenethylamine in mouse brain and urine after (−)- and (+)-deprenyl administration. *J. Pharm. Pharmacol.*, 33:739–741.

98. Phillips, F., Crisp, A. H., McGuinness, B., Kalucy, E. C., Chen, C. M., Koval, J., Kalucy, R. S., and Lacey, J. H. (1975): Isocaloric diet changes and electroencephalographic sleep. *Lancet*, II:723–725.

99. Porikos, K. P., and Van Itallie, T. B. (1984): Efficacy of low-calorie sweeteners in reducing food intake: Studies with aspartame. In: *Aspartame Physiology and Biochemistry*, edited by L. D. Stegink and L. J. Filer, Jr., pp. 273–286. Marcel Dekker, New York.

100. Price, M. T., Olney, J. W., Lowry, O. H., and Buchsbaum, S. (1981): Uptake of exogenous glutamate and aspartate by circumventricular organs but not other regions of brain. *J. Neurochem.*, 36:1774–1780.

101. Ranney, R. E., Mares, S. E., Schroeder, R. E., Hutsell, T. C., and Radzialowski, F. M. (1975): The phenylalanine and tyrosine content of maternal and fetal body fluids from rabbits fed aspartame. *Toxicol. Appl. Pharmacol.*, 32:339–346.

102. Rehfeld, J. F. (1981): Four basic characteristics of the gastrin-cholecystokinin system. *Am. J. Physiol.*, 240:G255–G266.

103. Reynolds, W. A., Bauman, A. F., Stegink, L. D., Filer, L. J., Jr., and Naidu, S. (1984): Developmental assessment of infant macaques receiving dietary aspartame or phenylalanine. In: *Aspartame Physiology and Biochemistry*, edited by L. D. Stegink and L. J. Filer, Jr., p. 405. Marcel Dekker, New York.

104. Reynolds, W. A., Parsons, L., and Stegink, L. D. (1984): Neuropathology studies following aspartame ingestion by infant nonhuman primates. In: *Aspartame Physiology and Biochemistry*, edited by L. D. Stegink and L. J. Filer, Jr., pp. 363–378. Marcel Dekker, New York.

105. Roak-Foltz, R., and Leveille, G. A. (1984): Projected aspartame intake: Daily ingestion of aspartic acid, phenylalanine, and methanol. In: *Aspartame Physiology and Biochemistry*, edited by L. D. Stegink and L. J. Filer, Jr., pp. 201–205. Marcel Dekker, New York.

106. Rubin, R. A., Ordonez, L. A., and Wurtman, R. J. (1974): Physiological dependence of brain methionine and S-adenosylmethionine concentrations on serum amino acid pattern. *J. Neurochem.*, 23:227–231.

107. Schwartz, J. C., Lampart, C., and Rose, C. (1972): Histamine formation in rat brain in vivo: Effects of histidine loads. *J. Neurochem.*, 19:801–810.

108. Scriver, C. R., and Clow, C. L. (1980): Phenylketonuria: Epitome of human biochemical genetics. *N. Engl. J. Med.*, 303:1336–1342.

109. Sershen, H., and Lajtha, A. (1979): Inhibition pattern by analogs indicates the presence of ten or more transport systems for amino acids in brain cells. *J. Neurochem.*, 32:719–726.

110. Shambaugh, G. E., III, and Koehler, R. A. (1981): Fetal fuels. IV. Regulation of branched-chain amino and keto acid metabolism in fetal brain. *Am. J. Physiol.*, 241:E200–E207.

111. Shannon, H. E., Cone, E. J., and Yousefnejad, D. (1982): Physiologic effects and plasma kinetics of β-phenylethylamine and its N-methyl homolog in the dog. *J. Pharmacol. Exp. Ther.*, 223:190–196.

112. Sjoerdmsa, A., Engelman, K., Spector, S., and Udenfriend, S. (1965): Inhibition of catecholamine synthesis in man with alpha-methyl tyrosine, an inhibitor of tyrosine hydroxylase. *Lancet*, 2:1092–1094.

113. Smith, I., Clayton, B. W., and Wolff, O. H. (1975): New variant of phenylketonuria with progressive neurological illness unresponsive to phenylalanine restriction. *Lancet*, I:1108–1111.

114. Stegink, L. D. (1984): Aspartate and glutamate metabolism. In: *Aspartame Physiology and Biochemistry*, edited by L. D. Stegink and L. J. Filer, Jr., p. 47. Marcel Dekker, New York.

115. Stegink, L. D. (1984): Aspartame metabolism in humans: Acute dosing studies. In: *Aspartame Physiology and Biochemistry*, edited by L. D. Stegink and L. J. Filer, Jr., pp. 509–553. Marcel Dekker, New York.

116. Stegink, L. D., Filer, L. J., Jr., Baker, G. L., and Brummel, M. C. (1979): Plasma and erythrocyte amino acid levels of adult humans given 100 mg/kg body weight aspartame. *Toxicology*, 14:131–140.

117. Stegink, L. D., Filer, L. J., Jr., Baker, G. L., and McDonnell, J. E. (1979): Effect of aspartame loading upon plasma and erythrocyte amino acid levels in phenylketonuric heterozygotes and normal adult subjects. *J. Nutr.*, 109:708–717.

118. Stegink, L. D., Koch, R., Blaskovics, M. E., Filer, L. J., Jr., Baker, G. L., and McDonnell, J. E. (1981): Plasma phenylalanine levels in phenylketonuric heterozygous and normal adults administered aspartame at 34 mg/kg body weight. *Toxicology*, 20:81–90.

119. Sved, A. F., Fernstrom, J. D., and Wurtman, R. J. (1979): Tyrosine administration reduces blood pressure and enhances brain norepinephrine release in spontaneously hypertensive rats. *Proc. Natl. Acad. Sci. USA*, 76:3511–3514.

120. Tephly, T. R., and McMartin, K. E. (1984): Methanol metabolism and toxicity. In: *Aspartame Physiology and Biochemistry*, edited by L. D. Stegink and L. J. Filer, Jr., p. 111. Marcel Dekker, New York.

121. Udenfriend, S. (1963): Factors in amino acid metabolism which can influence the central nervous system. *Am. J. Clin. Nutr.*, 12:287–290.

122. Uribe, M. (1982): Potential toxicity of a new sugar substitute in patients with liver disease. *N. Engl. J. Med.*, 306:173–174.

123. Van Woert, M. H., Rosenbaum, D., Howieson, J., and Bowers, M. B. (1977): Long-term therapy of myoclonus and other neurologic disorders with L-5-hydroxytryptophan and carbidopa. *N. Engl. J. Med.*, 296:70–75.
124. Wade, L. A., and Katzman, R. (1975): Rat brain regional uptake and decarboxylation of L-DOPA following carotid injection. *Am. J. Physiol.*, 228:352–359.
125. Weindl, A. (1973): Neuroendocrine aspects of circumventricular organs. In: *Frontiers in Neuroendocrinology*, edited by W. F. Ganong and L. Martini, pp. 3–32. Oxford University Press, New York.
126. Williams, M. (1984): Adenosine—a selective neuromodulator in the mammalian CNS? *Trends Neurosci.*, 7:164–168.
127. Winter, C. G., and Christensen, H. M. (1964): Migration of amino acids across the membrane of the human erythrocyte. *J. Biol. Chem.*, 239:872–878.
128. Wu, P. H., and Phillis, J. W. (1982): Uptake of adenosine by isolated rat brain capillaries. *J. Neurochem.*, 38:687–690.
129. Wurtman, R. J., and Fernstrom, J. D. (1975): Control of brain monoamine synthesis by diet and plasma amino acids. *Am. J. Clin. Nutr.*, 28:538–647.
130. Wurtman, R. J., Moskowitz, M. A., and Munro, H. N. (1979): Transsynaptic control of neuronal protein synthesis. In: *The Neurosciences: Fourth Study Program*, edited by F. O. Schmitt and F. G. Norden, pp. 897–909. MIT Press, Cambridge.
131. Yogman, M. W., and Zeisel, S. H. (1983): Diet and sleep patterns in newborn infants. *N. Engl. J. Med.*, 309:1147–1149.
132. Yokogoshi, H., Roberts, C. H., Caballero, B., and Wurtman, R. J. (1984): Effects of aspartame and glucose administration on brain and plasma levels of large neutral amino acids and brain 5-hydroxyindoles. *Am. J. Clin. Nutr.*, 40:1–7.
133. Zeisel, S. H., Blusztajn, J. K., and Wurtman, R. J. (1979): Brain lecithin biosynthesis: Evidence that bovine brain can make choline molecules. In: *Nutrition and the Brain, Vol. 5*, edited by A. Barbeau, J. H. Gowdon, and R. J. Wurtman, pp. 47–55. Raven Press, New York.
134. Zlokovic, B. V., Begley, D. J., and Chain, D. G. (1983): Blood-brain barrier permeability to dipeptides and their constituent amino acids. *Brain Res.*, 271:65–71.
135. Appendix E: Estimating distributions of daily intake of monosodium glutamate (MSG). (1976): In: *Estimating Distribution of Daily Intake of Certain GRAS Substances*. Committee on GRAS List Survey—Phase III, Food and Nutrition Board, Division of Biological Sciences, Assembly of Life Sciences, National Research Council, National Academy of Sciences, Washington, D.C.
136. Evaluation of consumer complaints related to aspartame use (1984): Centers for Disease Control (CDC).
137. Dried Soup Mixes (This is soup?) (1978): *Consumer Reports*, November, pp. 615–619.
138. *Federal Register*, Vol. 46, No. 142, July (1981), p. 38290.

Subject Index

Subject Index